Essentials of

Maternal Fetal

Medicine

Essentials of
Maternal Fetal
Medicine

Graham Gaylord Ashmead, M.D., Editor
Associate Professor of Developmental Reproductive
Biology and Department of Radiology
Case Western Reserve University
Cleveland, OH

Director of Fetal Diagnostic Center
MetroHealth Medical Center
Cleveland, OH

George B. Reed Jr., M.D., Associate Editor
Kaiser Permanente
Gilroy, CA

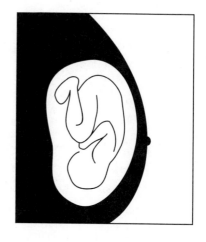

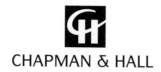

CHAPMAN & HALL

I(T)P® International Thomson Publishing
New York • Albany • Bonn • Boston • Cincinnati • Detroit • London • Madrid • Melbourne
Mexico City • Pacific Grove • Paris • San Francisco • Singapore • Tokyo • Toronto • Washington

Cover Design: Andrea Meyer, emDASH inc.

Copyright © 1997
Chapman & Hall

Printed in the United States of America

For more information, contact:

Chapman & Hall
115 Fifth Avenue
New York, NY 10003

Chapman & Hall
2-6 Boundary Row
London SE1 8HN
England

Thomas Nelson Australia
102 Dodds Street
South Melbourne, 3205
Victoria, Australia

Chapman & Hall GmbH
Postfach 100 263
D-69442 Weinheim
Germany

International Thomson Editores
Campos Eliseos 385, Piso 7
Col. Polanco
11560 Mexico D.F.
Mexico

International Thomson Publishing-Japan
Hirakawacho-cho Kyowa Building, 3F
1-2-1 Hirakawacho-cho
Chiyoda-ku, 102 Tokyo
Japan

International Thomson Publishing Asia
221 Henderson Road #05-10
Henderson Building
Singapore 0315

1 2 3 4 5 6 7 8 9 10 XXX 01 00 99 98 97

Library of Congress Cataloging-in-Publication Data

Essentials of maternal fetal medicine / [edited by] Graham G. Ashmead, George B. Reed, Jr.
     p.   cm.
   Includes bibliographical references and index.
   ISBN 0-412-08681-6 (alk. paper)
   1. Pregnancy—Complications.   2. Obstetrics.   3. Perinatology.   I. Ashmead, Graham G., 1951-   . II. Reed, G.B. (George B.) [DNLM: 1. Prenatal Diagnosis.   2. Fetal Diseases.   3. Genetic Screening—in pregnancy.   4. Pregnancy Complications—etiology.   5. Genital Neoplasms, Female.   WQ 209 M425 1997]
RG571 M33   1997
618.3—dc20
DNLM/DLC   96-35128
for Library of Congress   CIP

British Library Cataloguing in Publication Data available

To order this or any other Chapman & Hall book, please contact **International Thomson Publishing, 7625 Empire Drive, Florence, KY 41042.** Phone: (606) 525-6600 or 1-800-842-3636. Fax: (606) 525-7778, e-mail: order@chaphall.com.

For a complete listing of Chapman & Hall's titles, send your requests to
Chapman & Hall, Dept. BC, 115 Fifth Avenue, New York, NY 10003.

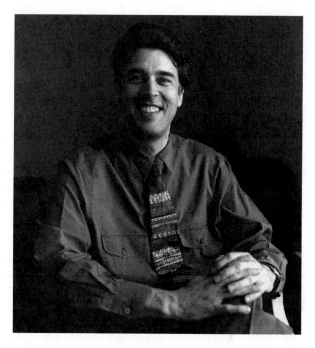

Photograph by LeRoy Dierker

Graham Gaylord Ashmead, M.D., Editor

Associate Professor
 of Developmental Reproductive Biology
 and Department of Radiology
Case Western Reserve University

Director of the Fetal Diagnostic Center
MetroHealth Medical Center

To my daughter Alexandra with love, and to her generation with hope.

Graham Ashmead, M.D.

To the past and present faculty and staff in Obstetrics, Pediatrics, and Pathology.

George Reed, M.D.

ACKNOWLEDGMENTS

The writing of this book would not have been possible without the help of many others. My deep appreciation goes to the excellent contributors who were generous enough to share their knowledge and expertise in the chapters of this book and to suffer through the multiple editorial revisions. My thanks goes also to the many medical students, residents, fellows, and attending physicians who inspired and made suggestions to improve this book. In particular, Carol Crowe, Kelly Donahue and Irwin Schafer were kind enough to review and improve the chapter on genetics. James Clapp and LeRoy Dierker provided continual moral support and philosophical guidance.

Caryl Lecznar tirelessly compiled the many manuscripts and without her efforts this book would not exist in its present form. Sonographers William Stepanchak, Barbara Cipiti, Susan Touma, and Diane Schulte helped obtain the ultrasound illustrations for this book. The cytogenetics laboratory technicians, Karla Zilch and Cindy Moore, provided samples of karyotopes. David Dunsmore, Vincent Messina, and LeRoy Dierker were kind enough to provide photographs and illustrations.

My thanks goes also to my clinical colleagues at MetroHealth Medical Center, including the staff of the Fetal Diagnostic Center, for their support and forbearance. Finally, I want to especially recognize my fellow editor, George Reed, who encouraged me to come up with the initial concept for this book.

Contents

Part II: IN UTERO FETAL DIAGNOSIS AND MANAGEMENT

Part III: MATERNAL-FETAL COMPLICATIONS DURING PREGNANCY

Part V: LABOR, DELIVERY, NEONATAL MANAGEMENT
AND PATHOLOGY

Foreword

The philosophies of one age have become the absurdities of the next, and the foolishness of yesterday has become the wisdom of tomorrow.

Sir William Osler (1849–1919)

Health care has undergone remarkable changes since I began my clinical experience at the Albert Einstein College of Medicine over 35 years ago. Tremendous progress has been made in the science and art of maternal-fetal medicine over the three plus decades of my career as a clinician, educator, and researcher in obstetrics and gynecology. For example, powerful antibiotics and medications are available now that were unknown then. Prenatal diagnosis by amniocentesis was in our hands a blind procedure, providing limited information at significant risk. Fetal procedures undreamed of during my early training, such as cordocentesis and embryoscopy, can provide detailed information on fetal morphology, physiology, and genetics. Fetuses are now routinely and safely evaluated with non-invasive real-time high-resolution and color Doppler ultrasound. Three-dimensional ultrasound evaluation of the fetus is available at certain high-risk referral centers. Medicines that cross the placenta to treat fetal cardiac arrhythmias or goiter and fetal surgery for bladder outlet obstruction or diaphragmatic hernia have changed the fetus from a passive passenger into a patient. Most exciting is the progress in preventing poor pregnancy outcomes. For example, preconception folate supplementation and good preconception glucose control of diabetes can prevent fetal neural tube or cardiac anomalies. Prenatal zidovudine (AZT) can prevent or reduce the in utero transmission of human immunodeficiency virus (HIV) to fetuses. Advances in the management of insulin-dependent diabetes mellitus during pregnancy have dramatically improved the outcomes for diabetic mothers and their babies. Within the next decade the human genome will have been mapped, permitting precise diagnosis to improve both prenatal diagnosis and therapy outcomes. I believe that future advances in maternal-fetal medicine will dwarf the remarkable changes I have been fortunate enough to witness during my long medical career.

In my opinion, the real challenge for the future is to provide excellent and humane care for everyone. In America, despite the remarkable technical progress in medicine there remains a national division of opinion as to whether health insurance coverage should be extended to large numbers of Americans—almost 40 million in 1995—who do not currently enjoy its benefits. I hope that my four children and five grandchildren will share a future where the best of prenatal care is available for all mothers and their babies. This book, edited by Graham Ashmead, one of my former maternal-fetal medicine fellows, and coauthored by many mutual friends and colleagues, should help medical students, residents, and clinicians interested in maternal-fetal medicine provide good clinical care and bring that bright future closer.

Leon I. Mann, M.D.
Chairperson, Department of Reproductive Biology, MetroHealth Medical Center
Professor, Department of Reproductive Biology, Case Western Reserve University School of Medicine
Senior Vice President, Medical Affairs, Metro-Health Medical Center
Chief of Staff, MetroHealth Medical Center
Associate Dean, Case Western Reserve University, School of Medicine

Contributors

SAEID B. AMINI, PhD, MBA
Department of Epidemiology and Biostatistics
Case Western Reserve University
Cleveland, OH

GRAHAM G. ASHMEAD, MD
Department of Obstetrics and Gynecology
MetroHealth Medical Center
Cleveland, OH

JOSEPHINE WYATT-ASHMEAD, MD
Department of Pathology
MetroHealth Medical Center
Cleveland, OH

KHALID M. ATAYA, MD
Department of Obstetrics and Gynecology
MetroHealth Medical Center
Cleveland, OH

WILLIAM D. BONEZZI, MD
Jacobson, Maynard, Tuschman & Kalur Co
Cleveland, OH

PATRICIA L. COLLINS, PhD, MD
Department of Obstetrics and Gynecology
MetroHealth Medical Center
Cleveland, OH

MARSHA D. COOPER, MD
Department of Medicine
Providence Hospital and Firelands Community
  Hospital
Sandusky, OH

STEPHEN P. EMERY, MD
Department of Obstetrics and Gynecology
MetroHealth Medical Center
Cleveland, OH

JOHN R. FISGUS, MD
Department of Anesthesia
MetroHealth Medical Center
Cleveland, OH

MONICA T. FUNDZAK, BSN, RNC, NNP
Maternal/Child Nursing
MetroHealth Medical Center
Cleveland, OH

PRABHCHARAN GILL, MD
Division of Maternal Fetal Medicine
Aultman Hospital
Canton, OH

MICHAEL T. GYVES, MD
Department of Obstetrics and Gynecology
St. Lukes Medical Center
Cleveland, OH

NANCY E. JUDGE, MD
Department of Obstetrics and Gynecology
MacDonald Women's Hospital
Cleveland, OH

MICHAEL A. KREW, MD
Department of Obstetrics and Gynecology
Aultman Hospital
Canton, OH

CAROL A. LINDSAY, MD
Department of Obstetrics and Gynecology
MetroHealth Medical Center
Cleveland, OH

MING-XU LU, MS
Maumee, OH

SANGITHAN J. MOODLEY, MD
Department of Obstetrics and Gynecology
Fairview General Hospital
Cleveland, OH

JOHN J. MOORE, MD
Department of Neonatology
MetroHealth Medical Center
Cleveland, OH

ALICE S. PETRULIS, MD
Department of Medicine
MetroHealth Medical Center
Cleveland, OH

ELLIOT H. PHILIPSON, MD
Department of Obstetrics and Gynecology
Cleveland Clinic Foundation
Cleveland, OH

MOSTAFA A. SELIM, MD
Department of Obstetrics and Gynecology
Division of Gynecologic Oncology
MetroHealth Medical Center
Cleveland, OH

YOGESH G. SHAH, MD
Department of Obstetrics and Gynecology
Fairview General Hospital
Cleveland, OH

ABDELWAHAB D. SHALODI, MD
Department of Obstetrics and Gynecology
Division of Gynecologic Oncology
MetroHealth Medical Center
Cleveland, OH

DIANA SMIGAJ, MD
Department of Obstetrics and Gynecology
Providence Yakima Medical Center
Yakima, WA

Part I

GENETICS AND PHYSIOLOGY OF PREGNANCY

1

Genetics

Graham G. Ashmead

INTRODUCTION

The purpose of this chapter is to cover the fundamental concepts of medical genetics and to illustrate them with examples. Because medical genetics is rapidly changing, a basic knowledge of the principles of inherited conditions is essential for those providers caring for pregnant women. Up to 7% of perinatal deaths and 25% of congenital anomalies are due to chromosomal abnormalities. Most congenital anomalies (65–75%) are currently attributed to multifactorial causes due to a combination of genetic and environmental influences. Up to 50% of pediatric inpatient and 12% of adult admissions are a result of complications related to congenital anomalies or genetic disorders. Genetic disorders account for 40% of childhood deaths.[1,2]

Providers with special interests in pregnancy need to have a strong understanding of human genetics and to know when it is appropriate to refer patients for further consultation with subspecialists in reproductive genetics. Obstetricians have been held liable for failure to offer prenatal testing, prenatally diagnose a genetic disorder, advise of fetal genetic risks, explain abnormal prenatal test results, or provide prenatal test results in a timely fashion. Indications for prenatal counseling include: advanced maternal age; previous child with a chromosomal abnormality; elevated maternal serum alpha-fetoprotein (MSAFP); abnormal multiple marker screening [(MSAFP, human chorionic gonadotropin (hCG)], and unconjugated estriol); family history of a genetic or a multifactorial disorder; multiple spontaneous abortions; exposure to a teratogen; or presence of a fetal anomaly.[1-3]

DEVELOPMENT AND TERATOGENS

The study of abnormal embryonic and fetal development is called dysmorphology (teratology). Significant congenital anomalies occur in 3% of the population and in more than half, the causes of the congenital anomalies are not known.

Teratogens are environmental agents that produce abnormal growth and development. They are recognized to be responsible for a small number of individuals born with anomalies. Other causes of anomalies include chromosome abnormalities, single-gene disorders, and multifactorial factors. Important points to consider in evaluation of potential teratogenesis include: the teratogen involved, dose, stage of development at exposure, and the sensitivity or threshold of mother and conceptus. Teratogen exposure in the first 2 weeks of embryogenesis usually results either in complete loss of the

Table 1-1. Human Embryonic and Fetal Development in Days

Development	Days
Blastula	4–6
Implantation	6–7
Preembryo	1–14
Neural plate	18–20
First heartbeats	22
Oral plate perforation	24
Anterior neuropore closed	24–25
Mesonephros	25
Thyroid appears	27
Upper limb bud	27–29
Posterior neuropore closed	26–27
Lung bud appears	28
Lower limb bud appears	29–30
Eye pigment	34–35
Heart septation complete	46–47
Oral palate closed	56–58
Physiologic gut herniation reduced	60
Total gestational time	267

Source: Adapted from ref. 5.

pregnancy or in an unaffected fetus. Teratogen exposure during embryonic organogenesis can produce major structural abnormalities in affected developing organs. After organogenesis is complete in the fetal period (13 weeks), teratogens tend to cause reduction in organ size rather than structural defects. See Table 1-1.

Animal studies have been used to evaluate potential teratogens, but the results may be misleading. For example, thalidomide in rats and mice did not cause malformations later documented in human fetuses while corticosteroids caused cleft palate in mice but not in human fetuses. Counseling regarding teratogenic exposure should be performed in a sensitive manner and patients should be referred to a health care provider such as a genetic counselor with special expertise in teratology and birth defects. See Table 1-2 for a list of documented teratogens.[4,5]

BASIC GENETICS

Modern molecular genetics began in 1953 when James Watson and Francis Crick recognized the three-dimensional double helix nature of deoxyribonucleic acid (DNA). Knowledge of the structure of DNA led to an understanding of how genetic information is stored and how genetic material is transmitted and replicated. See Figures 1-1–1-5.

DNA is a macromolecule consisting of a linear array of deoxyribonucleotides. Each deoxyribonucleotide is composed of a nitrogeneous base, a sugar (deoxyribose) and a phosphate. The nitrogenous bases in a strand of DNA are linked to their adjacent bases by the sugar and phosphate groups and to their paired complementary bases on the opposite strand of DNA by hydrogen bonds. The nucleotide base pairs in DNA are adenine with thymine (A-T) and guanine with cytosine (G-C). Genetic information in the DNA is encoded by the order of the linear sequence of the nucleotide base pairs. Nucleotide triplets (codons) of A-T or G-C base pairs correspond to a specific amino acid. A series of codons code for a sequence of amino acids and form a polypeptide. A gene can be defined as a portion of DNA that codes for a particular polypeptide. One gene forms one polypeptide, but several polypeptides may be needed to form a protein.

The two helical complimentary polynucleotide chains of DNA serve as a template for the formation of a new chain of DNA or for transmitting information. The most common form of DNA consists of two DNA chains wound together in a right-handed fashion (B DNA) with major and minor grooves between the chains. The less common left-handed DNA (Z DNA) has only one size groove and may serve specialized functions. The phosphate group of one DNA sugar is linked at position C5 (5' carbon) by a phosphate diester bridge to the hydroxyl group at position C3 (3' carbon). The DNA nucleotide chain is therefore polar and has "ends" referred to as 5' and 3'. By convention, the sequence of nucleotide bases is written in the direction from the 5' to the 3' end. Formation of new DNA from old DNA occurs only from the 5'–3' end but not in the 3'–5' direction. The two strands of DNA are weakly held together by the noncovalent hydrogen bonds between the nucleotide base pairs. The two strands of DNA are easily separated (denaturation) by mild heating or many agents but reunite with cooling (renaturation). A single strand of DNA will only bind (hybridize) with a complementary segment of DNA. The property of DNA hybridization only occurring with complementary sequences is used in many of the tests of gene analysis of genetic disorders.

Genetic information from DNA is first transmitted by a process known as *transcription*. In transcription the sequence of nucleotide bases is transferred from DNA to a complementary strand of messenger ribonucleic acid (RNA, mRNA). Coding segments are called exons. Noncoding segments called introns are removed from the mRNA in humans before the mRNA leaves the cell nucleus to become a template to make proteins. The mRNA is then "translated." In translation the nucleotide codons of the mRNA are used to create a sequence of amino acids to form proteins. This is done by another kind of RNA called transfer RNA (tRNA). Each amino acid has its own tRNA. The tRNA has a binding site for a specific amino acid and a recognition site (anticodon) for the codon on the mRNA. Translation or protein synthesis in multicellular organisms (eukaryocytes) occurs outside of the cell nucleus in ribosomes (rRNA) in the cytoplasm. Translation ends when a stop codon is reached. The polypeptide then leaves the ribosome and forms a protein or gene product.[6-8]

In general, genetic disorders are due to an alteration in DNA structure resulting in a defective gene product (a protein). There are three different mutations involving single nucleotides (point mutations): substitution, deletion, and insertion. A substitution may alter a codon to produce the wrong amino acid but not affect the reading frame (missense). For example, in sickle cell anemia on the short arm of chromosome eleven a single base in the sixth codon of the β-globin gene has a substitution point mutation of adenine to thymine. The codon guanine-adenosine-guanine (GAG) is changed to guanine-thymine-guanine (GTG). As a result a valine rather than glutamic acid is incorporated into the β-globin, resulting in an abnormal hemoglobin. This point mutation has spontaneously occurred at least five times in equatorial Africa and the Middle East. The mutation conferred partial protection for the heterozygote with sickle cell trait against malaria that flourished in those areas with the rise of agriculture. A nonsense mutation can be a single base substitution resulting in a chain-termination codon. Other point mutations such as an insertion or deletion can result in a shift of the reading frame causing the subsequent sequence to no longer code for a functional gene product (frameshift). Mutations can also consist of much larger deletions or duplications involving several exons and even several genes. A recently discovered type of mutation described later in this chapter involves abnormal numbers of repetitive triple nucleotide repeat sequences. In the 3 million kilobases (kb) of nucleotides per haploid genome forming the 50,000 genes in each human, there are probably four or five major defective mutations.[9,10]

Chromosomal Disorders

The DNA forming the human genetic code is stored in the cell nucleus in structures called chromosomes. The cell DNA, not counting the DNA present in cell mitochondria, is arranged in 80–300 million DNA base pairs per chromosome. The normal human number (diploid) of chromosomes in somatic cells is 46. Human chromosomes consist of 22 pairs called autosomes and two sex chromosomes (XX or XY). A normal female has two X chromosomes in each somatic cell, one inherited from each of her parents while a normal male has an X chromosome from his mother and a Y chromosome from his father. See Figure 1-5 for chromosomes prior to being arranged in a karyotype and Figure 1-6 for a normal male karyotype. Mitochondrial DNA is present in the 100,000 mitochondria in the cell cytoplasm and is inherited through the mother. Certain rare disorders are now known to be associated with mitochondrial DNA mutations and occur when there is a threshold of abnormal mitochondria.

Table 1-2.   Documented Teratogens

Agent Drug or Chemical	Effects	Comments
Alcohol	Growth retardation, microcephaly, major and minor malformations	6 drinks (6 oz) per day gives a 40% risk of fetal alcohol syndrome (FAS)
Androgens	Pseudohermaphroditism in females	Dose and timing dependent, minimal brief exposure risk
Anticoagulants (warfarin and dicumarol)	Hypoplastic nose, bony abnormalities, growth retardation	Risk 25% in first trimester
Antithyroid (iodide, propylthiouracil, methimazole)	Hypothyroidism, fetal goiter	Fetal goiter may hyperextend head, hydramnios
Chemotherapeutic (methotrexate, aminopterin)	Spontaneous abortions, anomalies	Cytotoxic drugs are potentially teratogenic
Diethylstilbestrol (DES)	Vaginal adenosis, abnormal cervix and uterus, infertility, rare adenocarcinoma	Vaginal adenosis in 50% exposed before 9 weeks, 25% male, abnormalities
Lead	Abortions and stillbirths	Abnormal fetal central nervous system (CNS)
Lithium	Congenital heart disease (CHD), Ebstein anomaly	2% incidence of CHD in first trimester
Organic mercury (Minimata disease)	Cerebral atrophy, mental retardation	Occurs even in third trimester (fish and grain contamination)
Phenytoin (Dilantin)	Growth deficiency, mental retardation, microcephaly	10% have full syndrome, 30% have some manifestations
Streptomycin	Hearing loss, eighth nerve damage	Histologic changes in inner ear in animals
Tetracycline	Enamel hypoplasia, incorporated into bone	No known effect unless after first trimester
Thalidomide	Anotia and microtia days 21–27, bilateral limb anomalies days 27–40, other anomalies	20% of children whose mothers used thalidomide were affected
Trimethadione (Tridione) and paramethadione (Paradione)	Cleft lip or palate, cardiac, microcephaly, ophthalmologic, growth retardation, mental retardation	60–80% defects or spontaneous abortion with first-trimester exposure, syndrome identified
Valproic acid (Depakene)	Neural tube defects	1–2% neural tube defects if exposed prior to neural tube closure
Vitamin A (retinoic acid, Accutane, tretinoin, isotretinoin)	Abortions, craniofacial, central nervous system and cardiac defects, cleft palate	23% of women treated in first trimester had fetuses with major malformations (over half had intellectual deficits by age 5)

There are a large variety of chromosomal disorders both in number and structure. Chromosome anomalies are seen in 1/200 live births and in 50–70% of first-trimester miscarriages. Trisomy 21 (Down syndrome), trisomy 18 (Edward's syndrome), trisomy 13 (Patau syndrome), and some sex chromosome disorders increase in incidence with advancing maternal age. The most common is Down syndrome (1/800 liveborn infants) usually due to maternal nondisjunction in meiosis I. Women with trisomy 21 (47,XX,+21) are fertile and about 30% of their offspring will have Down syndrome. Genetic counseling and prenatal testing should be offered to all women who will be 35 years or older by their estimated date of confinement (EDC). See Table 1-3. In general, the prenatal risk for all chromosomal disorders is roughly twice the maternal age-related risk for Down syndrome. A mother with a liveborn with Down syndrome has a recurrence risk of at least 1%. The recurrence risk for other chromosomal tri-

Table 1-2.   Continued

Infectious Agent	Effects	Comments
Cytomegalovirus (CMV)	Microcephaly, growth retardation, brain damage, hearing loss	0.1/1000 newborns have severe defects (0.5–1.5% of newborns colonized)
Herpes simplex virus types I and II	Microcephaly, intracranial calcifications, eye defects and vesicular skin lesions, intrauterine growth retardation and prematurity	Neonatal infection is usually acquired by delivery through an infected cervix or ruptured membranes and may be prevented by cesarean section. Acyclovir at term may prevent recurrence.
Parvovirus B19 (erythema infectiosum)	Microphthalmia, fetal hydrops, aplastic anemia	MSAFP may increase prior to fetal hydrops. Hydrops due to aplastic anemia can be treated in utero with cordocentesis blood transfusions. Fetal hydrops can also have spontaneous recovery.
Rubella	Cataracts, deafness, cardiac, all organs	50% malformations with first-trimester exposure, 6% organ damage mid-pregnancy, vaccine virus does not appear to harm fetus
Syphilis	Hydrops or demise with severe infection; skin, teeth, and bone abnormalities with mild infection	Severity depends on duration of infection, penicillin treatment can stop progression of fetal damage
Toxoplasmosis	Possible effects on all organs, severity depends on duration	Initial infection must occur during pregnancy to place fetus at risk, can treat during pregnancy with pyrimethamine and sulfadiazine
Varicella (Chickenpox, also herpes zoster or shingles)	Possible effects on all organs, skin scarring and muscle atrophy	Low frequency of congenital varicella, zoster immunoglobulin available for newborns and also vaccine

Radiation	Effects	Comments
X-ray therapy	Microcephaly, mental retardation	Medical diagnostic radiation (less than 10 rads) has little or no teratogenic risk

Source: Adapted from refs. 4 and 5.

somies is unknown but is probably about 1%. A mother with a prior pregnancy with Turner syndrome (45,X) does not have an increased risk for future infants with Turner syndrome. The most common chromosome abnormality in spontaneous abortuses is Turner syndrome. See Tables 1-4 and 1-5. See Figures 1-7, 1-8 and 1-9 of abnormal karyotypes. Advanced paternal age (>55 years old) is not a major risk factor for aneuploidy but it is a risk for autosomal-dominant mutations and structural chromosome abnormalities.

Another chromosome abnormality is a translocation or rearrangement of chromosomal seg-ments. A balanced translocation occurs when there is no loss or gain of genetic material. Even though patients with balanced translocations may have the correct amount of genetic material, they are at risk for having offspring with monosomies and trisomies. A balanced translocation can be Robertsonian, with centromeric fusion of two acrocentric chromosomes (13, 14, 15, 21, or 22) or a reciprocal translocation between two non-homologous chromosomes. The most common Robertsonian translocation t(14q;21q) involves fusion of the long arms of chromosome 14 and 21 and occurs in 1/1000 live births. The risk of a maternal carrier with

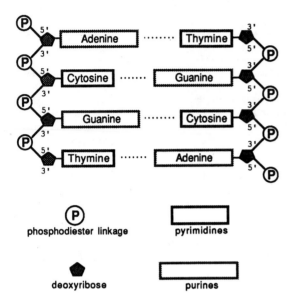

phosphodiester linkage   pyrimidines

deoxyribose   purines

Figure 1-1. The complementary structure of double stranded-DNA. (From ref. 28.)

t(14q;21q) having a child with Down syndrome is 10–15% and a paternal carrier is 2%. Five percent of Down syndrome is due to a Robertsonian translocation and in half the cases, the translocation is due to a new mutation.

Inversions are another kind of chromosomal abnormality and occur when a segment of chromosome material is inverted between two break points. As with translocations, parents with an inversion may produce offspring with partial trisomies and monosomies. A paracentric inversion involves breaks in only one arm of a chromosome. A pericentric inversion is an inversion that occurs across a centromere. Eight percent of maternal and 4% of paternal pericentric inversions result in unbalanced offspring.[1,3]

Mendelian Disorders

A single gene abnormality on either an autosome or a sex chromosome can cause a Mendelian disorder. Over 4000 traits are established and 10,000 are presumed to be inherited as Mendelian disorders. Mendelian disorders can be recessive or dominant. An allele is a DNA sequence or gene occupying the same site (locus) on two paired (homologous) chromosomes.

An autosomal-recessive (AR) disorder will be expressed when each parent has one allele with a mutation (heterozygous) and the affected offspring two alleles with mutations (homozygous), one from each parent. There is a 25% chance of heterozygous parents having an affected (homozygous) child. Males and females are equally affected. The risk of an affected individual having offspring with an AR disorder is dependent on the chance that his or her partner is a carrier for the abnormal gene (i.e., how rare the disease is). Every human being is thought to be heterozygous for 8–10 deleterious AR genes. Consanguinity increases the risk of sharing common genes and so of having a child affected with an AR disorder. Autosomal-recessive disorders include sickle cell disease, cystic fibrosis, Tay-Sachs disease, and phenylketonuria (PKU).

An autosomal-dominant (AD) disorder will be expressed with just one mutated gene (heterozygous) present. The probability of an AD disorder being transmitted from a parent to a child is 50%. Dominant disorders tend to code for proteins that are either structural in nature or are involved in rate-limiting steps in metabolic pathways. Examples of autosomal dominant disorders include achondroplasia, Marfan syndrome, Huntington disease, myotonic dystrophy, and adult polycystic kidney disease. Usually a child with a dominant disorder will have an affected parent. Possible explanations for a child affected with a dominant disorder not having an affected parent include a new mutation, incomplete penetrance, variable expression, and gonadal mosaicism.

A new mutation of a dominant disorder is a spontaneous first-time occurrence in a child with unaffected parents. The parental risk of having another child with the same dominant disorder is usually the same as the population risk for a new occurrence of the disorder. Parental gonadal mosaicism can sometimes account for an otherwise normal couple having several children affected with an apparently new mutation AD disorder.

Penetrance is the chance that a genotype will be expressed as the expected phenotype. Incom-

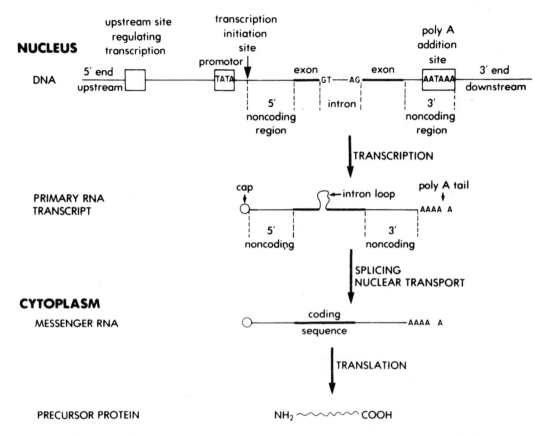

Figure 1-2. Eukaryotic gene structure and the pathway of gene expression. (From ref. 28.)

plete penetrance is commonly seen with autosomal disorders. An unaffected patient with both an affected parent and an affected child with an AD disorder most likely has incomplete penetrance.

Expressivity describes the degree of expression of a gene. Marfan syndrome for example is an AD disorder with varying expression. One individual with Marfan syndrome may only manifest tall stature and long digits while another may have the more severe manifestations of dislocation of the lens or aortic dissection. Distinguishing between a new mutation, gonadal mosaicism, incomplete penetrance, and expressivity requires taking a careful genetic history and evaluation of family members.

X-linked disorders can be recessive or dominant. Because males (46,XY) (unlike females, 46,XX) have only one X chromosome, an ab-

normal gene on an X chromosome causes disease in all affected males. Females with an abnormal recessive gene on an X chromosome are generally affected only if both of their X chromosomes are affected (homozygous) or if most of their normal X chromosomes are inactivated (Lyonization). In X-linked inheritance all daughters of an affected male are carriers and there is no male to male transmission.

In the heterozygous female, X-linked dominant traits are expressed. X-linked dominant disorders in males tend to be lethal while females usually have milder disease. X-linked dominant disorders in females are less severe because of random inactivation of the abnormal X chromosome in half of a female's cells, permitting expression of the normal gene by the other normal X chromosome. Examples of X-linked recessive disorders include glucose 6-phosphate

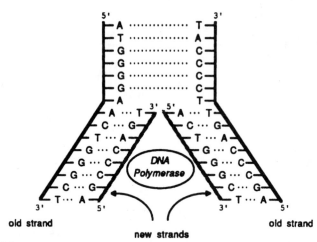

Replication

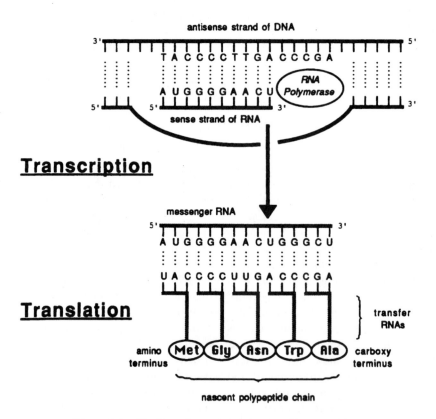

Transcription

Translation

Figure 1-3. The flow of genetic information. (From ref. 28.)

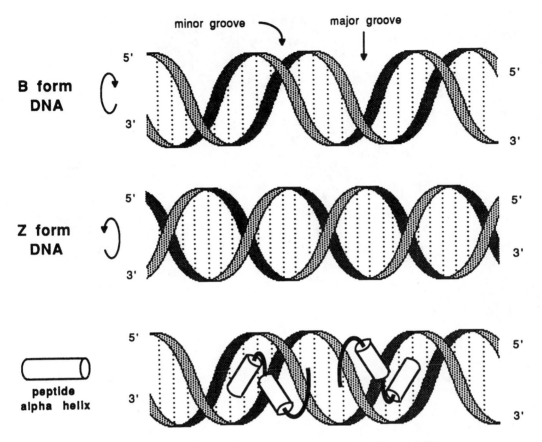

Figure 1-4.   Three-dimensional structures of DNA helices. (From ref. 28.)

dehydrogenase (G6-PD), Duchenne muscular dystrophy, and hemophilia. Hypophosphatemic (vitamin D-resistant) rickets, ornithine transcarbamylase (OTC) deficiency, and Kennedy disease (spinal and bulbar muscular atrophy) are examples of X-linked dominant disorders.[1,3,8]

Multifactorial Disorders

Multifactorial disorders are due to a combination of two or more genes (polygenic) and environmental influences. Characteristics of multifactorial disorders are: (1) an incidence of 1/1000–2/1000 births, (2) usually affects one organ system, (3) after one child has a disorder, the recurrence risk is 2–5% for future siblings, (4) the more severe the anomaly, the higher the recurrence risk, and (5) as the degree of relatedness decreases, the recurrence risk rapidly decreases. Examples of multifactorial disorders include neural tube defects, congenital heart disease, cleft lip or palate, diaphragmatic hernia, pyloric stenosis, omphalocele, renal agenesis, posterior urethral valves, Müllerian fusion defects, hypospadias, club feet, limb reduction defects, and dislocated hip.[1,3]

Uniparental Disomy

Uniparental disomy is a mode of inheritance with unequal contributions of genetic material from each parent. Two copies of a chromosome are inherited from one parent and no copies from the other parent. For example, this can occur when maternal meiotic nondisjunction is followed by loss of the paternal copy of a trisomic chromosome in early embryonic development. Because there is not both a maternal and a paternal copy of a chromosome there may be different patterns of gene expression depending on

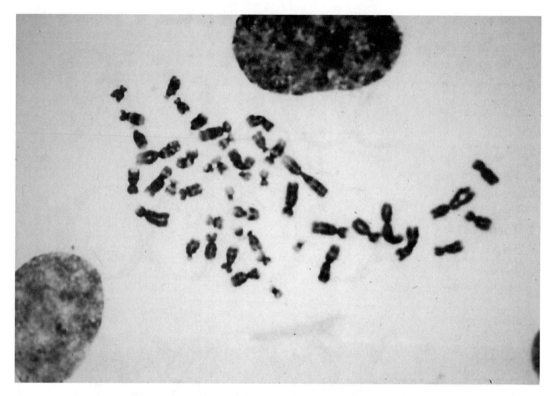

Figure 1-5. Chromosomes prior to being sorted into a karyotype.

the parent of origin (imprinting). For example, Prader-Willi and Angelman syndrome are two distinct genetic disorders that can result from imprinting or uniparental disomy. Prader-Willi syndrome can occur with paternally derived and Angelman syndrome with maternally derived deletions on chromosome 15 (imprinting). Prader-Willi and Angelman syndromes can also occur due to uniparental disomy if both chromosome 15's come from the mother (Prader-Willi) or from the father (Angelman).[3]

Triple Repeat Mutations

Several common genetic diseases are due to an amplification of normally occurring triple nucleotide repeat sequences. Triple repeat mutations can manifest themselves at an earlier age or with greater severity in successive generations. The phenomenon of increased risk with successive generations in a pedigree is known as *anticipation*. Triple repeat mutation genetic disorders include fragile X syndrome, Huntington disease, myotonic dystrophy, and Friedreich's ataxia.

Fragile X syndrome is an example of a triple repeat mutation that is X linked and is the most common inherited form of mental retardation (1/1500 males, 1/2500 females). Females with fragile X syndrome show variable penetrance, with 75% having some degree of mental retardation. All males with fragile X are affected with mental retardation, dysmorphic facial features, and macroorchidism. The name fragile X came about because the X chromosomes of affected males were prone to breakage under conditions of thymidine stress in culture.

Fragile X syndrome is associated with an abnormally increased number of the nucleotide sequence cytosine-guanine-guanine (CGG) at a gene on the X chromosome (Xq27.3) identified in 1991 as FMR-1. The CGG repeats occur just

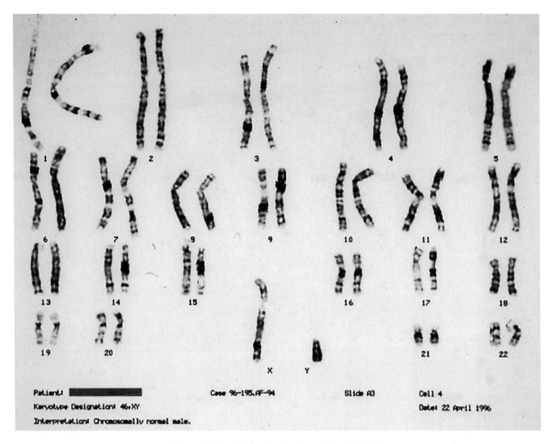

Figure 1-6. Normal male karyotype (46,XY).

before the gene FMR-1 gene (at the 5' end) and abnormal numbers of CGG repeats prevent the formation of stable RNA copies of the FMR-1 gene. The FMR-1 gene product is normally present in many tissues including the brain. Absence of the FMR-1 gene product results in the fragile X syndrome.

Normal individuals have about 30 repeats of CGG at this site. Individuals at risk (premutation) for having offspring with fragile X syndrome have 52–200 CGG repeats. In families with fragile X syndrome, the length of CGG repeats is unstable and increases during DNA meiosis and mitosis. Individuals with more than 200 CGG repeats (up to 1500) have the full fragile X syndrome. The change from premutation to full mutation occurs only with transmission of the abnormal fragile X chromosome from the mother.[3,11]

PREGNANCY AND COUNSELING

Genetic counseling should be offered to parents with risk factors so that they will understand the possibilities, limitations, and risks of prenatal testing. Ideally counseling should occur prior to conception or even premarital. Early assessment of risks may be especially helpful if the parents had a prior abnormal child, a family history of a genetic or congenital defect, exposure to teratogens, or if they are at risk for congenital anomalies because of an underlying disorder such as seizures or diabetes mellitus. Preconception glucose control of insulin-dependent diabetes mellitus may prevent fetal anomalies.[12] Folate supplementation before conception (4 mg/day) in patients who had a previous child with a neural tube defect (NTD) can prevent up to 72% of recurrent NTDs. It is now recom-

Table 1-3.   Incidence of Trisomy 21 in Liveborns and Fetuses in Relationship to Maternal Age

Maternal Age in Years	Incidence Trisomy 21 at Birth	Incidence Trisomy 21 at Amniocentesis (16 Weeks)	Incidence Trisomy 21 at Chorionic Villus Sampling (9–11 Weeks)
15–19	1/1250	—	—
20–24	1/1400	—	—
25–29	1/1100	—	—
30	1/900	—	—
31	1/900	—	—
32	1/750	—	—
33	1/625	1/420	—
34	1/500	1/325	—
35	1/350	1/250	1/240
36	1/275	1/200	1/175
37	1/225	1/150	1/130
38	1/175	1/120	1/100
39	1/140	1/100	1/75
40	1/100	1/75	1/60
41	1/85	1/60	1/40
42	1/65	1/45	1/30
43	1/50	1/35	1/25
44	1/40	1/30	1/20
45 and over	1/25	1/20	1/10

From ref. 27. Reprinted with permission.

mended that all women take 0.4 mg per day of folate prior to and in the early months of pregnancy.[13]

A history of the patient should include the medical backgrounds of the patient, her partner, and their biologic relatives. A three-generation pedigree by a genetic subspecialist can identify additional genetic risks over 40% of the time in

Table 1-4.   Chromosome Abberations: Spontaneous Abortions

Type	Frequency (%)
Aneuploidy	
45,XO	20
Autosomal monosomy	<1
Autosomal trisomy total	52
Trisomy 16	16
Trisomy 18	3
Trisomy 21	5
Trisomy 22	5
Other trisomies	23
Triploidy	16
Tetraploidy	6
Structural rearrangements	4

Source: From ref. 27. Reprinted with permission.

patients referred for routine amniocentesis for advanced maternal age. The age of onset of medical disorders and causes of any deaths should be determined. The patient should be evaluated for a family history of mental retardation, birth defects, pregnancy losses, consanguinity, teratogens and ethnic background. Prospective carrier screening can be offered for certain AR disorders such as sickle cell anemia for African-Americans (carrier rate 1/11), cystic fibrosis for Caucasians (carrier rate 1/22), Tay-Sachs for Ashkenazic Jews (carrier rate 1/30), α-thalassemia for Asians, and β-thalassemia for Italians, Greeks, and Asians.[14]

Prenatal evaluation for fetal Down syndrome risk because of advanced maternal age is a major indication for genetic counseling. Because 80% of trisomy 21 occurs in women under 35 years of age, only 20% of all cases of Down syndrome can be detected if evaluation is limited to mothers with advanced maternal age. Fortunately the biochemical markers alpha-fetoprotein (AFP), hCG, and unconjugated estriol (uE3) can improve screening for chromosome abnormalities. AFP is a glycoprotein with a mo-

Table 1-5. Chromosome Abberations—Outcome of 10,000 Conceptions

Outcome	Conceptions	Spontaneous Abortions	Percent (%)	Live Births
Total	10,000	1500	15	8500
Normal karyotype	9200	750	8	8450
Abnormal karyotype	800	750	94	50
Triploid or tetraploid	170	170	100	—
45,XO	140	139	99	1
Trisomy 16	112	112	100	—
Trisomy 18	20	19	95	1
Trisomy 21	45	35	78	10
Trisomy, other	209	208	99.5	1
47,XXY, 47,XXX, 47,XYY	19	4	21	15
Unbalanced rearrangements	27	23	85	4
Balanced rearrangements	19	3	16	16
Other	39	37	95	2

Source: From ref. 27. Reprinted with permission.

lecular weight of 70,000 that is synthesized in the fetal embryonic yolk sac, gastrointestinal tract, and liver. Fetal serum AFP is highest at 15–24 weeks of gestation and can be measured in fetal blood (milligram levels) by cordocentesis, amniotic fluid (microgram levels) by amniocentesis, and in maternal serum (nanogram levels). See Figures 1-10 and 1-11. Results are reported in multiples of the median (MoM) to standardize interpretation between laboratories.

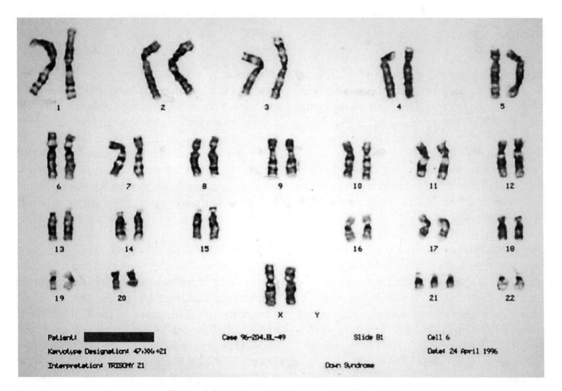

Figure 1-7.   Trisomy 21 karyotype (47,XX,+21).

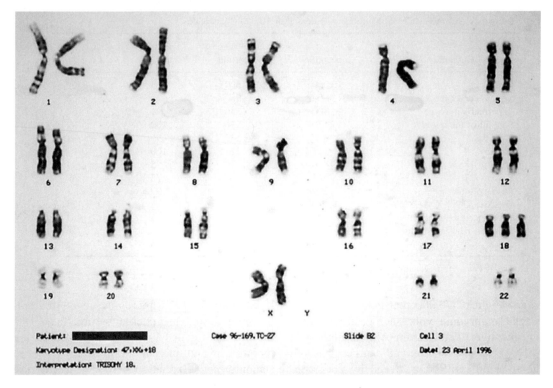

Figure 1-8. Trisomy 18 karyotype (47,XX,+18).

Race, maternal weight, multiple pregnancy, insulin-dependent diabetes mellitus, and fetal estimated gestational age (EGA) all affect evaluation of MSAFP. Low maternal serum AFP (MSAFP) is associated with Down syndrome and combined with maternal age can predict 50% of Down syndrome.[15–17] hCG is higher and unconjugated estriol (uE3) lower in pregnancies with Down syndrome. All three markers are lowered in trisomy 18.[18]

Combining MSAFP, hCG, and estriol in what is termed multiple marker screening has a sensitivity of 60% in predicting either trisomy 21 or trisomy 18 when performed between 15 and 22 weeks gestation. The ability of multiple markers to predict other aneuploidies is unknown. All patients should be offered a maternal serum multiple marker screening between 15 and 20 weeks gestation.

According to Vintzileos, experienced sonographers can identify more than 80% of fetuses with trisomy 21, 18, or 13 in the second trimester of pregnancy by antenatal ultrasound evaluation for fetal structural anomalies or abnormal biometry. In experienced hands, second-trimester ultrasonography may be used to adjust the need for genetic amniocentesis.[19,20] See Chapter 3 for ultrasound findings associated with chromosome abnormalities. See Figure 1-12 for a management plan using multiple markers to screen for chromosomal abnormalities.[21]

A neural tube defect (anencephaly or spina bifida) is a multifactorial disorder that results from failure of the neural tube to properly close during days 22–28 of embryogenesis. A neural tube defect (NTD) occurs in the United States in 1–2 of every 1000 live births, and over 90% of NTDs occur in families with no history of a prior NTD. See Table 1-6 for risk factors for a NTD. An elevated MSAFP (over 2.0–2.5 MoM or multiples of the median) can predict

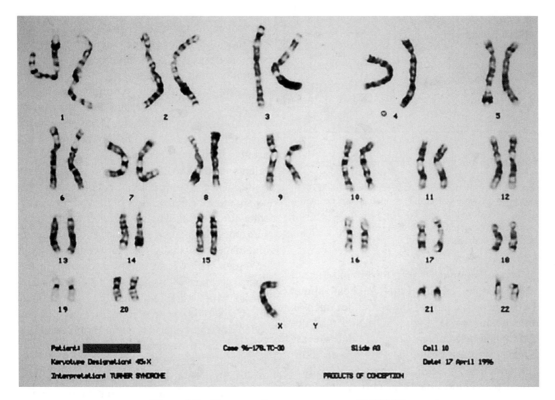

Figure 1-9.   Turner syndrome or monosomy X (45,XO).

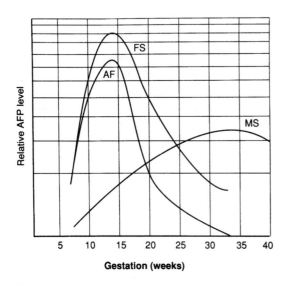

Figure 1-10.   Relative values of alpha-fetoprotein (AFP) in fetal serum (FS), amniotic fluid (AF), and maternal serum (MS) in a normal singleton pregnancy. (From ref. 21. Reprinted with permission.)

80–90% of fetuses with an open NTD. Closed NTDs may not elevate MSAFP and an elevated MSAFP can also occur with multiple gestation, many fetal anomalies (omphalocele, gastroschisis, teratoma), and fetal demise.[22]

A screening MSAFP for NTD should be performed between 15 and 20 weeks gestation and an elevated MSAFP should be repeated in 1–2 weeks gestation. Correct assignment of fetal EGA is critical as normal MSAFP levels change greatly with EGA and an incorrect EGA can lead to an incorrect evaluation of MSAFP. If the repeat MSAFP is still elevated, an ultrasound should be performed to confirm the fetal EGA and to evaluate the fetus for anomalies. An amniocentesis can be performed to evaluate the amniotic fluid for elevated amniotic AFP and for acetylcholinesterase (AChE). A normal AChE indicates that the elevated levels of AFP may be due to some other reason than a NTD. An elevated AChE suggests a fetal NTD or other anomaly.

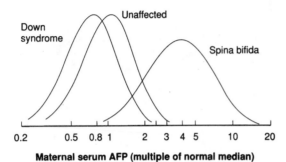

Maternal serum AFP (multiple of normal median)

Figure 1-11.   Maternal serum alpha-fetoprotein (AFP) levels at 16–18 weeks of gestation in singleton pregnancies measured in multiples of normal median for Down syndrome, normals, and spina bifida. (From ref. 21. Reprinted with permission.)

A careful comprehensive ultrasound (Level II) should be performed of the fetal head, spine, and abdomen to evaluate for anomalies such as hydrocephalus, cystic hygroma, neural tube defect, omphalocele, or gastroschisis that are associated with an elevated MSAFP. Even if no fetal anomalies are seen on ultrasound evaluation and the amniocentesis is normal, a markedly elevated MSAFP can indicate a pregnancy at high risk for stillbirth, low birthweight, congenital anomalies, and neonatal death. All patients should be offered MSAFP screening either as part of multiple-marker screening or separately. See Figure 1-13 for a diagram of a management plan for an elevated MSAFP.[21,22]

PREGNANCY IN WOMEN WITH GENETIC ABNORMALITIES

Advances in our knowledge and medical care can allow women who have a genetic disorder to become pregnant. However these women may not only have an increased risk of transmitting their disorder, but they also have an impaired ability to maintain their pregnancy. Some examples include women with PKU, Marfan syndrome, and cystic fibrosis (CF).

Mental retardation, microcephaly, intrauterine growth retardation, and congenital heart disease can occur in the nonphenylketonuric offspring of PKU women who do not adhere to

a low-phenylalanine diet. PKU women should start the low phenylalanine diet prior to pregnancy and should be maintained on the diet throughout their pregnancy.

Patients with Marfan syndrome having an aortic root dilation of greater than 40 mm on echocardiography should avoid pregnancy because of the high risk for life-threatening cardiovascular complications (over 50% death rate). Patients with Marfan syndrome should have prepregnancy counseling, echocardiography, and should be referred to a high-risk (Level III) center for pregnancy care. Women with Marfan syndrome who have minimal cardiovascular involvement can usually tolerate pregnancy well.

Women with CF are advised to avoid or terminate a pregnancy if their forced vital capacity is less than 50% predicted. Pregnant women with CF should be treated with antibiotics as needed for pulmonary infections, bronchodilators, and chest physical therapy. Women with CF who continue their pregnancy should be followed with a team approach consisting of their obstetrician, pulmonologist, nutritionist, anesthesiologist, and neonatologist.[1,9]

GENETIC PROCEDURES

Aminocentesis for prenatal diagnostic genetic testing at 15–20 weeks gestation is the gold standard. The risk of fetal loss after amniocentesis is probably less than 0.5% and the risk benefit ratio is considered favorable for mothers who will be age 35 or greater on their EDC. Chorionic villus sampling (CVS) performed between 9 and 12 weeks gestation has a risk probably 0.6–0.8% higher than amniocentesis and does not allow amniotic fluid evaluation of AFP to screen for NTD and other fetal anomalies. There may be an increased risk of limb and other anomalies with CVS performed before 9 weeks gestation or by an inexperienced operator. Early genetic amniocentesis at less than 15 weeks gestation (usually 12–14 weeks) has a fetal loss rate similar to CVS and permits amniotic fluid evaluation for anomalies. Other techniques of obtaining genetic material include

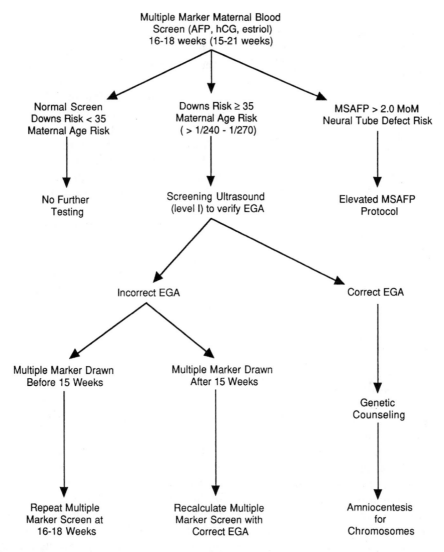

Figure 1-12. Antenatal management plan for abnormal multiple-marker screening at MetroHealth Medical Center, Cleveland, OH. The biochemical markers alpha-fetoprotein (AFP), human chorionic gonadotropin (hCG), and unconjugated estriol (uE3) are evaluated together to improve screening for chromosome abnormalities. EGA = estimated gestational age.

embryoscopy, fetoscopy, and cordocentesis. Preimplantation evaluation has been successfully performed for single-gene disorders by isolating fertilized blastulas or preembryos (up to 14 days postconception), sampling the blastomere(s) in vitro for a rapid genetic assessment and subsequently reimplanting the genotypically normal biopsied preembryos into the uterine cavity to continue the pregnancy to term.[23] A variety of ethical, economic, and legal is-

sues are raised by preimplantation diagnosis, but the technique has the advantage of permitting only those preembryos without the genetic defect to be placed in the uterus.[24] Maternal blood screening of fetal cells (red blood cells, lymphocytes, and trophoblast elements) for fetal chromosome abnormalities is still an experimental technique which may in the future obviate the need for invasive procedures for prenatal diagnosis. Genetic procedures,

Table 1-6.   Relative Risks of Neural Tube Defects (NTD) in the United States

Risk Factor	Incidence per 1000 Live Births
No family history	1
Positive paternal family history	5
Positive maternal family history	10
One prior infant with NTD	20
Insulin-dependent diabetes	20
One parent with NTD	30
Two prior infants with NTD	60

From ref. 21. Reprinted with permission.

risks, and benefits are more fully described in Chapter 4.

CONCLUSION (MANAGEMENT = COUNSEL AND TIMING)

Pregnancy genetic counseling should encompass the risks of the condition, prognosis, treatment options, prenatal testing, and management options. The time constraints of prenatal testing including the medical and legal availability of abortion services should be discussed. Viability in the United States is defined as 24 weeks gestation from the last menstrual period (LMP). After viability, a patient may no longer have the option of pregnancy termination even for a documented fetal structural or chromosome abnormality. It is imperative that prenatal counseling and testing be performed in a timely fashion prior to 20–22 weeks gestation in order to preserve a patient's full options. A few fetal conditions with both a certain prenatal diagnosis and no hope for meaningful survival such as anencephaly can be terminated at any point in gestation at a few specialized centers.

The best method of managing a patient with an abnormal fetus is a team approach. The team should involve the parents, referring health care provider and appropriate high risk (Level III) in house specialists. Specialists may include a geneticist, sonologist, perinatologist, neonatologist, pediatric surgeon, pediatric medical subspecialists, clinical genetics counselor, and nursing and social services.[1,2,14]

State of the Art

New diagnostic technology has revolutionized the field of genetics. Some of the new techniques are restriction enzymes, Southern blot analysis, restriction fragment length polymorphisms (RFLP), polymerase chain reactions (PCR), dot blots, and fluorescence in situ hybridization (FISH). See Table 1-7.

Restriction enzymes permit cutting up the large human genome into smaller manageable pieces ranging from several kilobases (kb) to 1000 kb. The restriction enzymes recognize specific DNA sequences and are named for the bacteria from which they were derived. For example, EcoR1 which recognizes the sequence GAATTC (cuts between G and A) refers to *Escherichia coli* strain R and was the first enzyme identified in the organism.

In Southern blotting (named for E. M. Southern), genetic disorders are evaluated at the level of the DNA. Southern blotting is a labor intensive technique requiring 5–10 μg of DNA that determines the size, basic structure, and presence of a gene. DNA is extracted from the nucleus of cells, cut by restriction enzymes, fractionated by agarose gel electrophoresis, stained with ethidium bromide, the DNA is split into single strands with alkali, transferred and fixed to a nylon membrane (Southern blot) and hybridized with a DNA probes. If pairing with the DNA probe does not occur, the DNA being analyzed does not have the gene structures in the probe. Southern blotting permits evaluation either of genetic patterns in families or precise identification of specific DNA abnormalities. The Northern blot technique identifies RNA and the Western blot protein. Dot blot analysis is a simpler method used with allele-specific probes to determine simply if a specific gene sequence is present. See Figure 1-14.

Restriction fragment-length polymorphisms (RFLP) are genetic variations which are often normal in individuals that result when differing fragments of DNA are cut by restriction enzymes and evaluated by the Southern blot technique. The polymorphisms do not themselves cause the genetic disorder but they may provide

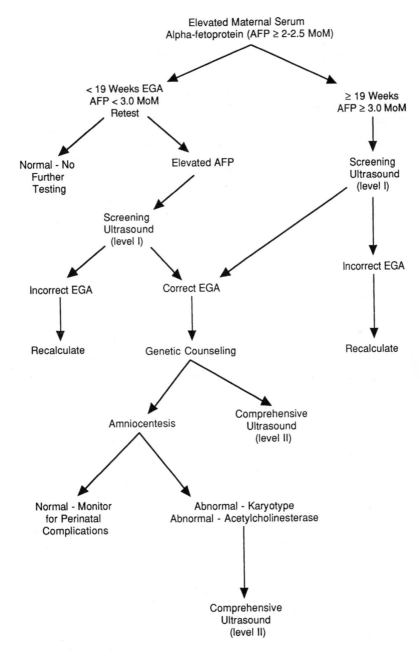

Figure 1-13. Antenatal management plan for an elevated MSAFP at MetroHealth Medical Center, Cleveland, OH. MoM = multiples of the median; MSAFP = maternal serum levels of alpha-fetoprotein.

Table 1-7.   Molecular Genetic Technologies

Genetic Technology	Material	Comment
Restriction enzymes (endonucleases)	DNA	Allows cleavage of a specific fragment of DNA, essential for cloning
Southern blot	DNA (5–10 μg)	Is used to study genetic disorders at DNA level (named for E. M. Southern), labor intensive; identifies presence, size and basic structure of a gene
Northern blot	RNA	Identifies a specific sequence RNA
Western blot	Protein	Identifies a specific protein
Restriction fragment-length polymorphisms (RFLP)	DNA	Polymorphisms on Southern blot; may not cause a genetic disorder but serve as diagnostic markers; detailed family histories may be needed for RFLP to be informative
Polymerase chain reaction (PCR)	DNA (0.1–1 μg)	Allows exponential amplification of small amounts of DNA (one cell) of known sequence; has greatly facilitated rapid genetic diagnosis (cystic fibrosis, Duchenne, hemophilia, Lesch-Nyhan)
Dot blot	DNA	Determines whether or not a gene is present, usually used for allele-specific probes (point mutations)
Fluorescence in situ hybridization (FISH)	DNA	Fluorescein-tagged probes can rapidly identify certain specific chromosome abnormalities (trisomy, monosomy, sex chromosome abnormalities)

Source: From ref. 8. Reprinted with permission.

diagnostic markers that can assist in diagnosing the presence or absence of a genetic disease.

Polymerase chain reaction (PCR) requires smaller amounts of DNA (0.1–1 μg) and is a much simpler and faster process than the Southern blot technique. The DNA to be analyzed is denatured, annealed, and hybridized with known DNA primers over many cycles. Each cycle doubles the amount of DNA of interest and in the customary 30 cycles the original DNA is amplified over one million times. Typically PCR fragments are several kilobases in length. PCR, however, unlike Southern blotting, requires that the sequence of the gene to be identified be known.

Fluorescence in situ hybridization (FISH) is a new DNA technique combining molecular genetics and cytogenetics. Fluorescein-tagged DNA probes are hybridized to specific chromosomes. FISH can be performed on interphase uncultured cell preparations, reducing turn around time since cultured cells can be passed by. FISH can diagnose a trisomy if three hybridization signals are seen in interphase cells instead of the normal two. FISH can screen for X-linked disease by determining the fetal sex with X- and Y-specific probes. FISH can rapidly diagnose chromosomal abnormalities that can be identified by chromosomal probes including trisomy 21, 18, 13, Turner syndrome, and sex chromosome abnormalities.[3,8]

Future of Prenatal Diagnosis and Fetal Therapy

The human genome project began in 1989 with completion scheduled for the year 2005. The federally funded project has over a 100 million dollar annual budget to map and identify the human, mouse, nematode, and fruit fly genome. Once this project is complete humans will be able to read their own genetic blueprint. Knowledge of the human genome should permit the understanding, diagnosis and treatment of genetic disorders. Knowledge of the animal genome should aid in the understanding of human gene structure, regulation, and function. This new knowledge will result in new drugs, therapies, and cures for genetically related medical disorders. It will be possible for prenatal diagnosis and treatment of disorders such as diabetes mellitus, muscular dystrophy, and

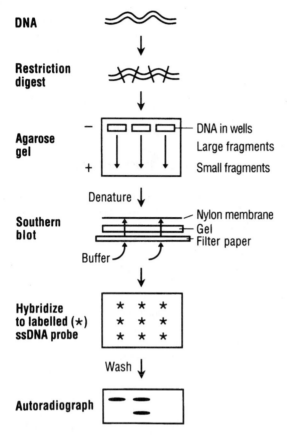

DNA

Restriction digest

Agarose gel

- DNA in wells
Large fragments
Small fragments
+

Denature ↓

Southern blot

Nylon membrane
Gel
Filter paper

Buffer

Hybridize to labelled (*) ssDNA probe

Wash ↓

Autoradiograph

Figure 1-14. Southern blot technique. SSDNA = single stranded deoxyribonucleic acid. (From ref. 8.)

cystic fibrosis. Ethical concerns however have already arisen including discrimination in health insurance, employment and society against those predisposed to genetically related disorders. Hopefully our profession, society, and culture will be wise enough to handle both the rapid advances in genetic knowledge and the legitimate concerns of a humane society.[7,25,26–28]

REFERENCES

1. Rossiter JP, Johnson TR. Management of genetic disorders during pregnancy. *Obstet Gynecol Clin North Am* 1992;19:801–813.

2. Cohn GM. The genetic history: What every OB must know. *OBG Management* April 1996:62–68.

3. Precis V: *An update in Obstetrics and Gynecology.* Danvers, MA: ACOG, 1994.

4. American College of Obstetricians and Gynecologists, *Teratology.* ACOG Technical Bulletin 84. Washington, DC: ACOG, 1985.

5. Shepard TH. *Catalog of Teratogenic Agents,* 8th ed. Baltimore: Johns Hopkins University Press, 1995.

6. Passarge E. *Color Atlas of Genetics.* New York: Thieme, New York, 1995.

7. Green ED, Waterson RH. The human genome project: Prospects and implications for clinical medicine. *JAMA* 1991;226:1966–1975.

8. American College of Obstetricians and Gynecologists, *Genetic Technologies.* ACOG Technical Bulletin 208. Washington, DC: ACOG, 1995.

9. Nance WE. Statement of the American Society of Human Genetics on cystic fibrosis carrier screening. *Am J Hum Genet* 1992;51:1443–1444.

10. Steinberg MH. Genetic modulation of sickle cell anemia. *Proc Soc Exp Biol Med* 1995;209:1–13.

11. Jain K. DNA diagnosis: Fragile X syndrome. *Genetics Lett* 1993;3:1–3.

12. Goldman JA, Dicker D, Feldberg D, et al. Pregnancy outcome in patients with insulin dependent diabetes mellitus with preconception diabetic control: A comparative study. *Am J Obstet Gynecol* 1986;155:293–297.

13. Wald N. Prevention of neural tube defects: Results of the medical research council vitamin study. *Lancet* 1991;338:131–137.

14. Rubin SP, Malin J, Maidman J. Genetic counseling before prenatal diagnosis for advanced maternal age: An important medical safeguard. *Obstet Gynecol* 1983;62:155–159.

15. Merkatz IR, Nitowsky HM, Macri JN, et al. An association between low maternal serum α-fetoprotein and fetal chromosomal abnormalities. *Am J Obstet Gynecol* 1984;148:886–894.

16. Palomaki GE, Haddow JE. Maternal serum α-fetoprotein, age and Down syndrome risk. *Am J Obstet Gynecol* 1987;156:460–463.

17. Hershey DW, Crandall BF, Perdue S. Combining maternal age and serum α-fetoprotein to predict the risk of Down syndrome. *Obstet Gynecol* 1986;68:177–180.

18. Kellner LH, Weiss RR, Weiner Z, et al. The advantages of using triple-marker screening for

chromosomal abnormalities. *Am J Obstet Gynecol* 1995;172:831–836.

19. Vintzileos AM, Egan JFX. Adjusting the risk for trisomy 21 on the basis of second-trimester ultrasonography. *Am J Obstet Gynecol* 1995; 172:837–844.

20. Vintzileos AM, Guzman ER, Smulian JC. The role of second trimester ultrasonography in detecting chromosomal abnormalities. *Female Patient* 1996;21:53–61.

21. American College of Obstetricians and Gynecologists, *Alpha-Fetoprotein*. ACOG Technical Bulletin 154. Washington, DC: ACOG, 1991.

22. Waller KD, Lustig LS, Cunningham GC, et al. Second trimester maternal serum alpha-fetoprotein levels and the risk of subsequent fetal death. *N Engl J Med* 1991;325:6–10.

23. Tarin JJ, Handyside AH. Embryo biopsy strategies for preimplantation diagnosis. *Fertil Steril* 1993;59:943–952.

24. Robertson JA. Ethical and legal issues in preimplantation genetic screening. *Fertil Steril* 1992; 57:1–11.

25. White R, Lalouel JM. Chromosome mapping with DNA markers. *Sci Am* 1988;258:40–48.

26. Albrecht B. Researcher sees benefits risks of genetic mapping. Report of Cleveland City Club lecture by Francis S. Collins, Director of National Center for Human Genetic Research. Cleveland, OH: *The Plain Dealer*, April 20, 1996, p. 128.

27. Thompson MW, McInnes RR, Willard HF. *Thompson & Thompson: Genetics in Medicine*. 5th ed. Philadelphia: Saunders, 1991.

28. Emery AEH, Rimoin DL. *Principles and Practice of Medical Genetics*, 2nd ed., 2 vols. New York: Churchill Livingston, 1990.

BIBLIOGRAPHY

Emery AEH, Rimoin DL. *Principles and Practice of Medical Genetics*, 2 vols., 2nd ed. New York: Churchill Livingstone, 1990.

Reed GB, Claireaux AE, Cockburn F. In Ashmead CG, Chambers SE, Driscoll SG, et al. (eds), *Diseases of the Fetus and Newborn: Pathology, Imaging, Genetics and Management*. 2 vols., 2nd ed. London and New York: Chapman & Hall, 1995.

Romero R, Pilu G, Jeanty P, et al. *Prenatal Diagnosis of Congenital Anomalies*. Norwalk, CT: Appleton & Lange, 1988.

Thompson MW, McInnes RR, Willard HF. *Thompson & Thompson: Genetics in Medicine*, 5th ed. Philadelphia: Saunders, 1991.

QUESTIONS
(choose the single best answer)

1. Indications for prenatal genetic counseling and an increased risk of chromosome abnormalities include all except:
   a. Maternal age 35 or greater at estimated date of confinement.
   b. Low maternal serum alpha-fetoprotein (MSAFP).
   c. Prior infant with monosomy X (45, X).
   d. Three or more spontaneous abortions.

2. All are true except that human teratogens:
   a. Cause effects dependent on dose, stage of embryogenesis, and sensitivity of mother and fetus.
   b. Are also teratogens in rats or mice.
   c. Cause reduction in organ size after organogenesis.
   d. Early in gestation can cause spontaneous abortions.

3. All are true except that the sickle cell disease disorder:
   a. Is a point mutation of adenine to thymine resulting in nonsense.
   b. Results in replacement of a valine for a glutamic acid in β-globin.
   c. Is an abnormality on the short arm of chromosome 11.
   d. In the Middle East, has historically provided a survival benefit for the heterozygote.

4. All are true except that trisomy 21:
   a. Occurs in about 1/800 live births.
   b. Has no increased recurrence risk (only maternal age risk) if the mother was less than 21 years of age.
   c. Will occur in 30% of the offspring of women with a 47,XX,21 karyotype.
   d. Does not significantly increase with advanced paternal age.

5. All of the following are true about alpha-fetoprotein except:
   a. Alpha-fetoprotein is measured in microgram

levels in maternal serum and milligrams levels in amniotic fluid.

b. Maternal serum levels are affected by race, maternal weight, multiple pregnancy, insulin-dependent diabetes mellitus, and estimated gestational age.

c. Low maternal serum alpha-fetoprotein combined with maternal age can predict 50% of Down syndrome.

d. Alpha-fetoprotein is a glycoprotein made in the fetal yolk sac.

6. An autosomal-recessive disorder is:

a. Unlikely to be in the genome of an average person.

b. Glucose 6-phosphate dehydrogenase disease.

c. Phenylketonuria.

d. Angelman syndrome.

2

The Physiology of Pregnancy

Nancy E. Judge

INTRODUCTION

Pregnancy triggers astounding physiologic changes, made more remarkable both by the number of systems affected and by the rate at which alterations occur. The complexity of these adaptations produces an overwhelming urge to group and explain them, often with strained attempts to identify evolutionary advantages for every facet of pregnancy. The survival benefits of volume expansion and hemodilution prior to an era of intravenous solutions and blood banks seem obvious. The life-preserving aspects of backaches and sinus congestion are less apparent, although the mechanisms by which these changes occur are fairly well understood.

More pragmatically, recognition of the differences between pregnant and nonpregnant patients permits physicians to order and interpret laboratory tests correctly, avoid unnecessary interventions, and respond to emergencies. Many physiologic pregnancy symptoms are confusing or alarming to patients and their caregivers. Labor and delivery represent the ultimate test of maternal homeostasis, but at any point during gestation, failure to adapt to the needs of pregnancy may jeopardize both mother and fetus.

Pregnancy impels the maternal organism through a series of changes that often appear to be against her immediate best interest, all for the sake of an eventual successful transition to the puerperium. Alterations include fluid retention, anemia, reduced exercise tolerance, modified maternal immunity, weight gain, joint laxity, gastrointestinal distress, varicose veins, and urinary stasis, among others. This chapter will address many of the best recognized, clinically significant alterations in maternal physiology.

CARDIOVASCULAR SYSTEM

Pregnancy has at least two inescapable requirements: (1) the fetal compartment must receive sufficient perfusion to permit development and waste elimination without seriously compromising its host, and (2) at the conclusion of gestation, evacuation of the uterine contents must occur. The latter is accompanied by blood loss of at least 500 cc. In spite of this substantial shift, maternal homeostasis must be maintained or loss of ability to care for the neonate might ensue. The fundamental solution to both problems is a massive increase in expendable volume, with additional modifications to circulate and oxygenate the new fluid load.

From the sixth week of gestation through the initial portion of the third trimester, maternal plasma volume increases dramatically, by 30–45% over prepregnancy values. The increase is achieved by hormonally mediated salt and water retention by the kidneys: (1) The corpus luteum and syncyctiotrophoblast produce a pharmacologic level of progesterone (20×) which, in combination with uterine metabolites, probably including nitric oxide, produce local and peripheral vasodilation.[1,2] (2) The dilated uterine circulation is a high-flow, low-resistance shunt, which directly increases vascular capacity. (3) Increased vascular capacity drops systemic arterial pressure and intraatrial pressure, triggering renal and atrial mechanisms for volume homeostasis. (4) The activation of the renal renin/angiotensin system to retain sodium and water is also enhanced by placental estrogens and probably other volume-active substances, such as atrial natriuretic factor and fetal dihydroepiandrosterone sulfate (DHEAS). (5) Renal retention of sodium and water is also directly increased by the extremely elevated levels of progesterone. Centrally, maternal thirst and consequent oral intake is increased as well.[2] The magnitude of volume expansion is dependent on a number of factors, including maternal habitus, lack of vascular disease, and fetal size and number, but peaks at about 6–8 L.[1]

Plasma expansion reaches a plateau in the third trimester, then regresses slightly toward term, with a net sodium increase of 500–1000 mEq.[3] Meanwhile, erythropoietin secretion increases, in response to both actual and dilutional anemia. The maternal red blood cell (RBC) mass eventually expands by 25%.[1] At delivery, the relative disproportion between plasma and RBC mass reduces the magnitude of hemoglobin and iron losses. Lower blood viscosity may also decrease the risk of placental infarction and prevent microtrauma and thrombosis in intervillous and other small vessels.[3] Maternal colloid production lags behind the volume expansion; the resulting gradual decline in oncotic pressure increases escape of fluids from the vasculature (''third spacing'') and contributes to dependent soft tissue edema. Although pulmonary capillary wedge pressure (PCWP) is not affected by pregnancy, the reduced gradient between the PCWP and colloid osmotic pressure (from 15 mm Hg to 10 mm Hg) during pregnancy favors the development of pulmonary edema after fluid overload and other stressors.[4,5]

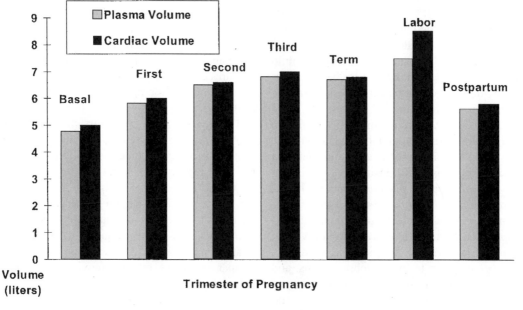

Figure 2-1.   Volume and output during gestation. (Adapted from refs. 3–5.)

Cardiac output (CO) increases from the fifth week of gestation, initially as a result of a faster pulse and later from greater volume per compression (increased by 20%). Late in pregnancy, CO reaches a plateau at 40–50% above baseline, then drops slightly towards prepregnancy values, echoing the volume curve.[1] By term, uterine blood flow has increased dramatically, from 100 mL/min to more than 700 mL/min; more than 90% of the added flow is targeted for the intervillous space. The low-pressure network of the intervillous bed drops the systemic vascular resistance (SVR) to 80% of prepregnancy values, an effect enhanced by systemic vasodilation. Simultaneously, venous pressures in the legs and other dependent sites increase up to 75% above prepregnancy levels. In response to reduced systemic arterial resistance, mean arterial blood pressures initially drop, with systolic and diastolic reductions of 25% and 35%, respectively, at midpregnancy, but return to within 15% of original values by term.[3] In spite of increased levels of angiotensin II and its precursors, vascular responsivity is usually decreased in normal pregnant women. During labor, blood pressures increase in response to elevated catecholamines and angiotensin II; normalization occurs during the first week postpartum. Cardiac output rises by 30% during labor, primarily from catecholamine-enhanced stroke volume (SV), although heart rate is increased after contractions. Peak CO occurs when massive fluid transfers from the uterine vascular bed are triggered by delivery of the placenta. Normalization may require 48–72 hours.[1,3,6]

The CO and SVR are exquisitely sensitive to postural cues during pregnancy. Hemodynamic values cannot be interpreted accurately without reference to the patient's position. A significant proportion of apparent disagreements in the literature regarding maternal cardiovascular findings may be attributable to positional effects.[1] Compression of the inferior vena cava (IVC) in the supine position by the enlarged uterus diverts venous return to the vertebral plexus, and from the paraspinal veins into the azygos and ovarian veins. Right atrial pressure drops, and IVC and femoral venous pressures rise. In almost half of pregnancies, aortic compression also occurs, with supine hypotension particularly pronounced in women with inadequate paravertebral collaterals (10% of the population). Stroke volume and CO routinely decrease by 25%, with a 20% drop in uterine perfusion in the supine position. In contrast, the left lateral position maximizes venous return and CO.[1,3,4]

The demands of pregnancy on the heart are similar to those of prolonged aerobic athletic training; but because there is no corresponding drop in heart rate, the net effect is modest cardiac strain. In fact, cardiac function in pregnancy is fostered only by the SVR-linked drop in afterload and marginal increases in pO_2. All else—the increased basal metabolic rate (BMR), heart rate, contractility, and preload, combined with decreases in hemoglobin and diastolic filling time—serves to undermine cardiac balance, placing pregnant women with preexisting heart disease in particular jeopardy. In healthy women, however, the cardiac reserve is more than sufficient to permit them to continue daily activities and to exercise without significant risk of ischemia.[1,3,7]

The left ventricle increases in size during diastole because of the increased preload; the rapid heart rate encourages a stable ventricular size during systole.[1] As a result of diaphragmatic elevation and altered ventricular filling, the heart shifts forward and to the left during pregnancy; the apex moves toward the fourth interspace and the midclavicular line. The first heart sound and the mitral-tricuspid split are accentuated. Exaggeration of the third heart sound and a physiologic fourth heart sound are common during intravascular volume expansion. The valve orifices increase slightly in diameter; tricuspid regurgitancy is thought to account for the Grade 1–2 early to mid-systolic murmur often found at the left sternal border, although increased flow through the mammary vessels may also contribute to the frequency of pregnancy-related murmurs. Valve diameters and left ventricular thickness remain above pregestational values for months after delivery.[3]

In addition to alterations in the physical examination, adaptations to pregnancy may affect

Table 2-1. Cardiovascular Alterations During Pregnancy

	Nonpregnant Value	Pregnancy Value
Increased		
Heart rate	60–80 bpm	70–90 bpm
Cardiac output	3–5 L/min	5–7 L/min
Stroke volume	35–80 cc/beat	55–100 cc/beat
LV end-diastolic volume	110–120 cc	120–140 cc
Total blood volume	4–6 L	6–8 L
Decreased		
Systemic vascular resistance	1500 dyne–cm sec^{-5}	800–1200 dyne–cm sec^{-5}
Pulmonary vascular resistance	60–100 dyne–cm sec^{-5}	50–90 dyne–cm sec^{-5}
Colloid oncotic pressure	28 mOsm	17–19 mOsm
Mean arterial pressure	72–95 mm Hg	60–85 mm Hg
Minimally altered		
Ejection fraction	60%	60–70%
PCWP	6–8 mm Hg	
LV stroke work index	40–50 g/m/m^{-2}	
CVP	2–7 mm Hg	

Adapted from refs. 3, 4, and 10, left lateral recumbency.

Abbreviations: CVP, central venous pressure; LV, left ventricular; PCWP, pulmonary capillary wedge pressure.

common diagnostic tests of cardiac status. Electrocardiographs (ECGs) usually demonstrate sinus tachycardia, with a shortened P-R interval. The QRS axis shifts to the right in the first trimester; the T-wave axis shifts leftward. Left-sided precordial leads and limb leads may show S-T segment depression and low-voltage T waves; Q waves may be seen in lead III, confusing evaluations for ischemia. Supraventricular arrhythmias are also more common during pregnancy. Echocardiography changes include mild left ventricular hypertrophy, increased cardiac mass (up to 50% over baseline), and more than 10% increases in aortic, mitral, and pulmonic valve areas, with frequent tricuspid regurgitation.[3,5] Serial increases in the myocardial fraction of the creatine kinase assay are usually used to confirm injury or infarction; both skeletal and myocardial isoenzymes are expressed in the uterus and the placenta. Overlap with diagnostic myocardial levels has been reported after vaginal delivery; lesser elevations follow cesarean section.[8] Fortunately, myocardial infarction rarely complicates pregnancy; other tests, such as lactate dehydrogenase isoenzyme levels and perfusional scans are not affected by pregnancy.

PULMONARY ADAPTATIONS TO PREGNANCY

Oxygen requirements increase by 40–60% during gestation, reflecting both fetal needs and increased maternal consumption.[9,10] O_2 demands rise by 40% during the first stage of labor and by 75% or more during the second stage, accentuated by energy expended in hyperventilation.[3] Ambient and maternal pulmonary arterial oxygen levels remain unchanged; respiratory rate does not vary significantly with pregnancy, and total lung volumes are unaltered. Just two compensations are substantially responsible for achieving adequate oxygenation. (1) Minute ventilation increases by 100–300%, through greater tidal volume (deeper breathing). Increased energy requirements of pregnancy generate 20% more CO_2; elevated CO_2 and progesterone sensitization of the respiratory centers stimulate respiration, thus increasing the tidal volume.[2,3,9] Most women describe breathlessness or more frequent sighing during pregnancy as subjective responses to increased respiratory drive. (2) The alveolar sacs are also more efficiently ventilated because there is reduced dilution of fresh air by depleted residual air once diaphragmatic elevation compresses residual lung volumes.[3,9] Hormonally stimulated capillary engorgement occurs in the nasal and oropharyngeal mucosa, producing more mouth breathing and a sense of dyspnea; paradoxically, airway conductance may be increased in larger airways beneath the larynx. Drying of the mucosa and capillary engorgement increases the susceptibility of nasopharyngeal tissues to trauma and bleeding.[3]

Anatomically, the diaphragm is driven upward approximately 4 cm by the increasing fundus and displaced gastrointestinal tract; in spite of this, its excursion is actually increased. The thorax widens, by 7 cm in circumference, but with increasing subcostal angulation; the dynamic chest wall excursion is decreased. The overall effect on lung volumes is a slight (5%) decrease in total lung capacity (TLC) from offsetting changes in tidal, expiratory reserve, and residual volumes. A marked (45%) increase in minute and alveolar ventilation compensates for similar increases in dead space. Flow loops are comparable to nonpregnant performance, suggesting minimal effects on small airways. The most noticeable respiratory effect is on the arterial blood gas (ABG) profile, in which mild hypocapnia (P_aCO_2 of 30 mm Hg) is largely offset by decreased bicarbonate levels, with a trend toward respiratory alkalosis.[3,9]

Maternal position also dramatically affects pulmonary function; upright position optimizes results. The supine position decreases functional reserve capacity to 70% of the upright volume; this may be below the closing capacity (the point at which small airways collapse) in some women, increasing susceptibility to hypoxia. Moreover, the enhanced oxygen needs of the fetus and mother double the rate at which asphyxia develops during inadequate ventilation. Maternal pulmonary adaptations to pregnancy resolve gradually over several months postpartum; additional conflicts in published data may reflect the use of puerperal normal values instead of prepregnancy levels.[3]

Oxygen consumption increases by 30–60 mL/min during pregnancy from the combination of maternal and fetal utilization. Vasolidation, collateral vessels and increased circulating volume respond to this demand, increasing blood flow to the uterus. Several adaptations maximize the delivery of oxygen to the fetus. Transfer is by simple diffusion, but is facilitated by increased maternal levels of 2,3-diphosphotidyl-glycerol (2,3-DPG)[10] This compound binds to hemoglobin and decreases its affinity for oxygen, improving oxygen release to tissues and fetal red blood cells. Fetal hemoglobin binds 2,3-DPG poorly compared to maternal hemoglobin A, increasing fetal avidity for oxygen and shifting the oxygen dissociation curve to the left, relative to the mother.[2,10] This advantage is decreased if the mother has received banked blood or has a hemoglobinopathy. Exposure to high altitude, anemia, fever, exercise, androgens, thyroid, and growth hormones increases the mother's levels of 2,3-DPG, shifting her oxygen dissociation curve further to the right, favoring oxygen release. Attachment of oxygen to red cells is also increased by lower levels of carbon dioxide (CO_2). The diffusion of CO_2 from the fetal to the maternal side is so rapid that low fetal levels enhance oxygen pickup. A final advantage for the fetus in its quest for oxygen is that fetal hemoglobin levels are about 50% greater than maternal values.[10,11]

RENAL FUNCTION DURING PREGNANCY

The maternal renal system responds to the need for retention of both salt and water, then handles the resulting massive increase in intravascular volume. Blood flow to the kidneys increases by up to 85% in normal patients, tapering to 65% at term, reflecting both redistribution of maternal flow toward the pelvis and previously described changes in intravascular volume.[3] Urine

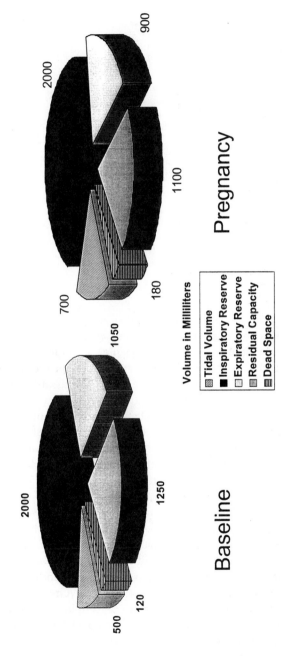

Figure 2-2. Lung volumes. (Adapted from refs. 3 and 9.)

Table 2-2. Pulmonary Alterations During Pregnancy

	Nonpregnant Value	Pregnancy Value
Increased		
Oxygen consumption	32 mL/min	58 mL/min
Respiratory quotient	0.76	0.83
Tidal volume	500 mL/min	700 mL/min
Minute ventilation	7.5 L	120–140 cc
Dead space	120 cc	180 cc
P-50 (dissociation constant)	26 mm Hg	30 mm Hg
Decreased		
Arterial CO_2 tension (P_aCO_2)	35–40 mm Hg	300 mm Hg
Residual volume	1200 mL	1000 mL
Total lung volume	5500 mL	5200 mL
Expiratory reserve volume	1000 mL	800 mL
Minimally altered		
Respiratory rate	12–18 breaths/minute	
pH	7.4	7.44
Arterial O_2 tension (P_aO_2)	100 mm Hg	103–107 mm Hg
Oxygen saturation	95%	
Vital capacity	4 L	

Adapted from refs. 3 and 9, seated position.

production increases, with noticeable changes in both volume and frequency of voiding. The resorption of sodium, chloride and water increases by 50%; at the same time, the glomerular filtration rate (GFR) increases by 50%, balancing resorption. The increased GFR correlates well with progesterone levels and may reflect higher renal plasma flow; alterations in oncotic and hydrostatic pressures may also contribute to the GFR.[12] A higher filtration rate is responsible for the 40% reduction in blood urea nitrogen (BUN) and creatinine. The GFR remains elevated during the first week postpartum, but returns to normal by the fourth week.[10,12]

Tubular resorption of uric acid is reduced by the increased filtration rate; after a first trimester drop to 50% of baseline, values return to normal by term.[5] Creatinine clearance increases from the sixth week of gestation, peaking at more than 130 mL/min during the second trimester before dropping back toward prepregnancy values.[3] Sodium increases by 1 g net during the course of pregnancy; potassium is retained by the proximal tubules in spite of high aldosterone levels (usually a cause of hypokalemia), and potassium losses from the distal tubule and loop of Henle. Calcium losses are increased in healthy women; gastrointestinal tract absorption exceeds calciuria, allowing maternal and fetal needs to be met without changing free serum values.[5] Serum osmolality drops by up to 10 mOsm without triggering antidiuretic hormone (ADH) secretion, possibly because of overriding effects of decreased blood pressure.[12] Glycosuria increases markedly during pregnancy in spite of increased proximal tubule absorption, higher insulin levels, and lower serum glucose values, because the volume load and hormonally impaired resorption affect the collecting tubules and loop of Henle. Increased urinary losses are also noted for a number of amino acids, including alanine, glycine, histidine, serine and threonine; the implication of this finding is uncertain.[5] Positional effects on renal function, as for cardiopulmonary studies, complicate comparisons of research data; circadian rhythms, changes in body/renal size, and greater variance in resorption and clearance of traditional markers add to difficulties in interpretation.[12]

Renal size increases by 30% during pregnancy. The combination of hormonal effects (progesterone) and mechanical obstruction of the ureters by pelvic vessels and gravid uterus produces reflux and hydronephrosis in a majority of patients, with a predilection for the right side.[3,5] These physical changes may promote the development of upper urinary tract infections during pregnancy, and certainly complicate interpretation of renal ultrasound and radiologic studies. Kidney size returns to normal by the first postpartum week, but hydronephrosis and hydroureters persist for up to 12 weeks longer. Pregnancy effects on the urethral angle appear modest. Even though urethral length and closing pressures are somewhat increased, pressure of the presenting part against the bladder, in combination with hormonally mediated relaxation of urinary tract musculature, increases the prevalence of stress urinary incontinence during pregnancy.[5,14]

GASTROINTESTINAL TRACT ADAPTATIONS TO PREGNANCY

Nearly all pregnant patients will experience unpleasant symptoms related to the gastrointestinal tract, particularly nausea and pyrosis. The most obvious alteration during pregnancy is obligatory and mechanical: the stomach is pushed up and leftward by the displaced gut and enlarged uterus; it then rotates rightward on its long axis. The altered location and shape tend to increase a tendency to hiatal hernia formation and promote reflux by increasing intragastric pressure

and reducing lower esophageal tone. Intragastric pressures correlate well with susceptibility to heartburn; esophageal tone is most likely decreased by progesterone, which also slows peristalsis and rate of transit throughout the intestinal tract.[3] Brush border enzyme activity is increased, probably increasing efficiency of nutrient and water absorption. Surprisingly, there is no clear relationship between these effects and constipation. Gastric pepsin secretion and acidity may be lessened through the thirtieth week of gestation; findings at term are in the nonpregnant range, however.[3,15] Gastric emptying slows during the first trimester, but rapidly returns to normal for the remainder of pregnancy, except at delivery. During labor, gastric volume and acidity rise and gastric emptying slows, delays are exaggerated by narcotics. These changes increase the potential for severe aspiration pneumonitis.[3] The etiologies of common complaints like nausea and vomiting (''morning sickness'') and of related conditions such as ptyalism and hyperemesis remain obscure, but are attributed to combined effects of several gestational hormones on central and end-organ sites. Increased hunger sensation is generally reported by the beginning of the second trimester. Taste sensation is also altered, possibly reflecting a combination of nasal engorgement and progesterone stimulated changes in saliva.

Numerous hepatic synthetic and metabolic activities are increased during pregnancy. In spite of no significant perfusional changes. Additionally, the liver undergoes hormonally me-

Table 2-3. Renal Changes in Pregnancy

	Prepregnancy	Pregnancy
Increased		
Creatinine clearance	90–110 mL/min	110–150 mL/min
Urinary protein (24 hours)	<150 mg/day	<300 mg/day
Decreased		
Serum creatinine	0.8–1.5 mg/dL	0.5–1.0 mg/dL
BUN	10–20 mg/dL	5–12 mg/dL
Uric acid	1.5–6.0 mg/dL	1.2–5.0 mg/dL

Source: Adapted from ref. 13.

Abbreviations: BUN, blood urea nitrogen.

diated fatty changes and a predictable second-trimester mechanical displacement. Hepatic production of globulins, coagulation proteins, and various binding and transport proteins are increased, along with triglycerides, cholesterol, low-density, and very-low-density lipoproteins, all in response to estrogen. Increased maternal cholesterol production is essential, as this compound, crucial for fetal neuroendocrine development, is not synthesized by the placenta. Liver enzymes generally demonstrate slightly increased values in pregnancy; both total and conjugated bilirubin may rise. Sharply elevated heat-stable alkaline phosphatase levels derive from placental, not hepatic production.[16]

Gallbladder emptying slows, with enlargement common by late pregnancy. Bile composition is affected by progesterone and estrogen, increasing saturation and decreasing the chenodeoxycholic acid pool. Stasis and stone formation are enhanced by these effects.[15,16]

As a result of estrogen-stimulated hepatic production of clotting factors and increased platelet turnover, pregnancy exhibits accelerated coagulability, offset by increased fibrinolysis. Decreased levels are noted only for antithrombin III (enhancing coagulability), Factor XI (thromboplastin accelerator), and Factor XIII (fibrin-stabilizing factor); the last is largely responsible for increased rates of fibrin degradation and measured increases in fibrin degradation products. Levels of Factor II (prothrombin), Factor V (proaccelerin), and platelet counts are usually unchanged during pregnancy; all the other clotting factors, plasminogen, and fibrinopeptide A are increased. Enhanced coagulation may be particularly important in controlling small placental bleeding sites and in secondary mechanisms of puerperal hemostasis. Postpartum, clotting times decrease even further; fibrinogen decreases, however and fibrinolysis markers dissipate. Up to 8 weeks will elapse prior to complete normalization of values.[3]

Overall levels of immunoglobulin G (IgG), immunoglobulin A (IgA), and immunoglobulin M (IgM) remain constant, but hepatic production of specific antibodies is altered. Pregnancy may result in mildly diminished immunocompetency, possibly reflecting isolation and maintenance of the fetal allograft. Antibody production against herpesvirus, measles, and influenza A is decreased; nonetheless, transmission of maternal IgG across the placenta occurs throughout pregnancy, providing passive neonatal immunity for polio, diphtheria, and measles, among others.[3,10] Leukocyte counts nearly double during pregnancy, rising throughout labor to 15,000/μL at delivery. Gradually, values drop below 10,000/μL at the end of the first postpartum week, and normalize after 6 weeks. Increases are in the form of immature polymorphonucleocytes (PMNs) with decreased chemotaxis and adherence. Consistent with these observations, the empirical incidence and severity of some infections seem increased during pregnancy; along with higher corticosteroid levels, these alterations in immunity may also account for the observation that autoimmune diseases may improve during pregnancy.[3,17]

METABOLIC, NUTRITIONAL, AND STRUCTURAL CHANGES

Increased caloric intake is needed to support the developing gestation; the resulting enlargement of the uterus, its contents, and host is one of the best recognized changes of pregnancy. Weight gain in normal pregnancy averages 17% of basal values, or about 12 kg, distributed in increases of 1–2 kg in the first trimester, and 4–6 kg in each subsequent trimester.[3] During the final month of gestation, the fetus normally gains approximately 0.25 kg per week. Uterine weight increases from 50 g to 1 kg; at term, the fetus averages 3.2 kg and placenta and amniotic fluid, 2–3 kg; the breasts gain 1 kg, 2.5 kg of fluid is retained, and at least 1.5 kg of hip and thigh fat deposition occurs. These weight gains occur in spite of a 15% increase in BMR, reflecting effects of fluid retention, increased appetite, and decreased activity. Supplemental intake averaging 300 kcal/day is required for fetal growth and fat stores. Fetal glucose requirements are about 25 g/day; alternative fuel sources include ketoacids and free fatty acids. Fetal and gestational protein needs total 30 g/day above baseline.[18] Calcium uptake from the gastrointestinal tract increases, but the fetal need for calcium to produce bones, muscles, and transmitters totals 1/50th of the maternal supply. Mild osteoporotic changes may occur in some mothers. Iron requirements of pregnancy total 1 g; 300 mg are for fetal red blood cell and tissue production and the remainder is needed for maternal red blood cell (RBC) mass. Additional folic acid is necessary for nucleic acid and protein synthesis, and neural and red cell development; vitamins B, C, D, E, and K are also required in amounts above basal values.[10] Without supplements, requirements which exceed dietary intake exhaust maternal stores; however, deficiency states severe enough to compromise outcome or well-being are not often identified in developed countries.

As pregnancy progresses, fluid shifts and dependent venous pressure result in labial edema and lower body puffiness; varicose veins and hemorrhoids appear in a significant number of women.[19] Venous stasis may also promote leg cramps. Uterine weight increases tension on supporting ligaments, stimulating smooth muscle activity and cramping. The weight of the gestation also affects the musculoskeletal system; compensation through increased lumbar lordosis and counterbalancing neck flexion are probably responsible for common complaints of back and shoulder discomfort. Exaggerated lordosis or gluteal edema may produce clinically significant sciatic nerve compression. Increased shoulder slumping occurs in response to increased breast weight and rib cage changes, but may result in brachial plexus traction and subsequent arm pain, weakness or numbness.[3] Fluid retention in the flexor retinaculum cuff of the wrist increases the severity of carpal tunnel symptoms. Heightened mobility of sacroiliac, sacrococcygeal, and pubic joints is noted by 30 weeks gestation, possibly as a result of relaxin.[2] The arches of the feet flatten; pedal length and width may increase permanently, most probably from sustained weight bearing and hormonal effects. Gait alterations occur as a result of pelvic

joint relaxation, flattened arches, and greater lordosis, but may also reflect distribution of recent weight gains.

Hormonal effects in the maternal skin are very noticeable. Skin perfusion increases by three to four times prepregnancy levels, associated with increasing skin turgor and skin temperature. Small vessels dilate and proliferate, with telangiectasias, spider angiomata formation, and palmar erythema, the latter two secondary to estrogen. Acrochordons (skin tags) may appear in response to increased levels of skin tag growth factor. With rapid weight changes and increased cortisol levels, striae ("stretch marks") appear at sites of linear collagen tears over the abdomen, hips and breasts in susceptible patients. Placental androgen stimulation of sebaceous and follicular glands increases the prevalence of hirsutisim and acne. Meanwhile, estrogen decreases the rate of hair growth but lengthens the duration of the growth phases, dropping the proportion of hair in the telogen (falling out) phase to below 10%. For several months postpartum, there is a 35% compensatory rise in telogen phase hair, responsible for the misperception that childbearing causes hair loss. Hyperpigmentation of skin and pigmented lesions during pregnancy is nearly universal, although whether these effects are from estrogen, progesterone, melanocyte stimulating hormone, melatonin, or adrenocorticotropic hormone (ACTH) is unclear. The linea alba and areolar regions increase in pigmentation; chloasma ("mask of pregnancy") occurs in more than 70% of women, accentuated by sun exposure.[20] Gingival hyperplasia and pyogenic granulomata are oral changes common in pregnancy; the latter lesions may also manifest on the vulva.[19] Most skin changes improve significantly postpartum; residual alterations in pigmentation, superficial varicosities, skin tags, hemorrhoids, and "stretch marks" occur to some extent in most women.

Neurologic changes of pregnancy are difficult to evaluate. Peripheral nerve symptoms rarely occur with vitamin deficiencies, but more frequently result from postural or edema-enhanced direct compression. Referred pain from sacral plexus stimulation in latter gestation may give rise to vaginal arching. Occasionally, prolonged pressure from fetal or extrinsic sources during delivery result in peroneal or femoral neuropathies, usually self-limited. Increased levels of progesterone, estrogen, prolactin, endorphins, and serotonin activity may combine to reduce sensitivity to physical discomfort, elevate mood, increase a sense of well-being, and decrease stress. By the third postpartum day, dropping estrogen and progesterone levels contribute to transient emotional lability and depressed affect (''the baby blues''). Increased sympathetic tone increases venous return from the lower extremities; catecholamine levels and endorphins both rise during labor. Pregnancy also tends to potentiate neuromuscular blockades with some specific agents, independent of mildly decreased cholinesterase levels. The venous pressure of the epidural space is increased, and cerebrospinal fluid (CSF) volume may be slightly decreased; otherwise, except for increases with pushing or contractions, CSF dynamics appear unaffected by pregnancy. Epidural pressures generally normalize within 6–12 hours after delivery.[3]

ALTERATION OF HORMONAL LEVELS

Nearly every hormonal system is affected by gestation. In addition to altered maternal production, there are new sites for hormone synthesis during pregnancy, including the decidua, myometrium, chorion, placenta, and fetus. Although maternal pituitary blood flow and pituitary size are markedly increased, not all pituitary hormones are increased. Growth hormone decreases, probably because of feedback from placentally produced variants like human chorionic somatotropin. Pituitary inhibition by placental progesterone and estrogen result in decreased follicle stimulating hormone (FSH) and luteinizing hormone (LH) levels with further suppression by inhibin production from the corpus luteum and placenta.[18,21,22] Prolactin, oxytocin, and thyrotropin production is increased.

The thyroid increases in size by up to 50% and increases production as a result of the influence of placental production of human chorionic gonadotropin (hCG) and human chorionic thyrotropin, but the levels of free (active) thyroid hormone remain unchanged because of increased protein binding.[10] Glucocorticoids are markedly increased and aldosterone more than doubles in response to elevations of ACTH and corticotropin-releasing hormone (CRH); the rise in the free level of cortisol is somewhat blunted by increased binding globulin production by the liver, but still reaches values 2.5 times normal. Insulin secretion is increased by the third month of gestation and peaks in the third trimester; in spite of this and increased fetal demands, serum glucose levels tend to rise as a result of human placental lactogen effects. Most hormone levels except for prolactin approach prepregnancy values within 72 hours after delivery.[3,18,21]

The decidual products include progesterone, prostaglandin, prolactin, relaxin, sulfatase, and $1,25\text{-}(OH)_2$-vitamin D. The syncytiotrophoblast is the more hormonally active placental cell line, secreting hCG from within 2–3 days after implantation, estrogens (particularly estriol from fetal precursors), progesterone, human placental lactogen, sulfatase, and aromatase.[10] Cytotrophoblast secretes stimulatory and inhibitory peptides and growth factors, including gonadotropin-releasing hormone (GnRH); it also produces somatostatin, prorenin, and may produce inhibin, growth hormone releasing factor, and angiotensin II. The cytotrophoblast does not make sulfatase or aromatase; the placenta does not synthesize cholesterol, 17-OH-progesterone, or prolactin.[2,18,22]

LABOR

The duration of pregnancy is 270 days from conception. Labor occurs after a prodrome of varying length, characterized by increased sensitivity to catecholamines, increasing endorphin secretion and an increased frequency of mild uterine contractions over baseline values.[10] Cervical position, consistency, and length are altered ("ripening"), with increased passage of cervical mucus of increasing liquidity ("mucus plug"). The latter is often accompanied by staining from disruption of small maternal vessels in the lower uterine segment and cervix ("bloody show"). Parturients may complain of vague back and lower abdominal discomfort. The last portion of these changes is the latent phase of labor, characterized by steady increases in contraction frequency, intensity, and duration, resulting in completion of cervical effacement and initial cervical dilation.[24]

The precise trigger for normal labor is unknown. Uterine gap junctions increase in number throughout gestation, perhaps in response to estrogen effects; gap junctions increase the speed and co-ordinate propagation of contractions.[2] Uterine muscle contracts when myosin binds to actin, induced by myosin light-chain kinase in the presence of ATP. The kinase is activated when intracellular calcium is bound to calmodulin. Oxytocin maintains intracellular calcium in the myometrial calcium/magnesium adenosine triphosphatase (ATPase) system, stimulating contractions; oxytocin also increases the number of prostaglandin receptors.[25] Although oxytocin receptors increase 100-fold by the last third of pregnancy, enhancing response to endogenous secretion, peak levels occur well after the onset of labor.[2] Fetal oxytocin secretion is also increased, before detectable rises in maternal levels, but without known fluctuations at labor onset. Prostaglandin secretion directly stimulates uterine contractions through release of calcium or prevention of reuptake; it also increases oxytocin receptors, water content, and distensibility of the cervical stromal tissues. Uterine distention may enhance decidual disruption and release of prostaglandins. As the fetus matures, its adrenal output is increased, possibly altering local estrogen and other steroid levels; local changes in membrane stability may release additional prostaglandin.[10]

Once labor begins, pressure from the membranes and presenting part and continued distention of the cervix result in further secretory pulses of oxytocin from the pituitary. Uterine massage, fetal movements, and mechanical

stretching may all increase contraction frequency. Contractions begin at the fundus and cornua and travel toward the cervix, waning as they proceed. Active labor succeeds the gradual changes of the latent phase, following a sinusoidal curve of cervical dilation and contraction intensity with up to 10 kg downward force.[10] Oxygen consumption rises; systolic and diastolic blood pressures increase and cardiac output is augmented. During contractions, uteroplacental perfusion decreases, recovering during relaxation. Pain may result from both tissue hypoxia and visceral sensory signals from cervical distention. The hypogastric nerves are the primary afferent initially, succeeded by somatic nerves of the cervix and vagina in latter stages.[26] Anxiety and pain increase CO, probably through catecholamine-mediated inotropic and chronotropic changes; conversely, analgesics diminish this effect. Circulating volume and CO are optimized by left lateral positioning during labor.[6,27] Culmination of active labor occurs at approximately 10 cm cervical dilation (corresponding to the fetal cephalic diameter), a combination of voluntary and involuntary expulsive efforts of the second stage then results in delivery of the infant.[10]

The third stage (placental delivery) is triggered by the sudden decrease in uterine size; the less elastic placenta shears away from the implantation site with a concomitant transfer of 300 mL of blood to the maternal circulation from constriction of uterine sinuses, balancing an average 500 mL blood loss. Hemostasis occurs first through mechanical compression of intramyometrial vessels by uterine musculature, and by prostaglandin-mediated vasoconstriction; continued decidual autolysis produces the lochial discharge.[10] The uterus gradually resumes its prepregnancy size over 4–6 weeks; alterations of both gap junction formation and calcium binding appear to persist for a number of years.

After initial blood loss and compensatory autotransfusion, plasma volume increases, as extracellular fluid reenters the vascular compartment and aortocaval compression is eliminated. Within 15 minutes after delivery, CVP and SVR rise; SV and CO increase by up to 75% above prepregnancy values within the first hour, making this period particularly hazardous for women with fixed valvular lesions or other risks for heart failure. During the next 24–48 hours, CO drops by 30%, with decreases in both the SV and heart rate.[5,6] Volume changes generally resolve by the second or third postpartum month; resolution of cardiac findings may require up to 6 months. Some hypertrophy and subtle alterations in contractility, CO, and SV are detectable 2 years postpartum.

LACTATION

Lactation occurs only after extensive hormonally mediated preparation of the breasts. Estrogen, progesterone, prolactin, and possibly hCG stimulate proliferation of the ductal system, lobules, alveoli, and secretory cells, contribute to breast enlargement. Initial production of colostrum by alveolar cells begins by the 20th week; however, full lactation does not begin until placental delivery triggers a drop in estrogen and progesterone. Colostrum is fat-free and contains one hundred times the energy content by volume of later milk. Breast milk has more lactose than colostrum or cow's milk, less protein, more fat, much less sodium, and an intermediate amount of calcium.[2]

Eventually, milk production may reach 1.5 L daily and require 500 kcal/day above normal intake. Sustained milk production requires adequate parathormone, growth hormone, thyroid hormone, and adrenal glucocorticoids to ensure sufficient calcium (more than 2 g daily), sodium, and nutrients. Suckling stimulates the release of oxytocin from the pituitary and maintains prolactin secretion at levels between 10 and 20 times prepregnancy values.[2] Prolactin promotes milk production in the alveoli; oxytocin contracts the myoepithelial cells of the milk ducts, transporting milk to the nipple for consumption. Eventually, milk ejection may occur in response to other stimuli, such as sight or sound of an infant, representing a conditioned reflex. During initial phases of lactation, GnRH is inhibited, decreasing LH, FSH, and estrogenic stimulation of the endometrium and vaginal glands. By 6 months postpartum or with weaning, ovulation usually returns.[10]

RESOLUTION OF PREGNANCY CHANGES

Almost all physiologic changes experienced during pregnancy eventually resolve. There appear to be several alterations enduring past the endpoint of most studies, as well as some tantalizing implications that deserve future investigation. Given the extended period of increased weight bearing, lasting alterations in the shape of the pelvic girdle and feet seem predictable. On a lifetime basis, the supporting ligaments of the pelvis may be compromised more frequently in parous patients; specific contributions of delivery route, perineal integrity, number and weight of infants, exercise, prophylatic, and corrective measures remain subjects for study. Longstanding changes in ureteral diameter and in bladder function occur in some, but not all women. Vaginal rugations are attenuated and the shape of the cervical os usually changes from a small circle to a patulous lateral line or ovoid. Uterine enlargement may occur after repeated pregnancies.[14] Labor progress remains somewhat accelerated in parous patients for years after the initial delivery, perhaps reflecting permanent changes in impulse conduction or calcium binding.

Residual weight gain after pregnancy and lactation varies, but is not usually excessive.[28] As with other scars, stretch mark striations fade, but remain hypopigmented, in contrast to the linea nigra and chloasmic areas, which may remain slightly darker. Ptotic changes in the breasts occur in most women and appear unrelated to the choice of feeding method. Without supplementation during pregnancy and lactation, iron reserves of most gravidas will remain depleted for more than a year; particularly in older patients, calcium losses from pregnancy and lactation may never be fully restored. From epidemiological data, parturients may retain a number of differences from nulliparous women, although causation is not established. Child-bearing and lactation appear somewhat protective against breast, ovarian, and endometrial cancers, subject to a number of limitations. Development of transient hypertension and glucose intolerance during gestation appears to have predictive value for later-onset disease; additionally, a positive correlation between parity and cardiovascular disease risk was recently reported.[29]

CONCLUSION

As insights about the relationship of heredity to physiology increase, it is likely that some of the variation in individual responses to pregnancy will be better predicted. More appropriate management choices may be made if we are able to anticipate specific limitations in a patient's ability to adapt to the demands of gestation and parturition. Increased recognition of and control for confounding experimental varaibles may lead to improvements in applying findings to clinical situations; moreover, the current rigorous process for approval of study designs will reward those who demonstrate a firm basis in physiology for their hypotheses. The accomplished physician of the future will undoubtedly be distinguished by the ability to integrate the latest advances in maternal physiology into research and practice.

REFERENCES

1. Duvekot JJ, Peeters LHH. Maternal cardiovascular hemodynamic adaptation to pregnancy. *Obstet Gynecol Surv* 1994;49(12):S1–S14.

2. Ganong WF. *Review of Medical Physiology.* East Norwalk, CT: Appleton & Lange, 1995.

3. Conklin KA. Physiologic changes of pregnancy. In Chestnut DH (ed), *Obstetric Anesthesia: Principles and Practice.* St. Louis: Mosby-Year Book, 1994:17–42.

4. Clark SL, Cotton DB, Lee W, et al. Central hemodynamic assessment of normal term pregnancy. *Am J Obstet Gynecol* 1989;161:1439–1442.

5. Monga M, Creasy RK. Cardiovascular and renal adaptation to pregnancy. In Creasy RK, Resnik R (eds), *Maternal-Fetal Medicine: Principles and Practice*, 3rd ed. Philadelphia: Saunders Company, 1994:758–767.

6. Robson SC, Dunlop W, Boys RJ, et al. Cardiac output during labor. *Br Med J (Clin Res Ed)* 1987;295:1169–1172.

7. Hunter S, Robson SC. Adaptation of the maternal heart in pregnancy. *Br Heart J* 1992;68:540–543.

8. Leiserowitz GS, Evans AT, Samuels SJ, et al. Creatine kinase and its MB isoenzyme in the third trimester and the peripartum period. *J Reprod Med* 1992;37:910–916.

9. DeSwiet M. Pulmonary disorders. In Creasy RK and Resnik R (eds), *Maternal-Fetal Medicine: Principles and Practice*, 3rd ed. Philadelphia: Saunders, 1994:891–904.

10. Guyton AC, Hall JE. *Textbook of Medical Physiology.* Philadelphia: Saunders, 1996.

11. Meschia G. Placental respiratory gas exchange and fetal oxygenation. In Creasy RK and Resnik R (eds), *Maternal-Fetal Medicine: Principles and Practice*, 3rd ed. Philadelphia: Saunders, 1994:288–297.

12. Duvekot JJ, Peeters LLH. Renal hemodynamics and volume homeostasis in pregnancy. *Obstet Gynecol Surv* 1994;49(12):830–839.

13. Burrow GN, Ferris TF. *Medical Complications During Pregnancy*, 4th ed. Philadelphia: Saunders, 1995.

14. Haadem K. The effects of parturition on female pelvic floor anatomy and function. *Curr Opin Obstet Gynecol* 1994;6:326–330.

15. Scott LD. Gastrointestinal disease in pregnancy. In Creasy RK, Resnik R (eds), *Maternal-Fetal Medicine: Principles and Practice*, 3rd ed. Philadelphia: Saunders, 1994:1027–1039.

16. Fallon HJ, Riely CA. Liver diseases. In Burrow GN, Ferris TF (eds), *Medical Complications During Pregnancy*, 4th ed. Philadelphia: Saunders Co., 1995:307–342.

17. Laros RK. Maternal hematologic disorders. In Creasy RK, Resnik R (eds), *Maternal-Fetal Medicine: Principles and Practice*, 3rd ed. Philadelphia: Saunders, 1994:905–933.

18. Genuth SM. The reproductive glands. In Berne

RM, Levy MN (eds), *Physiology*. St. Louis: Mosby-Year Book, 1993:980–1024.

19. Friedrich EG. *Vulvar Disease*, 2nd ed. Philadelphia: Saunders, 1983.

20. Rapini RP, Jordon RE. The skin and pregnancy. In Creasy RK, Resnik R (eds), *Maternal-Fetal Medicine: Principles and Practice*, 3rd ed. Philadelphia: Saunders, 1994:1101–1111.

21. Nader S. Other endocrine disorders of pregnancy. In Creasy RK, Resnik R (eds), *Maternal-Fetal Medicine: Principles and Practice*, 3rd ed. Philadelphia: Saunders Company, 1994: 1004–1025.

22. Yen SSC. Endocrinology of pregnancy. In Creasy RK, Resnik R (eds), *Maternal-Fetal Medicine: Principles and Practice*, 3rd ed. Philadelphia: Saunders, 1994:382–412.

23. Genuth S. The reproductive glands. In Berne RM, Levy MN (eds), *Physiology*, 3rd ed. St. Louis: Mosby-Year Book, 1993:980–1023.

24. Olson DM, Mijovic JE, Sadowsky DW. *Control of Human Parturition. Semin Perinatol* 1995; 19:52–63.

25. Huszar G. Physiology of the myometrium. In Creasy RK, Resnik R (eds), *Maternal-Fetal Medicine: Principles and Practice*, 3rd ed. Philadelphia: Saunders, 1994:133–139.

26. Brown DL. Spinal, epidural and caudal anesthesia: Anatomy, physiology, and technique. In Chestnut DH (ed), *Obstetric Anesthesia: Principles and Practice*. St. Louis: Mosby-Year Book, 1994:181–201.

27. Brownridge P. The nature and consequences of childbirth pain. *Eur J Obstet Gynecol Reprod Biol* 1995;59:S9–S15.

28. Parker JD. Postpartum weight change. *Clin Obstet Gynecol* 1994;37:528–537.

29. Ness RB, Harris T, Cobb J, et al. Number of pregnancies and the subsequent risk of cardiovascular disease. *N Engl J Med* 1993;328: 1528–1533.

QUESTIONS
(choose the best single answer)

1. Significant milk production does not begin until several days after delivery because:
   a. The mother may be jeopardized by the volume challenge necessary to provide adequate milk flow.
   b. Pituitary production of prolactin does not begin until the third postpartum day.
   c. Suppression of production by placental hormones is not eliminated until the third postpartum day.
   d. Suckling vigorous enough to release oxytocin does not occur until the baby is several days old.
   e. All of the above.

2. Maternal blood pressure rises during labor because:
   a. Mean arterial pressure in the left lateral position actually decreases during labor.
   b. Catecholamine release is the most likely etiology for the rise.
   c. Blood pressure rises to compensate for the drop in cardiac output at delivery.
   d. Supine positioning routinely used for delivery will cause renin-induced pressure increases.
   e. Mean arterial pressure rises as a result of rising pulmonary capillary wedge pressures.

3. The onset of labor is preceded by:
   a. A significant rise in cardiac output.
   b. A surge in nocturnal oxytocin secretion.
   c. A sharp increase in maternal and fetal prolactin levels.
   d. Progressive cervical dilation.
   e. None of the above.

4. Blood loss at time of delivery is well tolerated because:
   a. Maternal circulating volume is well above normal.
   b. Uterine constriction limits losses once delivery has occurred.
   c. Uterine constriction produces an "autotransfusion" back into the systemic circulation.
   d. Hemodilution limits the absolute amount of iron and hemoglobin lost.
   e. All of the above.

5. Maternal pulmonary function is enhanced during pregnancy by:
   a. Increased respiratory rate.
   b. Decreased levels of 2,3-DPG.
   c. Prolactin-stimulated respiratory drive.
   d. Decreased tidal volume.
   e. Increased minute ventilation.

Part II

IN UTERO FETAL DIAGNOSIS
AND MANAGEMENT

3

Ultrasound Diagnosis of Anomalies

Graham G. Ashmead

INTRODUCTION

Ultrasound offers a window into the womb and is essential to modern obstetrics. Ultrasound and other antenatal testing provide the obstetrician with two patients, the mother and the fetus. Although there are controversies about the appropriate use of antenatal ultrasound it is difficult to imagine practicing present-day obstetrics without it to help guide the management of abnormal pregnancies or provide maternal reassurance in normal pregnancies.

Diagnostic ultrasound can detect 70% of all major fetal malformations and more than 90% of structural-functional anomalies. Fetal anomalies result in 15–25% of all perinatal deaths—more deaths than prematurity in most medical centers. The risk of an anomaly in any pregnancy is 2%. In 70% of these anomalies, the cause is unknown. Numbers alone cannot describe the anguish of parents of a child afflicted with a major birth defect. Even if the infant survives, the potential costs and stresses to the parents, child, and society can be devastating. Diagnostic ultrasound provides early detection of fetal malformations, establishes perinatal management protocols, and helps determine if in utero fetal therapy is feasible.[1]

Physics of Ultrasound

Ultrasound is sound waves over 20,000 cycles/sec. The higher the ultrasound frequency the better the resolution but the shallower the penetration. Diagnostic obstetric ultrasonography is usually 3.5–5 MHz (megahertz) transabdominally in order to permit adequate imaging of the fetus through the maternal abdomen and 5–7.5 MHz transvaginally because of the closer access to the fetus and pelvic structures. Real-time ultrasonography permits evaluation of the active fetus and of any moving structures including fetal echocardiography. Transducers can be sector with a single head rotating in an arc, linear with crystals firing in a linear sequence, annular with transducers in rings, or curvilinear combining linear and sector properties. The major recent advance in real-time obstetric ultrasound has been the widespread use of specially designed probes for vaginal insertion and imaging.

Safety of Ultrasound

There is no evidence that clinical obstetric ultrasound can cause harm to a patient. Despite many in vitro and animal studies on the bioeffects of ultrasonography there is no independently reproduced evidence of a bioeffect of diagnostic ultrasound. A safe level has been arbitrarily defined as less than 100 mW/cm^2 and most diagnostic ultrasound produces energies not greater than 10–20 mW/cm^2 at the transducer head. As higher energy, outputs have been developed for fetal evaluation, ultrasound machines that monitor and display the power output can enable the sonographer to minimize the power exposure levels to the mother and fetus.

Indications for Ultrasound Studies

There are multiple indications for ultrasound in obstetrics and gynecology (Table 3-1). The type of examination may vary depending upon the indication. At the Fetal Diagnostic Center at MetroHealth Medical Center the current policy is that obstetric ultrasound should be performed for an indication and not for routine screening, nor determination of fetal sex nor maternal reassurance. In practice most obstetric patients at MetroHealth either present with or develop an appropriate indication for an obstetric ultrasound.

NORMAL ULTRASOUND

Obstetric ultrasound evaluations should be performed with real-time ultrasound scanners and the patient generally initially evaluated transabdominally with a full bladder. After emptying the patient's bladder, endovaginal ultrasound may be indicated early in gestation (first trimester) to document pregnancy, estimate gestational age, or evaluate fetal anatomy and later in gestation to examine the cervix (normal length > 3 cm) or determine placental location. A basic ultrasound (screening or Level I) to estimate gestational age is most accurate in the first trimester, decreases in accuracy through gestation and can be inaccurate (plus or minus 3 weeks) in the third trimester. Estimation of fetal gestational age should be based on menstrual dating if the menstrual dating is within the error range of the ultrasound dating. Fetal gestational age should not be changed solely based on an ob-

Table 3-1.   Indications for Ultrasonography During Pregnancy

Estimation of gestational age for patients with uncertain dates or verification of dates for patients who are to undergo scheduled elective repeat cesarean delivery, indicated induction of labor, or other elective termination of pregnancy
Evaluation of fetal growth
Vaginal bleeding of undetermined etiology in pregnancy
Determination of fetal presentation
Suspected multiple gestation
Adjunct to amniocentesis, chorionic villus sampling, cordocentesis or other special procedures
Significant uterine size/clinical dates discrepancy
Pelvic mass
Suspected hydatidiform mole
Adjunct to cervical cerclage placement
Suspected ectopic pregnancy
Adjunct to special procedures
Suspected fetal death
Suspected uterine abnormality
Intrauterine contraceptive device localization
Biophysical evaluation for fetal well-being
Observation of intrapartum events
Suspected polyhydramnios or oligohydramnios
Suspected abruptio placentae
Adjunct to external version from breech to vertex presentation
Estimation of fetal weight and/or presentation in premature rupture of membranes and/or premature labor
Abnormal serum alpha-fetoprotein value
Follow-up observation of identified fetal anomaly
Follow-up evaluation of placental location for identified "placenta previa"
History of previous congenital anomaly
Serial evaluation of fetal growth in multiple gestation
Evaluation of fetal condition in late registrants for prenatal care

Source: from ref. 37. Reprinted with permission.

stetric ultrasound obtained after 20 weeks gestation. A transabdominal ultrasound at 18–20 weeks gestation may be the best time to obtain a single ultrasound to provide accurate dating confirmation combined with adequate visualization of fetal anatomy. Normal ultrasounds in the second and third trimester, in addition to an estimation of fetal gestational age and a screen for fetal anatomy, should provide an estimation of fetal weight and weight percentile. For a description of basic, limited and first trimester ultrasound see Table 3-2.

Table 3-2. Ultrasound Examination Information: Basic Ultrasound, Limited Ultrasound, and First-Trimester Ultrasound

Basic or screening ultrasound
   Fetal number
   Fetal presentation
   Documentation of fetal life
   Placental location
   Assessment of amniotic fluid
   Assessment of gestational age
   Survey of fetal anatomy for gross malformations
   Evaluation for maternal pelvic masses
Limited ultrasound
   Assessment of amniotic fluid volume
   Fetal biophysical profile testing
   Ultrasound guided amniocentesis
   External cephalic version
   Confirmation of fetal life or death
   Localization of placenta in antepartum hemorrhage
   Confirmation of fetal presentation
First trimester ultrasound
   Presence or absence of an intrauterine sac
   Identification of embryo or fetus
   Fetal number
   Presence or absence of fetal cardiac activity
   Crown-rump length
   Evaluation of uterus and adnexal structures

Source: from ref. 37. Reprinted with permission.

Limited Ultrasound

A limited ultrasound examination may be indicated in certain situations to meet the urgent demands of clinical care. A limited ultrasound can improve care by assessing fetal viability, amniotic fluid volume, placentation, or fetal presentation in a high-volume labor and delivery service or office setting (see Table 3-3).

Screening (Level I) Ultrasound

Most obstetric patients will require a screening or basic (Level I) ultrasound. A basic ultrasound is performed when there is no suspicion of a fetal anomaly and is expected to be within the expertise of the office-based sonographer (see Table 3-4).

First-trimester ultrasound evaluations can be performed abdominally or vaginally. A gestational sac at 4–5 weeks is the first definitive sign of pregnancy, however, a pseudogestational sac can occur in 10–20% of patients with an

Table 3-3. Fetal Ultrasound Survey May Not Be Possible

Oligohydramnios
Hyperflexed position of the fetus
Engagement of the head
Compression of some fetal parts
Maternal obesity

Source: from ref. 37. Reprinted with permission.

Table 3-4. Basic or Screening (Level I) Ultrasound

1. Document fetal viability, number and presentation
2. Estimate amniotic fluid volume and do an amniotic fluid index (AFI) if necessary
3. Identify placental location and grade and placenta's relationship to the cervix
4. Assess gestational age:
   Biparietal diameter (BPD)/Head circumference (HC) at transverse plane of the head at the level of the thalami and cavum septi pellucidi
   Abdominal circumference (AC) transverse image of the abdomen at the level of the umbilical vein and stomach
   Femur length (FL) long axis view of the femur with crisp edge lines and acoustic shadow
5. Fetal anatomic survey views:
   Cerebellum plane to include the posterior fossa
   Transverse abdominal scan at the level of the kidneys: documenting normal renal parenchyma and renal pelvis
   Transverse view of the pelvis demonstrating bladder or longitudinal view of the lower fetal body demonstrating buttocks and bladder
   Transverse view of a section of umbilical cord demonstrating three vessels
   Video tape four chamber heart view for at least twenty seconds or if a video cassette recorder (VCR) is not available document M-mode tracing of fetal heart motion
6. Anatomy that should be visualized but need not be filmed routinely:
   Transverse and longitudinal views of the entire fetal spine: attempting to demonstrate skin edge
   Trace out all fetal extremities
   Evaluate the uterus and adnexal structures
   Evaluate fetal facial structures for any obvious defects, clefts or abnormalities
   Evaluate anterior fetal abdomen and cord insertion for any evidence of herniation of abdominal contents
   Evaluate the cerebral ventricles at the level of the glomus of the choroid plexus and the atria of the lateral ventricles. Normal range is 6–8 mm and over 11 mm is considered abnormal

ectopic pregnancy. The gestational sac when first seen may only be 2–3 mm in diameter and its mean diameter increases at approximately 1 mm/day during early pregnancy. Fetal cardiac activity can be seen when a fetal pole measures 5 mm or within 3–5 days after the pole measures 4 mm. Fetal heart motion can be detected at 6–7 weeks gestation transabdominally and 5–6 weeks transvaginally.[2,3]

The finding on ultrasound of an intrauterine pregnancy virtually excludes an ectopic pregnancy. The exception is a heterotopic or simultaneous intrauterine and extrauterine pregnancy, that occurs in 1:30,000 spontaneous pregnancies and 1:6000 assisted reproduction pregnancies. In a normal pregnancy a quantitative serum human chorionic gonadotropin (hCG) level will increase 66% every 48 hours or double every 3 days. A subnormal hCG rise can indicate an extrauterine pregnancy or a threatened intrauterine pregnancy. Because of different hCG standards, differing units and laboratory variation, physicians should determine at what level they can determine pregnancy (one author uses 935–2388 mIU/ml transvaginally and 3600 mIU/ml transabdominally by International Reference Preparation).[3]

A crown rump length (CRL) can be measured between 8 and 13 weeks and used to establish gestational age within 5 days in 95% of cases. In measuring the CRL it is important not to mistake the fetal yolk sac for the fetal head. A quick way to estimate the fetal age is to add 6.5 to the

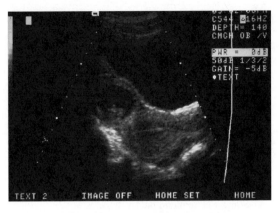

Figure 3-2.   Ectopic pregnancy.

CRL in centimeters to get the gestational age in weeks.[2,4] See Figure 3-1 for a transabdominal ultrasound of a CRL and Figure 3-2 for a transvaginal ultrasound of an ectopic pregnancy.

Obstetric ultrasounds are often used to determine gestational age. Common fetal measurements include CRL, biparietal diameter (BPD), head circumference, abdominal circumference, and femur length (Figures 3-3–3-5). An average of measurements may provide a more accurate reflection of gestational age than any single measurement although individual measurements may provide an insight into the fetal condition (small head with microcephaly, short limbs with dwarfism syndromes).

The BPD is the maximal distance between the two fetal parietal bones. It is measured along a line, most frequently in the transverse and coronal planes. The BPD is measured from outer

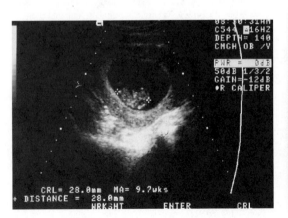

Figure 3-1.   Crown rump length.

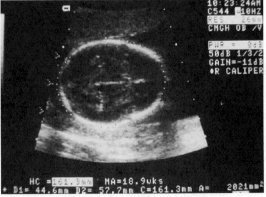

Figure 3-3.   Biparietal diameter.

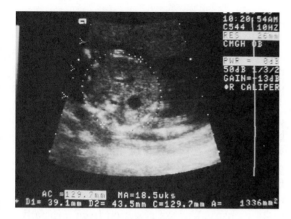

Figure 3-4. Abdominal circumference.

to inner edge on the largest perpendicular to the midline echo. The transverse sections are preferred because they rely on the axial resolution of the ultrasound beam and allow a better display of intracranial anatomy. The BPD should be perpendicular to the midline, in the correct plane and symmetrical. The thalamus or the cerebral peduncles, the cavum septi pellucidi, part of the falx and the insula with the middle cerebral artery can be observed at the correct level for the BPD. The head shape should be ovoid. If the cephalic index (biparietal diameter × 100/ occipital frontal diameter) is greater than 85 (brachiocephalic) or less than 75 (dolichocephalic) then the BPD may not be reliable. Common errors in measuring the BPD include asymmetry, too high a level (level of lateral ventricles), too low a level (level of skull base

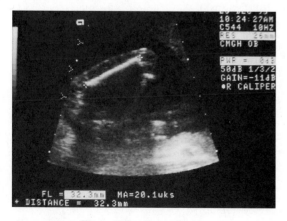

Figure 3-5. Femur length.

or petrous ridges), calipers not placed on a line perpendicular to midline, or too much pressure on the head deforming the BPD.

The head circumference (HC) can be used to determine gestational age, to diagnose microcephaly, and in the evaluation of intrauterine growth restriction (IUGR). An elevated HC/abdominal circumference (AC) ratio is consistent with asymmetric (head-sparing) IUGR. The HC should be measured in the plane of the BPD and the occipital frontal diameter (OFD) at the level of the thalamus and cavum septi pellucidi. The measurement should be followed by tracing the outer side of the skull without including the skin. The HC can be calculated from the BPD and OFD using the equation HC = (BPD + OFD) × 1.62.

The reason for measuring the fetal abdomen is to estimate the size of the fetus based on the size of the fetal liver. The fetal liver is affected in fetal growth retardation because of decreased liver glycogen storage. The AC is used to estimate fetal weight, calculate the HC/AC ratio, and assist in the diagnosis of microcephaly. The most important point in obtaining an AC is to achieve as round a section as possible. The approximate plane for the measurement of the AC can be chosen on the basis of the umbilical blood supply to the fetus. The appropriate plane of section for the AC shows a short tubular segment of the umbilical segment of the left portal vein roughly one third of the way posterior from the anterior abdominal wall. Too low an AC will show a section of the umbilical vein through its short axis along the abdominal wall and too angulated a level will show a portion of the left portal vein. The AC = (transverse diameter + anteroposterior diameter) × 1.57.[5]

Two main patterns of IUGR have been described. When animals are nutritionally deprived their offspring are symmetrically small and have decreased cerebral deoxyribonucleic acid (DNA). When uterine blood flow is mechanically compromised, there is asymmetrical IUGR with sparing of the brain. Asymmetrical IUGR is due to the preferential shunting of blood to the fetal brain in situations of inadequate nutrition or oxygenation. In symmetrical

IUGR (onset prior to 26 menstrual weeks gestation) the brain-sparing protective mechanisms have been overwhelmed. Campbell and Thomas found the HC/AC ratio allowed discrimination between symmetrical and asymmetrical IUGR. Small-for-gestational-age infants below the fifth percentile had HC/AC ratios greater than the 95th percentile in 71% of cases. Normal HC/AC ratios are 1.18 at 17 weeks, 1.11 at 29 weeks, 1.01 at 36 weeks, and 0.96 at 40 weeks.[6]

The femur length (FL) is useful in predicting gestational age, calculating fetal weight, evaluating IUGR, screening for chromosomal abnormalities, and in detecting skeletal dysplasias. One technique for obtaining a FL is follow the fetal spine to the fetal bladder, locate the iliac crests, identify the bright echo of the femur by the iliac crest, rotate the transducer till the femur is in view, and measure the FL when an acoustic shadow is cast and the femur length is longest. The FL should be measured from the major trochanter to the external condyle, not including the femoral head. Common errors in measuring the FL include incorrect plane (acoustic shadow not uniform), underestimation (foreshortening), or overestimation (including the femoral head or distal epiphysis). Hadlock et al. found that the femur length to abdominal circumference ratio (FL/AC) was constant at 0.21 ($\pm$0.02) after 21 weeks gestation and an elevated FL/AC ratio (0.24) can suggest length-sparing IUGR.[7]

Fetal growth can be evaluated by measuring growth over several weeks. The most accurate parameters are those measured in the first tri-mester and the least accurate are those in the third trimester (Table 3-5). The measurement error for instance of the biparietal diameter in the third trimester is plus or minus 3 weeks. Estimated fetal weight can be determined with a 95% confidence interval of 15–20% (1 standard deviation 7.5–10%). Estimated fetal weight equations are less accurate in determining fetal weight in the very-small or the very-large-for-gestational-age fetus. See Table 3-6 for fetal ultrasound equations.[4] Singleton live birthweights at the 10th, 50th, and 90th percentiles from 24 to 44 menstrual weeks gestation from a racially mixed inner city population delivering at MetroHealth Medical Center in Cleveland are listed in Table 3-7[8] (see Figure 3-37).

Doppler velocimetry studies of the uterine and umbilical arteries have good sensitivity in detecting fetuses that will develop the most severe forms of hypertensive disorders of pregnancy or IUGR but cannot be used to screen a low-risk population. Common Doppler calculations include: (1) S/D ratio = systolic velocity/diastolic velocity, (2) resistive index (RI) = (systolic − diastolic velocity/systolic velocity), and (3) pul-

Table 3-5.   Assessment of Gestational Age Variability

Parameter	Gestational Age (weeks)	Range (2 SD*) (days)
Crown-rump	5–12	±5
Biparietal diameter	12–20	±8
	20–30	±14
	>30	±21
Femur length	12–20	±7
	20–36	±11
	>36	±16

*SD = standard deviation.

Source: Adapted from ref. 38 with permission.

Table 3-6.   Common Obstetric Ultrasound Equations

GA from FL = 9.18 + (2.67 × FL) + (0.16 × [FL squared]).

GA from CRL = 5.3066 + (0.20943 × CRL) − (0.0021264 × CRL squared) + (0.000011206 * CRL cubed).

GA from BPD = 7.021 + (2.3179 × BPD) + 0.1111 × (BPD squared). The 10th and 90th percentile ranges are minus or plus 0.5576 + (0.1007 × BPD) + (0.0199 × [BPD squared]).

Total intrauterine volume = 0.5233 × height × width × length.

EFW from BPD and AD = (3.42928 × BPD × (AD squared)) + 41.218

EFW from BPD and AC = 10 ^ (1.2508 + (0.166 × BPD) + (0.046 × AC) − (AC × BPD × 2.646/1,000))

EFW from HC, AC & FL = 1.5662 − (0.0108 × HC) + (0.0468 × AC) + (0.171 × FL) + (0.00034 × HC squared) − (0.003685 × AC × FL)

Length measurements are in centimeters except the crown rump length (CRL) is measured in millimeters. GA = gestational age in weeks, FL = femur length, CRL = crown rump length, BPD = biparietal diameter, HC = head circumference, EFW = estimated fetal weight in grams, AD = abdominal diameter and AC = abdominal circumference.

Source: from ref. 4.

Table 3-7. Percentiles of Birth Weight, Mean and Standard Deviations for Birth Weights in Grams by Gestational Age in Menstrual Weeks for Over 60,000 Live Singleton Births at MetroHealth Medical Center in Cleveland

Age in Wks	N	10%	50%	90%	Mean ± SD
24	152	560	670	1065	753 ± 309
25	190	590	760	1240	870 ± 389
26	224	670	898	1400	986 ± 368
27	226	730	1000	1500	1096 ± 415
28	313	815	1170	1840	1290 ± 529
29	301	1010	1360	2370	1537 ± 597
30	406	1160	1560	2530	1712 ± 584
31	472	1270	1700	2620	1843 ± 572
32	662	1410	1865	2755	1995 ± 575
33	747	1555	2080	2825	2146 ± 516
34	1050	1765	2300	3030	2349 ± 514
35	1410	2000	2515	3220	2567 ± 524
36	2375	2150	2700	3350	2738 ± 504
37	3641	2340	2890	3540	2916 ± 488
38	6997	2510	3060	3655	3070 ± 462
39	9785	2660	3180	3775	3200 ± 450
40	16,289	2785	3320	3910	3336 ± 450
41	7163	2880	3430	4040	3446 ± 463
42	3623	2945	3520	4160	3540 ± 483
43	601	2930	3560	4240	3575 ± 505
44	101	3020	3500	4200	3557 ± 475

Source: adapted from ref. 8 with permission.

satility index (PI) = (systolic − diastolic velocity)/mean velocity. See Figures 3-6 and 3-7. The best cutoff value for an abnormal umbilical artery S/D ratio is greater than 5.4 at 19–24 weeks and 4.5 at 26–31 weeks and for the uterine artery respectively greater than 2.6 and 2.4.[9] Absent end-diastolic velocity of the umbilical artery is particularly ominous and can indicate severe fetal compromise that may result in fetal demise within days.[10] See Figure 3-8. Doppler velocimetry studies have also been useful in the evaluation of discordant twins (difference in BPD > 5 mm, estimated fetal weight > 25th percentile).[11] The precise obstetric use of Doppler velocimetry studies is controversial and each institution should consider developing its own curves of Doppler values and guidelines for clinical care.

Placental localization should be part of a basic ultrasound, and third trimester bleeding is an indication for assessing the location of the placenta. Transabdominal sonographic placental localization to rule out a placenta previa can be difficult because: (1) the cervix may not be seen,

(2) a posterior placenta can be hidden by a low vertex or presenting part and (3) the relationship of the placenta to the cervix changes during pregnancy. An overdistended bladder on transabdominal examination can cause a placenta to appear to be a previa, and emptying the bladder may help to identify the relationship between the cervix and placenta. A contracture in the lower uterine segment near the cervical os may appear to be a placenta previa. Term patients should be scanned to allow visualization of both the placenta and cervix. A fundal placenta does not rule out a previa. A careful transvaginal ultrasound or color Doppler studies may help in diagnosing or ruling out a placenta previa. Magnetic resonance imaging (MRI) may also help to diagnose a previa.

Because of changes in the lower uterine segment placenta previas in the second trimester may not be previas in the third trimester. Asymptomatic partial placenta previas in the second trimester can be ignored but symptomatic second trimester previas should be fol-

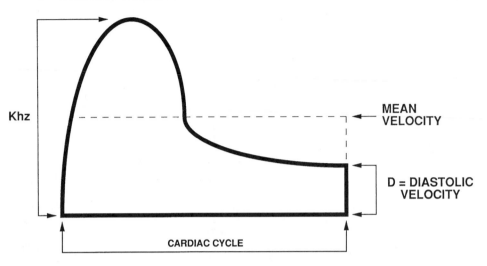

Figure 3-6.   Diagram of a systolic to diastolic ratio. PI (pulsatility index) = (systolic-diastolic)/mean; RI (resistance index) = (systolic-diastolic)/systolic; S/D = systolic/diastolic velocity.

lowed until the placenta changes position. Complete previas persisting after emptying the bladder should be followed with repeat ultrasound examinations until prior to delivery. Obstetric management of a placenta previa should not be based on an ultrasound more than 2 weeks old[2] (Figure 3-9).

Placental thickness after 23 weeks should be at least 15 mm and less than 50 mm. Grannum et al. classified the placenta into four grades as: (0) smooth chorionic plate, homogenous texture without echoes, (I) subtle indentations of plate, random echogenic areas in placenta, (II) basal echogenic densities, commalike densities, and (III) indentations of chorionic plate, echospared areas, irregular densities with acoustic shadowing. Grade 0 is seen prior to 28 weeks and rarely thereafter. Grade I is seen anytime and occurs in 40% of term placentas. Grade II is seen in 40% of term placentas. Grade III is seen in 20% of placentas and if seen prior to 36 weeks has been associated with premature senescence[12] (Figure 3-10). The value of placental grading in evaluating IUGR is unproven.[2]

Amniotic fluid cushions the fetus, facilitates lung development, and allows for proper fetal

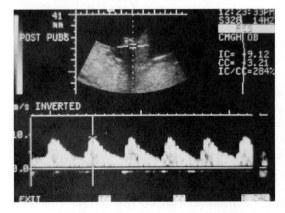

Figure 3-7.   Normal umbilical artery waveform.

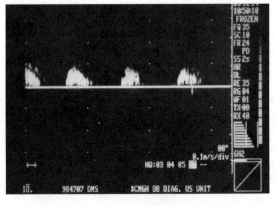

Figure 3-8.   Absent end-diastolic velocity.

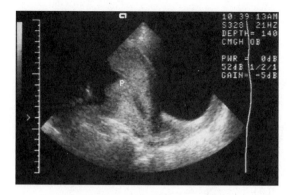

Figure 3-9. Complete placenta previa.

growth. Both oligohydramnios and polyhydramnios are associated with poor prognosis. Polyhydramnios can be diagnosed by an 8-cm pocket or by an elevated AFI using the four-quadrant technique. The AFI represents the sum of the largest vertical pocket of fluid measured in millimeters in four quadrants of the uterus while the patient is lying supine (roughly 50–200). See Figure 3-11 for AFI values through gestation. Decreased amniotic fluid volume can be useful in evaluation for IUGR.[2,13]

Frank Manning has used dynamic ultrasound imaging from 25 weeks onward to directly assess the fetus with the fetal biophysical profile (BPP) score. The biophysical score consists of five components each scored either a normal score of 2 or an abnormal score of 0. The five components are: fetal breathing movements (FBM), gross body movements (GBM), fetal

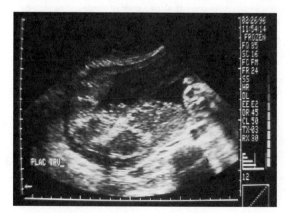

Figure 3-10. Grade 3 (III) placenta.

tone, reactive fetal heart rate (FHR), and qualitative AF volume.

A score of 2 for FBM requires 1 episode of FBM at least 30 seconds in 30 minutes of observation. A score of 2 for GBM requires 3 discrete body/limb movements in 30 minutes of observation. A score of 2 for fetal tone requires at least one episode of active extension with return to flexion of fetal limbs or trunk. A score of 2 for FHR requires a reactive FHR at least two episodes of FHR acceleration > 15 bpm of at least 15 seconds duration associated with fetal movement in 30 minutes. A score of 2 for qualitative AF volume requires at least one pocket of AF that measures at least 2 cm in two perpendicular planes.

Provided AF volume is normal a BPP score of 8/10 in any combination is considered as normal and no different than a score of 10/10. Manning states that most patients within 8 minutes will have scores of 2 each for all ultrasound-monitored variables and so Manning only recommends performing an NST in the 5% who do not score 8/8. All equivocal or abnormal BPP scores should include a full BPP with a non-stress test (NST). Manning recommends repeat BPP testing on a weekly basis except for patients who are postterm, diabetic, or alloimmunized—these patients should be seen at least twice weekly and as often as daily for patients with severe Rh disease. A good BPP score indicates that the fetal risk is low and intervention is only indicated for maternal or obstetric factors. Manning recommends inducing delivery in any postterm patient with an inducible cervix regardless of the BPP score and continued monitoring in a postterm patient with an unfavorable cervix. Severe deteriorating maternal disease (such as preeclampsia) with a normal BPP score, or oligohydramnios or an abnormal BPP score is an indication for delivery.

A BPP score of 10/10, 8/10 with normal fluid, or 8/8 with NST not done has an extremely low risk of fetal asphyxia with a perinatal mortality within 1 week without intervention of 1 per 1000 studies (false negative). A BPP score of 8/10 with abnormal fluid shows probable chronic fetal compromise with a perinatal mortality of

89 per 1000 studies (false negative) within 1 week. A BPP score of 6/10 with normal fluid is an equivocal test with possible fetal asphyxia and a variable perinatal mortality. This score can indicate delivery for a mature fetus or repeating the test within 24 hours for the immature fetus. A BPP of 6/10 with abnormal fluid indicates probable fetal asphyxia with a perinatal mortality of 89 per 1000 studies and that the fetus should be delivered for fetal indications. Worsening BPP scores can indicate increasing risk for perinatal mortality and the need for delivery for fetal indications (BPP of 4, 2, and 0 has a perinatal mortality of 91, 125, and 600, respectively, per 1000 within 1 week).[14]

Comprehensive (Level II) Ultrasound

A comprehensive ultrasound (Level II) is performed on patients at risk for having an abnormality and should be performed by an operator with experience and expertise. At MetroHealth Medical Center a comprehensive ultrasound is usually performed between 18 and 22 weeks gestation in order to allow adequate visualization of the fetus but still permit time for further diagnostic evaluation prior to viability (24 weeks). Because of the need for greater experience and higher-resolution equipment a comprehensive ultrasound may be best carried out in a regional perinatal center. A perinatal sonologist interpreting a comprehensive ultrasound has to (1) establish a reliable diagnosis, (2) evaluate the prognosis of the abnormality in late pregnancy, and (3) exclude other anomalies or chromosomal abnormalities. Follow-up examinations depend on the maternal and fetal conditions. A perinatologist performing a comprehensive ultrasound can provide a perinatal evaluation and make recommendations regarding management for the mother and fetus.[1]

FACIAL AND NECK ANOMALIES

Careful ultrasound evaluation of the fetal face and neck, especially tangential views, can detect cleft lip, cleft palate, tumors, goiter, nuchal thick-

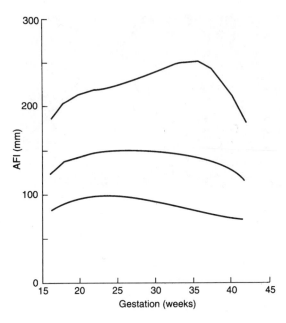

Figure 3-11. Amniotic fluid index (AFI) from normal patients. Upper, middle, and lower lines represent the 95th, 50th, and 5th percentile, respectively. (Adapted with permission from ref. 13.)

ening (associated with Down syndrome), and cystic hygromas.[1] See Figures 3-11–3-14. Pretorius and Nelson found that three-dimensional ultrasonography, by creating surface-rendered images of the fetal face, improved visualization of 24 of 27 fetuses from 10 to 39 weeks gestation and facilitated the diagnosis of facial abnormalities such as cleft lip and holoprosencephaly.[15]

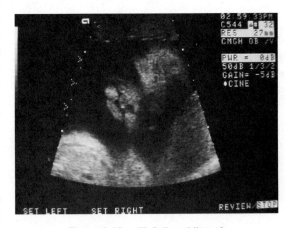

Figure 3-12. Cleft lip—bilateral.

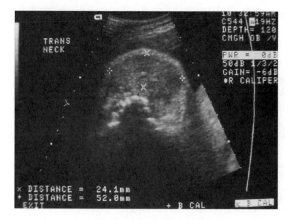

Figure 3-13. Fetal goiter.

Nuchal fold thickening is 6 mm or greater measured from the outer edge of the skull to the skin edge at the level of the posterior fossa, cerebellum, and thalami between 15 and 20 weeks. Nuchal fold thickening has been associated with trisomy 21 but has a sensitivity of at best 39%. Nuchal translucency, a small membrane 3 mm thick or greater without septations from the skull down to L1 to L2, has been noted in the fetus between 11 and 14 weeks on endovaginal probe and is strongly associated with trisomy 21. Cystic hygromas with cystic pouches on either side of the neck have been seen with trisomy 21 but are more characteristic of Turner syndrome (monosomy X).[16,17] A measured to expected ear ratio of 0.8 or less in 418 fetuses from 20 to 28 weeks gestation was 75% sensitive and 98% specific (8.5% positive predictive

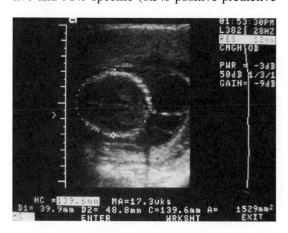

Figure 3-14. Cystic hygroma.

Table 3-8. Ultrasound Findings that May Increase the Risk of Trisomy 21 (Down Syndrome) > 1:270

First trimester
  Nuchal translucency > or = 3 mm
Second trimester (16–20 weeks)
  Nuchal fold > or = 6 mm
  Short ear (observed/expected < 0.8)
  Femur length, observed/expected < 0.91
  BPD/femur > 2 S.D.
  Humeral length, observed/expected < 0.90
  Femur + humerus, observed/expected < 0.90
  Femur + humerus/foot < or + 1.75
  Echogenic bowel
  Pyelectasis > 4 mm
  Hypoplasia of 5th mid-phalangeal digit
  Major structural malformation
  Choroid plexus cysts

value) in the general population in detecting trisomy 21.[18] See Table 3-8 for ultrasound findings associated with genetic abnormalities.

Occasionally neck masses such as cystic hygromas, tumors, or goiter can compress the esophagus and interfere with fetal swallowing, leading to polyhydramnios and premature labor. A neck mass may also compress the trachea and interfere with respiration after birth with a mortality rate that can exceed 20%. Delivery of a fetus with a large neck mass is best done at a tertiary center with appropriate karyotype, thyroid, immunology, or other workup and with a team approach to management. In utero diagnosis and therapy may be appropriate for symptomatic fetal goiter. If the fetal neck mass is large enough the delivery should be by a controlled cesarean section. A neonatologist or pediatric surgeon skilled in intubation or performing an emergency tracheotomy should be available in the delivery room in case the neck mass should prevent the infant from breathing.[1,19,20]

CRANIOSPINAL AND NEURAL ANOMALIES

The fetal cranium can be successfully examined at 11–12 weeks gestation transabdominally and

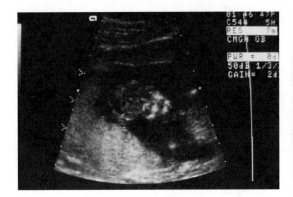

Figure 3-15.   Anencephalic.

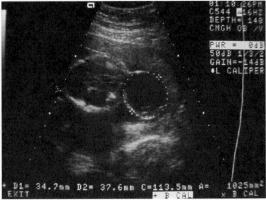

Figure 3-17.   Encephalocele.

even earlier transvaginally. Fetal craniospinal defects detected by ultrasound, arranged in rough embryological occurrence, include anencephaly, spina bifida, encephalocele, iniencephaly, holoprosencephaly, absent cerebellum, Dandy-Walker malformation, hydrancephaly, porencephaly, microcephaly, and hydrocephaly[1] (Figures 3-15–3-18).

The most striking fetal neural abnormality is anencephaly which occurs in less than 1 per 1000 births. Anencephaly can be diagnosed at 11 weeks in gestation and should not be missed on ultrasound at 16 weeks gestation. Late in gestation an anencephalic with a head low in the pelvis may be difficult to evaluate. Elevation of the head can reveal the classic absent cranial vault, angiomatous stroma, large tongue, and prominent orbits. Anencephaly is a lethal disorder and an indication for termination at any gestation, even after "viability" at 24 weeks.

Hydrocephalus occurs in 2.5 per 1,000 births and can be diagnosed on ultrasound by ventricular enlargement which usually precedes cranial enlargement. An elevated lateral ventricle to bihemispheric ratio can provide the diagnosis although increased fluid may initially be seen in the third or fourth ventricle depending on the etiology of the hydronephrosis. A lateral ventricle to bihemispheric ratio greater than 0.33 after 20 weeks of gestation may be suggestive of hydrocephalus. It may take several serial ultrasound evaluations during pregnancy to diagnose hydrocephalus. Hydrocephalus can be diagnosed on one ultrasound if (1) the biparietal diameter is greater than 95% for gestational age, (2) cystic areas replace the normal brain pattern, and (3) other morphometric measurements are appropriate for gestational age. The diagnosis of

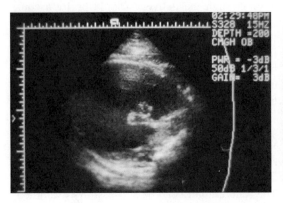

Figure 3-16.   Hydrocephalus.

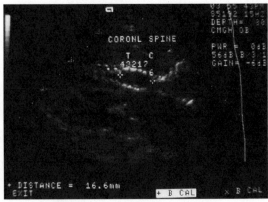

Figure 3-18.   Meningomyelocele.

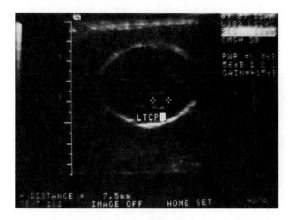

Figure 3-19. Choroid plexus cyst.

hydrocephaly can be ruled out if the width of the atrial portion of the lateral ventricle is less than 1 cm.[21]

Amniocentesis or cordocentesis should be performed to detect chromosomal abnormalities which may occur in up to 11% of fetuses with hydrocephalus. Vesicoamniotic shunts have not proven useful with hydrocephalus and so prenatal ultrasound diagnosis should be directed toward the timing and mode of delivery rather than in utero therapy.

After a diagnosis of hydrocephalus the spinal anatomy should be carefully studied as neural tube defects can occur in 25% of fetuses with hydrocephalus. Most fetuses with open spina bifida have an abnormality of the posterior fossa termed Arnold-Chiari type II malformation where the cerebellar vermis herniates into the cisterna magnum. Nicolaides et al. have reported the abnormal view of the cerebellum as the "banana" sign and the associated pinched-in frontal lobes as the "lemon" sign.[22] The skin edge over the spine should be evaluated in order to detect open neural tube defect. A characteristic splaying of the spine can be seen in neural tube defects, usually in the lumbar sacral area. Prognostic signs include the level of the defect, number of vertebrae involved, presence of hydrocephalus, or other anomalies. Over 80% of neural tube defects can be detected on ultrasound and over 90% when combined with alpha-fetoprotein screening. The best mode of delivery is not clear but vaginal delivery with a

neural tube defect may traumatize the defect.[23] Periconceptual folic acid supplementation (4 mg/day 1 month prior to conception) can decrease the first recurrence of neural tube defects by more than 70%.[24]

Many other cranial abnormalities have been diagnosed antenatally. Choroid plexus cysts have been detected in 1% of fetuses in midgestation and are reported to increase the fetal risk for trisomy 18 and trisomy 21. Patients with fetuses with choroid plexus cysts should be offered genetic counseling[25] (Figure 3-19). Antenatal diagnosis of agenesis of the corpus callosum is considerably rarer (70 cases in the literature) but because of a 1 in 10 risk of fetal aneuploidy parents should be offered fetal karyotyping.[26]

CARDIAC ANOMALIES

The incidence of congenital fetal heart disease is roughly 8/1000 births. Fetal cardiac anomalies that have been diagnosed antenatally on ultrasound include: atrial septal defect, ventriculoseptal defect, mitral atresia, Ebstein's anomaly, transposition of the great vessels, hypoplastic left or right ventricle, and hypertrophic cardiomyopathy. Indications for a fetal echocardiographic evaluation include a family history of congenital cardiac anomalies, maternal diabetes mellitus, maternal lithium ingestion, maternal collagen vascular disease, or an abnormal fetal heart noted on basic ultrasound.

A basic ultrasound of the fetal heart should include a four-chamber view of the heart at the level of the inflow tracts. A four chamber view should detect up to 90% of major congenital heart malformations. The four-chamber view allows the examination of the right and left atrial and ventricular chambers, the tricuspid and mitral valves, the walls and septa of the heart, and the foramen ovale. The heart should occupy about a third of the chest cavity in the four-chamber view, the ventricles should be about equal in size, and the flap of the foramen ovale should be in the left atrium. Inability to obtain a normal four-chamber view of the fetal heart in an otherwise normal ultrasound evaluation can suggest a fetal cardiac abnormality. If possible, in addition to the four-chamber view the left and right ventricular outflow tracts should be identified to rule out a transposition of the great vessels, tetralogy of Fallot, or other abnormality.

During evaluation of the fetal heart a shift of the normal heart position, cardiac or chest masses, pleural effusions, or bowel in the chest should be looked for and the fetus screened for diaphragmatic hernia, cystic adenomatoid malformation, and other major anomalies in the fetal chest. A thoracic circumference should be measured at the level of the four-chamber heart. A thoracic to abdominal circumference (TC/AC) ratio of less than 80% should suggest the possibility of fetal pulmonary hypoplasia.

Because the fetal heart is a complex structure in continual motion the antenatal diagnosis of congenital heart disease requires experience and excellent equipment. High-resolution real-time imaging, M (motion) mode, Doppler velocimetry, and color directional flow imaging can facilitate diagnosis and analysis of fetal cardiac anomalies and arrythmias. A pediatric cardiologist working in consultation with a perinatal sonologist can add to the interpretation of fetal echocardiography. Obtaining a fetal karyotype should be considered in fetuses with cardiac malformations because of the increased risk of chromosomal abnormalities. Correct cardiac diagnosis allows therapy of arrythmias in utero,

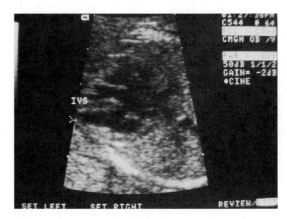

Figure 3-21.   Cardiac cross sections of double-outlet right ventricle (DORV).

early delivery of a fetus in distress, delivery at a tertiary center with appropriate cardiac support, and maternal reassurance[1,27,28] (Figures 3-20–3-25).

GASTROINTESTINAL TRACT ANOMALIES

Fetal gastrointestinal tract abnormalities account for 15–20% of anomalies and antenatal ultrasound has detected fetal omphalocele, gastroschisis, diaphragmatic hernia, umbilical hernia, duodenal atresia, jejunal atresia, meconium peritonitis, and colonic obstruction. The most helpful antenatal ultrasound finding in fetal gastrointestinal tract malformations, especially

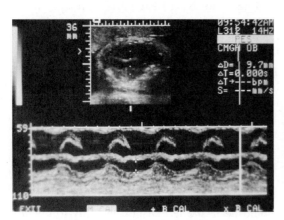

Figure 3-20.   Ebstein's anomaly of the heart.

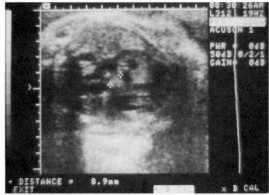

Figure 3-22.   Multiple rhabdomyomas of heart (tuberous sclerosis).

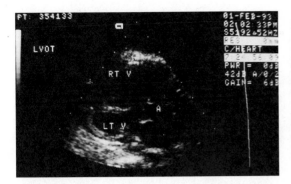

Figure 3-23. Tetralogy of Fallot.

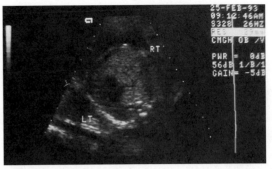

Figure 3-25. Cystic adenomatoid malformation of the lung.

esophageal and duodenal atresia, is polyhydramnios.

Omphalocele and gastroschisis occur in less than 1/2500 births. Ultrasound differentiation between omphalocele and gastroschisis is important because major malformations and chromosomal abnormalities are common with omphalocele but rare with gastroschisis. If a sac covers the gastrointestinal malformation, or if liver or heart is in the defect, the malformation is probably an omphalocele. At MetroHealth Medical Center a fetus with a large omphalocele is usually delivered by cesarean section to prevent rupture or injury of the malformation while the mother of a fetus with an isolated gastroschisis is advised to consider a vaginal delivery. Accurate prenatal diagnosis of a gastrointestinal malformation permits delivery in at tertiary cen-

ter specializing in high-risk obstetrics and pediatric surgery[1,29] (Figures 3-26 and 3-27).

RENAL ANOMALIES

Approximately 3% of the population has a kidney or ureter anomaly. Renal or urinary tract anomalies detected on prenatal ultrasound include hydronephrosis, obstructive uropathy, renal agenesis (1/1000 births), and polycystic kidney disease (1/50,000 births). A key finding on antenatal ultrasound is oligohydramnios. Oligohydramnios, however, can make fetal renal evaluation extremely difficult. In hydronephrosis the dilated renal pelvis (anteroposterior > 1 cm) is usually one half or more the thickness of the kidneys. The ratio of the normal kidney circumference to abdominal circumference is 0.27–0.30 throughout gestation and increased

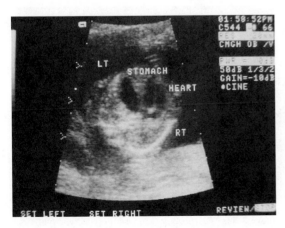

Figure 3-24. Diaphragmatic hernia.

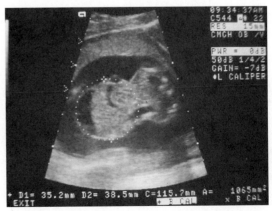

Figure 3-26. Omphalocele.

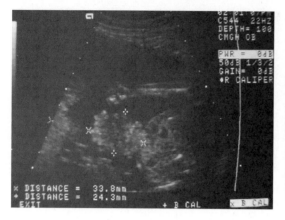

Figure 3-27.   Gastroschisis.

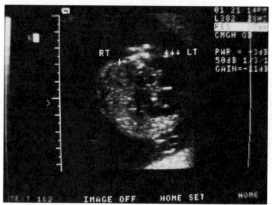

Figure 3-29.   Normal right kidney with left multicystic kidney.

ratios (0.4 or greater) suggest renal pathology such as infantile polycystic kidney disease or dysplastic kidneys[1,30,31] (Figures 3-28 and 3-29). Bilateral multicystic or polycystic fetal kidney disease are fatal conditions. Unilateral fetal renal disease needs careful evaluation but is much less ominous provided the AF volume is normal.

SKELETAL OR LIMB ANOMALIES

Limb malformations seen on ultrasound include achondroplasia, achondrogenesis, diastrophic dwarf, thanatophoric dwarf, limb reduction deformity, osteogenesis imperfecta, phocomelia, absent radius or ulna, and clubfoot. On ultrasound the absence of limbs (amelia), partial absence (meromelia), shortened limbs, defective

mineralization (achondrogenesis), and spontaneous fractures (osteogenesis imperfecta) can be identified. High-resolution ultrasound can allow evaluation of the fetal digits, absent digits, and rockerbottom feet (trisomy 18 and 18-p). Clubfoot (talipes equinovarus) can be diagnosed if the tibia, fibula, and foot are in the same view. Clubfoot is often seen with oligohydramnios and if present with normal amniotic fluid can be suggestive of a chromosomal abnormality or arthrogryposis[1,32] (Figures 3-30 and 3-31).

OTHER ANOMALIES

Normally two arteries and one vein should be seen on a longitudinal or cross-sectional view of

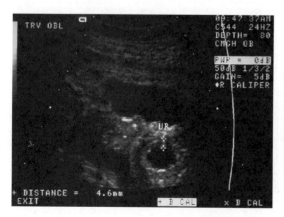

Figure 3-28.   Bladder outlet obstruction.

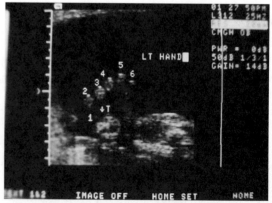

Figure 3-30.   Polydactyly (short rib polydactyly syndrome).

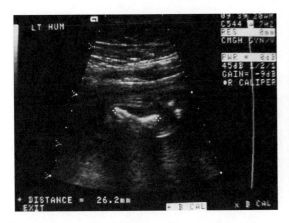

Figure 3-31. Osteogenesis imperfecta limb fracture.

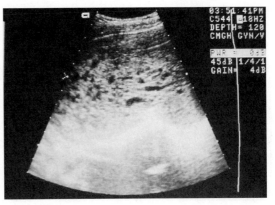

Figure 3-33. Molar pregnancy.

the umbilical cord. A single umbilical artery can be seen in 1% of singletons and has been associated with multiple other anomalies.[33] In MetroHealth Medical Center's Fetal Diagnostic Center an isolated umbilical artery without other anomalies on ultrasound appears a benign variant. Sinstral (counterclockwise) umbilical cord coiling occurs in 95% of fetuses and fetuses with noncoiled umbilical vessels may have increased anatomic abnormalities[34] (Figures 3-32–3-34).

CONCLUSIONS

Diagnosing subtle fetal anomalies on ultrasound requires an attentive, patient, experienced observer and a thorough examination. Roughly

99% of basic ultrasounds and 80–90% of comprehensive ultrasounds reveal no fetal malformations. The credit for diagnosing a fetal malformation on ultrasound should be attributed to the initial sonographer who suspects a lesion. Once one fetal anomaly has been detected the fetus should be thoroughly evaluated for other possible abnormalities. If a fetal abnormality is suspected it is important, in order to preserve the option of pregnancy termination, to have an early comprehensive ultrasound evaluation prior to fetal viability at 24 weeks gestation.

After a fetal abnormality has been diagnosed there are five therapeutic options: (1) selective abortion, (2) correction after term delivery, (3) preterm delivery for early neonatal therapy, (4) prophylactic delivery and (5) therapy in utero. Management is made more complicated because the two patients, mother and fetus, may have interests that conflict. The best results in diag-

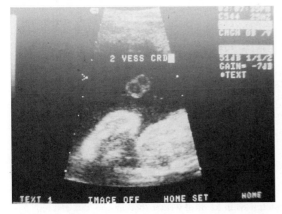

Figure 3-32. Abnormal two-vessel umbilical cord.

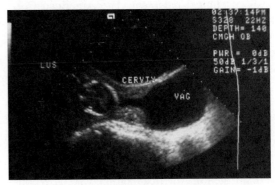

Figure 3-34. Dilated cervix.

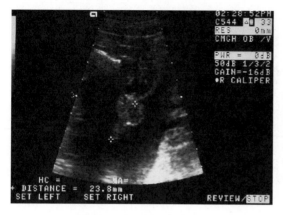

Figure 3-35. Normal male.

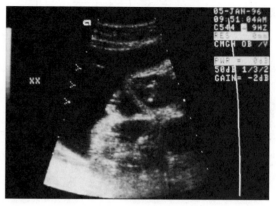

Figure 3-36. Normal female.

nosing and managing a patient with an abnormal or malformed fetus diagnosed on ultrasound can be obtained by a team approach involving the parents, referring health care provider, sonologist, sonographer, perinatologist, neonatologist, pediatric medical subspecialists, pediatric surgeon, cytogenetic specialists, genetic counselor, and social service.[1]

Role of Ultrasound Screening in Pregnancy

The randomized prospective 1993 Routine Antenatal Diagnostic Imaging with Ultrasound (RADIUS) study[35,36] of 15,151 pregnant women at low risk for perinatal outcomes did not show any benefit of routine ultrasound screening. This study concluded that screening sonography did not improve perinatal outcome as compared with the selective use of ultrasonography on the basis of clinical judgment. The American College of Obstetrics and Gynecology (ACOG) has agreed with the RADIUS findings and has concluded that although obstetric ultrasound studies are routinely performed in Europe, American centers have not been able to show the benefit of routine sonography. Arguments for routine screening include the detection of anomalies, multiple gestation, precise dating, and decreased perinatal mortality rate.[2] When the success of routine ultrasound screening in other countries is duplicated in America then the RADIUS conclusions may need to be reevaluated.

Future of Ultrasound

High-risk obstetric patients with clinical indications for ultrasound will continue to have access to ultrasonographic studies but patients with uncomplicated pregnancies desiring ultrasounds for reassurance or to identify gender

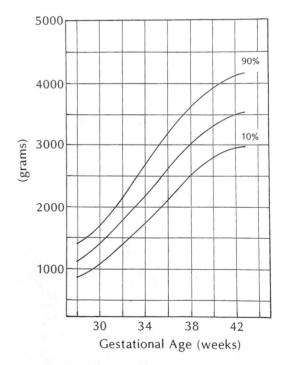

Figure 3-37. Birth weights and gestational ages at MetroHealth Medical Center (bottom, middle, and top lines = 10th, 50th, and 90th percentile, respectively).

may have to share in the cost of medically unindicated studies (Figures 3-35 and 3-36).

Ultrasound technology is changing and digital image enhancement, computerization, storage, and retrieval are with us now. Three-dimensional ultrasound holds great promise for the future and is already in clinical use. Doppler techniques to precisely evaluate regional fetal and placental blood flow are on the horizon. Although technology is no longer widely adopted without verifying its usefulness, the trend for the future in maternal-fetal medicine in America is for increased use of ultrasound and other noninvasive technologies that enhance clinical care and establish the fetus as a patient of a perinatologist.

REFERENCES

1. Ashmead GG, Ashmead JW. Ultrasound in the antenatal diagnosis of fetal anomalies. *Postgrad Obstet Gynecol* 1986;23:1–6.

2. American College of Obstetricians and Gynecologists. Ultrasonography in pregnancy. *ACOG Technical Bulletin 187*. Washington, DC: ACOG, 1993.

3. American College of Obstetricians and Gynecologists. Gynecologic ultrasonography. *ACOG Technical Bulletin 215*. Washington, DC: ACOG, 1995.

4. Ashmead GG, Barth RA. A pocket computer program for obstetric ultrasound calculations. *Am J Perinatol* 1986;3:69–73.

5. Ott WJ. Clinical application of fetal weight determination by real-time ultrasound measurements. *Obstet Gynecol* 1981;57:758–762.

6. Campbell S, Thomas A. Ultrasound measurement of the fetal head to abdomen ratio in the assessment of growth retardation. *Br J Obstet Gynaecol* 1977;165–174.

7. Hadlock FP, Deter RL, Harrist RB, et al. A date independent predictor of intrauterine growth retardation. *AJR* 1983;141:979–983.

8. Amini SB, Catalano PM, Hirsch V, et al. An analysis of birth weight by gestational age using a computerized perinatal data base, 1975–1992. *Obstet Gynecol* 1994;83:342–352.

9. Todros T, Ferrazzi E, Arduini D, et al. Performance of doppler ultrasonography as a screening test in low risk pregnancies: Results of a multicentric study. *J Ultrasound Med* 1995;14:343–348.

10. Ashmead GG, Lazebnik N, Ashmead JW, et al. Normal blood gases in fetuses with absence of end-diastolic umbilical artery velocity. *Am J Perinatol* 1993;10:67–70.

11. Gerson AG, Wallace DM, Bridgens NK, et al. Duplex doppler ultrasound in the evaluation of growth in twin pregnancies. *Obstet Gynecol* 1987;70:419–423.

12. Grannum PA, Berkowitz RL, Hobbins JC. The ultrasonic changes in the maturity of the placenta and their relation to fetal pulmonary maturity. *Am J Obstet Gynecol* 1979;133:915–922.

13. Moore TR. Superiority of the four quadrant sum over the single deepest pocket technique in ultrasonographic identification of abnormal amniotic fluid volumes. *Am J Obstet Gynecol* 1990;163:762–767.

14. Manning FA. Dynamic ultrasound-based fetal assessment: The fetal biophysical profile. *Clin Obstet Gynecol* 1995;38:26–44.

15. Pretorius DH, Nelson TR. Fetal face visualization using three dimensional ultrasonography. *J Ultrasound Med* 1995;14:349–356.

16. Sanders RC. Ultrasonic clues to the detection of chromosomal anomalies. *Obstet Gynecol Clin North Am* 1993;20:455–481.

17. Pandya PP, Brizot ML, Kuhn P, et al. First-trimester fetal nuchal translucency thickness and risk for trisomies. *Obstet Gynecol* 1994;84:420–423.

18. Awwad JT, Azar GB, Karam KS, Nicolaides KH. Ear length: A potential marker for Down syndrome. *Int J Gynaecol Obstet* 1994;44:233–238.

19. Tanaka M, Sato S, Naito H, et al. Anaesthetic management of a neonate with prenatally diagnosed cervical tumor and upper airway obstruction. *Can J Anaesth* 1994;41:236–240.

20. Polk DH. Diagnosis and management of altered fetal thyroid states. *Clin Perinatol* 1994;21:647–662.

21. Filly RA, Cardoza JD, Goldstein RB, et al. Detection of fetal CNS anomalies. A practical level of effort for a routine sonogram. *Radiology* 1989;172:403–408.

22. Nicolaides KH, Campbell S, Gabbe SG, et al. Ultrasound screening for spina bifida: Cranial and cerebellar signs. *Lancet* 1986;2:72–74.

23. Chervenak FA, Duncan C, Ment L, et al. Perinatal management of meningomyelocele. *Obstet Gynecol* 1984;63:376–380.

24. Rose NC, Mennuti MT. Periconceptual folic acid supplementation as a social intervention. *Semin Perinatol* 1995;19:243–254.

25. Snijders RJ, Shawa L, Nicolaides KH. Fetal choroid plexus cysts and trisomy 18: Assessment of risk based on ultrasound findings and maternal age. *Prenat Diagn* 1994;14:1119–1127.

26. Gupta JK, Lilford RJ. Assessment and management of fetal agenesis of the corpus callosum. *Prenat Diagn* 1995;15:301–312.

27. Kleinman CS, Hobbins JC, Jaffe CC, et al. Echocardiographic studies of the human fetus: Prenatal diagnosis of congenital heart disease and cardiac dysrhythmias. *Pediatrics* 1980;65:1059–1067.

28. Copel JA, Pilu G, Greene J, et al. Fetal echocardiographic screening for congenital heart disease: The importance of the four-chamber view. *Am J Obstet Gynecol* 1987;157:648–656.

29. Carpenter MW, Curci MR, Dibbins AW, et al. Perinatal management of ventral wall defects. *Obstet Gynecol* 1984;64:646–651.

30. Grannum P, Bracken M, Silverman R, et al. Assessment of fetal kidney size in normal gestation by comparison of the ratio of kidney circumference to abdominal circumference. *Am J Obstet Gynecol* 1980;136:249–254.

31. Dalton M, Romero R, Grannum P, et al. Antenatal diagnosis of renal anomalies with ultrasound. *Am J Obstet Gynecol* 1986;154:532–537.

32. Hobbins JC, Bracken MB, Mahoney MJ. Diagnosis of fetal skeletal dysplasias with ultrasound. *Am J Obstet Gynecol* 1982;142:306–312.

33. Byrne J, Blanc WA. Malformations and chromosome anomalies in spontaneously aborted fetuses with single umbilical artery. *Am J Obstet Gynecol* 1985;151:340–342.

34. Strong TH. Trisomy among fetuses with noncoiled umbilical blood vessels. *J Reprod Med* 1995;40:789–790.

35. Crane JP, LeFevre ML, Winborn RC, et al. A randomized trial of prenatal ultrasonographic screening: Impact on the detection, management, and outcome of anomalous fetuses. *Am J Obstet Gynecol* 1994;171:392–399.

36. Ewigman BG, Crane JP, Frigoletto FD, et al. Effect of prenatal ultrasound screening on perinatal outcome. *N Engl J Med* 1993;329:821–827.

37. Ultrasonography in Pregnancy. *ACOG Technical Bulletin*, No. 187, December 1993. (Adapted from U.S. Dept. of Health and Human Services, Diagnostic ultrasound in pregnancy. National Institute of Health Publication No. 84-667. Bethesda, MD: National Institute of Health, 1984.)

38. Iams JD, Gabbe SG. Intrauterine growth retardation. In Iams JD, Zuspan FP, Quilligan EJ, eds. *Manual of obstetrics and gynecology*, 2nd ed. St. Louis: Mosby, 1990:165–172.

BIBLIOGRAPHY

Reece EA, Goldstein I, Hobbins JC, eds. *Fundamentals of Obstetric and Gynecologic Ultrasound.* Norwalk, CT: Appleton & Lange, 1994.

Reed GB, Claireaux AE, Cockburn F, et al., (eds). *Diseases of the Fetus and Newborn: Pathology, Imaging, Genetics and Management*, 2nd ed., 2 vols. New York: Chapman & Hall, 1995.

Romero R, Pilu G, Jeanty P, et al., eds. *Prenatal Diagnosis of Congenital Anomalies*. Norwalk, CT: Appleton & Lange, 1988.

QUESTIONS
(choose the best single answer)

1. A safe fetal exposure energy level for obstetric ultrasound is:
   a. Less than 100 mW/cm^2.
   b. Not more than 10 mW/cm^2.
   c. 200 mW/cm squared at the transducer head.
   d. Because of proven ultrasound bioeffects there is no safe level.
2. A crown rump length is:
   a. Most accurate at less than 6 weeks gestation.
   b. Usually has an error >5 days.
   c. Most accurate between 8 and 13 weeks.

d. Unreliable because of frequent confusion between the fetal head and yolk sac.
3. Genetic abnormalities are least associated with:
   a. Short ears (measured to expected <0.8).
   b. Nuchal thickening (15–20 weeks).
   c. Nuchal translucency (11–14 weeks).
   d. Dolichocephaly (20–24 weeks).
4. A normal biparietal diameter is one with:
   a. A lateral ventricle to bihemispheric ratio over 33% after 20 weeks.
   b. A cephalic index of 85–95.
   c. A view of the insula and middle cerebral artery.
   d. A cephalic index of 65–75.
5. A gastroschisis:
   a. Usually has a covering membrane or sac.
   b. If an isolated defect, can usually be safely delivered vaginally.
   c. Often has a chromosome abnormality.
   d. Is usually associated with other malformations.

4

Antenatal Invasive Diagnosis and Therapy

Graham G. Ashmead

INTRODUCTION

The notion that the fetus is a patient, medically, legally, and ethically is a recent concept. Historically the fetus was viewed as a homunculus. During this century, the noninvasive imaging technique of ultrasound or sonography and other modes of antenatal testing have enabled obstetricians to monitor the fetus in utero. These technologies, whether invasive or noninvasive, have enabled physicians to alter the course of fetal disease in utero. Severe fetal Rh disease is now routinely treated in utero by administration of blood transfusions by cordocentesis. Fetal hypothyroidism may be prevented by giving in utero thyroid hormone via amniocentesis or cordocentesis. The fetus has even been removed from the uterine amniotic sac to surgically repair a congenital defect such as congenital diaphragmatic hernia. After repair, the fetus is returned to the womb to complete its gestation. The practice of antenatal invasive diagnosis and therapy is advancing rapidly and supports the notion that the fetus is a patient.

History

Midtrimester amniocentesis was introduced in the 1960s and chorionic villus sampling in the 1980s. By the 1990s prenatal testing has grown to include maternal triple marker blood screening (alpha-fetoprotein, human chorionic gonadotropin, unconjugated estriol) for fetal neural tube defects, Down syndrome (trisomy 21), trisomy 18, Turner syndrome (monosomy X). In addition, improved high-resolution ultrasonography is able to detect fetal structural defects and as an adjunct to evaluate the fetus by cordocentesis and skin biopsy.

Changing Environment

Current technology has made it (progressively) easier to detect diseases earlier than the last decade and antenatal screening is now the standard of obstetric care. Improvements in obstetric ultrasound have enabled physicians to successfully perform early antenatal diagnostic procedures on fetuses at risk for diseases or chromosomal abnormalities.

EARLY ANTENATAL DIAGNOSTIC PROCEDURES

Early antenatal procedures include: (1) routine amniocentesis at greater than 15 weeks gestation, (2) early amniocentesis at 14 weeks or less gestation, (3) chorionic villus sampling at 9–12 weeks gestation, and (4) embryoscopy at 4–10 weeks gestation.

Routine Amniocentesis

Amniocentesis with continuous ultrasound guidance is a routine procedure from 15 weeks gestation onward. Routine amniocentesis for antenatal diagnosis is usually performed from 15 to 20 weeks gestation. Indications for amniocentesis include: advanced maternal age (greater than or equal to 35 years of age at delivery); a previous child with a chromosome abnormality; a parental chromosome abnormality; carrier state for a metabolic or other disease (sickle cell, Tay-Sachs disease, cystic fibrosis, Duchenne's disease); a prior child with a neural tube defect; abnormal maternal serum screening (alpha-fetoprotein, unconjugated estriol, chorionic gonadotropin); or other condition that can be diagnosed antenatally with amniotic fluid. See Table 4-1 for a list of indications.[1]

Routine amniocentesis at MetroHealth's Fetal Diagnostic Center is performed under continuous ultrasonographic guidance using a 22-gauge needle after first obtaining a screening or Level 1 ultrasound. The ultrasound is used to document fetal viability, determine gestational age by multiple morphometric measurements (biparietal diameter, femur length), evaluate for fetal anomalies, and determine the most appropriate site for the amniocentesis. The patient's abdomen is prepared prior to the procedure with an antiseptic solution such as betadine. In order to maintain aseptic technique while scanning sterile gel is applied to the maternal abdomen and a sterilized transducer cover or plastic baggie is placed over a sector transducer. The amniocentesis is performed under continuous ultrasound guidance in order to: (1) prevent injuring the fetus, (2) avoid lacerating the umbilical cord or unnecessarily traversing the placenta, and (3) to successfully obtain amniotic fluid. An initial 0.5 cc is discarded in order to decrease the risk of maternal cell contamination. Thirty cubic centimeters of amniotic fluid are obtained for a fetal karyotype, alpha fetoprotein, or other testing. With multiple gestations a blue dye (indigo

Table 4-1. Indications for Amniocentesis at MetroHealth Medical Center (Cleveland, OH)

Antenatal diagnosis
  Advanced maternal age
  Family history
  Prior fetal anomaly or chromosome abnormality
  Abnormal maternal screening (triple check: AFP, hCG, uE3)
  Abnormal ultrasound
  Risk for Tay-Sachs disease, sickle cell disease, thalassemia(s)
Rh disease
  Rapid fetal blood typing by polymerase chain reaction (48 hours)
  Optical density 450 nm
Pulmonary maturity
  Lecithin to sphingomyelin (L/S) ratio
  Phosphatidyl glycerol
Infection
  TORCH titers
  Chorioamnionitis
Therapeutic
  Twin-to-twin transfusion syndrome
  Thyroid hormone
  Antiarrythmic drugs

Abbreviations: TORCH, toxoplasmosis, other, rubella, cytomegalovirus, and herpes simplex virus.

carmine 0.08%) can be injected (1–5 mL) after each amniocentesis to mark the sac already entered. As long as each successive amniocentesis yields clear fluid the same sac has not been entered twice.[1,2] Obtaining brownish fluid at the time of amniocentesis may reflect old intraamniotic blood and an increased risk for a poor outcome. In order to minimize the risk of fetal loss, no more than two needle insertions (except with multiple gestations) should be performed at the same session. The risk of fetal loss after routine amniocentesis has been reported as high as 1% but in experienced hands can be 0.3%.[3] RhoGAM® (Rh$_0$(D)immune globulin) should be administered after the procedure (300 μg) to unsensitized rhesus-negative women. Patients should refrain from vigorous activity after an amniocentesis. Common complications (1–3%) after amniocentesis include bleeding, vaginal leaking, tenderness, fever, or cramping (Tables 4-2 and 4-3). Cytogenetics results can be available in days for preliminary results (trisomy 21

Table 4-2. Technique of Amniocentesis in the Fetal Diagnostic Center at MetroHealth Medical Center (Cleveland, OH)*

1. Counsel the patient and obtain written informed consent.
2. Ultrasound prior to amniocentesis to determine: viability, number of fetuses, gestational age, anomalies, placentation, amniotic fluid pockets, and site for amniocentesis.
3. Prep the patient's abdomen with antiseptic solution and drape the area for amniocentesis.
4. Use sterile technique: transducer cover or "baggie" for real-time sector or curvilinear ultrasound transducer (3.5–5 Mhz) and gloves for operator and guiding sonographer.
5. Place 22-gauge spinal needle into amniotic fluid pocket under continuous ultrasound guidance using a freehand technique following the needle tip and avoiding the fetus, umbilical cord, and if possible the placenta.
6. No more than two passes per session.
7. Remove appropriate amount of amniotic fluid depending on the studies and clinical indication (for cytogenetics discard first 0.5 cc, then 1 cc per week before 15 weeks and 30 cc after 15 weeks).
8. Check on ultrasound for bleeding, bradycardia, or other complications, show the mother the fetal heart motion after the amniocentesis and monitor on fetal heart rate monitor for 15–30 minutes if after viability (24 weeks).
9. Administer RhoGAM® (300 μg) if the patient is Rh negative and unsensitized.
10. Provide discharge counseling, instructions, and follow-up on results.

*Patient discharge instructions following an amniocentesis procedure performed prior to viability (less than 24 weeks gestation) in the Fetal Diagnostic Center at MetroHealth Medical Center.

Table 4-3. Patient Discharge Instructions Following an Amniocentesis Procedure Performed Prior to Viability (Less than 24 Weeks Gestation) in the Fetal Diagnostic Center at MetroHealth Medical Center (Cleveland, OH)*

1. Bleeding: Contact a physician if you have vaginal bleeding more than spotting or lasting longer than 24 hours.
2. Vaginal leaking: Contact a physician if you have leaking of fluid from vagina that continues after bedrest for several hours.
3. Tenderness: You may have soreness at the amniocentesis site but contact a physician if the soreness does not subside within a day or two or if the soreness increases.
4. Fever: Take your temperature twice a day (every morning and evening) for a week or if you feel warm, have chills or flulike symptoms and contact a physician if your temperature is 38°C or 100.4° F.
5. Cramping: You may have cramping after the procedure but the cramping should subside within the next day. If the cramping continues or increases contact a physician.
6. Physical activity: Avoid strenuous activity, do not lift any heavy objects (anything over 5 lb), refrain from sexual intercourse and orgasm for 2 days.

or 18, monosomy X) up to a week or longer for a final karyotype.

The technique for amniocentesis after fetal viability (24 weeks gestation) is similar to amniocentesis earlier in gestation except that fetal heart rate monitoring for 15–30 minutes may be advisable before and after the procedure to assess the fetus. Depending on the clinical situation it may be prudent to perform an amniocentesis after viability in close proximity to a labor and delivery unit in case a profound bradycardia or other evidence of fetal distress should occur after the procedure.

Second- and third-trimester amniocentesis is usually done for pulmonary maturity studies, detection of amnionitis, evaluation of blood group isoimmunizations or treatment for hydramnios.[1] Interpretation of pulmonary function maturity studies are dependent on the normal values and experience of a particular laboratory but maturity may be evaluated by measurement of amniotic fluid lecithin (L), sphingomyelin (S), and phosphatidylglycerol (PG). Fetal pulmonary maturity in a nondiabetic patient is suggested by an L/S ratio greater than 2.0 in amniotic fluid not contaminated by blood or meconium. Pulmonary maturity is more reliably indicated in the presence of phosphatidyl glycerol (PG) regardless of the presence of blood or meconium.[4] A positive amniotic fluid culture can lead to the diagnosis of chorioamnionitis, as also can a positive Gram stain, decreased amniotic fluid glucose levels, or the presence of leukocyte esterase. See Table 4-4 for a list of antibodies causing in utero hemolytic disease that may indicate an amniocentesis for evaluation of isoimmunization. If the father is a heterozygote for an antigen that the mother has developed antibodies against, then DNA analysis

Table 4-4.   Antibodies Causing Hemolytic Disease*

Blood Group System	Antigens Related to Hemolytic Disease	Severity of Hemolytic Disease
CDE	D	Mild to severe
	C	Mild to severe
	c	Mild to severe
	E	Mild to severe
	e	Mild to moderate
Lewis		Not a proven cause of hemolytic disease of the newborn
		Not a proven cause of hemolytic disease of the newborn
Kell	K	Mild to severe with hydrops fetalis
	k	Mild to severe
Duffy	Fy^a	Mild to severe with hydrops fetalis
	Fy^b	Not a cause of hemolytic disease of the newborn
Kidd	Jk^a	Mild to severe
	Jk^b	Mild to severe
MNSs	M	Mild to severe
	N	Mild
	S	Mild to severe
	s	Mild to severe
Lutheran	Lu^a	Mild
	Lu^b	Mild
Diego	Di^a	Mild to severe
	Di^b	Mild to severe
Xg	Xg^a	Mild
P	$PP_1P^k(Tj^a)$	Mild to severe
Public	Yt^a	Moderate to severe
	Yt^b	Mild
	Lan	Mild
	En^a	Moderate
	Ge	Mild
	Jr^a	Mild
	Co^a	Severe
Private antigens	Co^{a-b}	Mild
	Batty	Mild
	Becker	Mild
	Berrens	Mild
	Evans	Mild
	Gonzales	Mild
	Good	Severe
	Heibel	Moderate
	Hunt	Mild
	Jobbins	Mild
	Radin	Moderate
	Rm	Mild
	Ven	Mild
	$Wright^a$	Severe
	$Wright^b$	Mild
	Zd	Moderate

Source: Modified from ref. 30.

*Conditions listed as mild can be treated like ABO incompatibility. Patients with all other conditions should be monitored as if they were sensitized to D.

by polymerase chain reaction (PCR) of amniotic fluid may be indicated and can rapidly determine (48 hours) if the fetus is at risk for isoimmunization. Spectrophotometric evaluation of the amniotic fluid has been used since the mid-1960s to assess the severity of in utero erythroblastosis. The optical density at 450 nm (delta OD 450) is plotted against gestational age on a Liley graph and used to assist in management. Contamination of amniotic fluid by meconium or red cells can alter spectrophotometric analysis at 450 nm and interpretation of the Liley graph. In addition, the Liley graph and fetal hematocrit may be poorly correlated prior to 26 weeks gestation. See Figure 4-1 for a Liley graph and Figure 4-2 for a management plan incorporating the Liley graph.[5]

Hydramnios resulting in premature labor or maternal respiratory compromise can be alleviated by slow decompression by amniocentesis. The "stuck twin" syndrome where one twin has hydramnios and the other oligohydramnios can be relieved 60% of the time by amniocentesis decompression of the twin with hydramnios. There are reports of up to 5 L of amniotic fluid removed per therapeutic amniocentesis. Often the amniotic fluid reaccumulates around the twin with oligohydramnios.

Other rare indications for amniocentesis include amnioinfusion, obtaining cytogenetics after stillbirth and the administration of in utero medications. Amnioinfusion (80 cc normal saline) for patients with oligohydramnios can be helpful to diagnose anomalies on ultrasound,

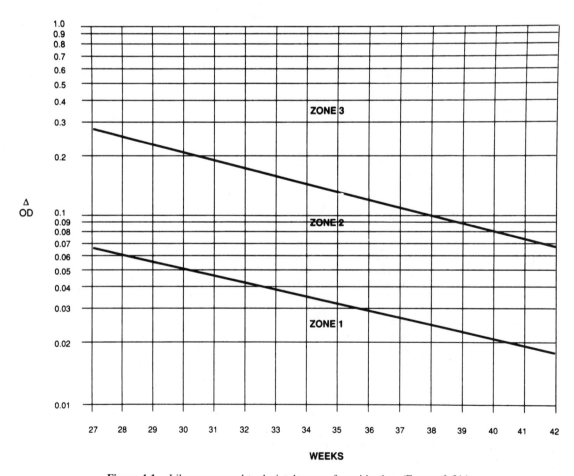

Figure 4-1.   Liley curve used to depict degrees of sensitization. (From ref. 31.)

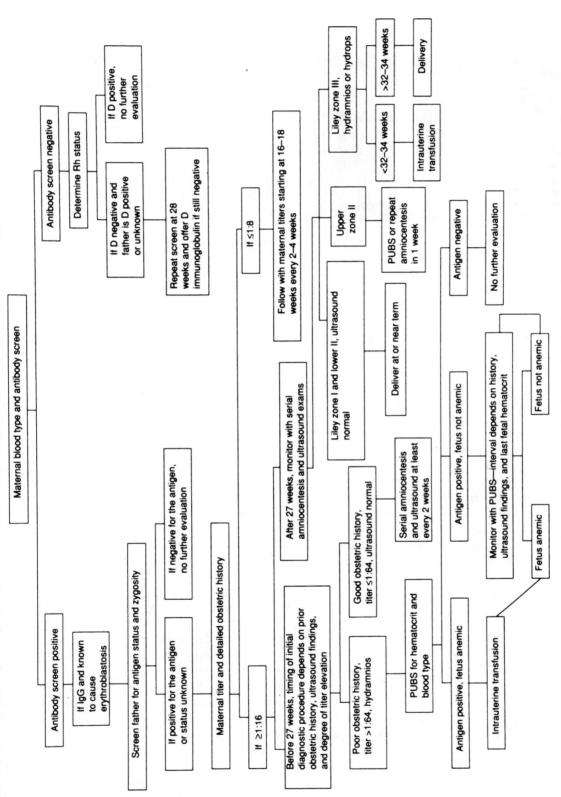

Figure 4-2. Management plan for isoimmunization. (From ref. 5. Reprinted with permission.)

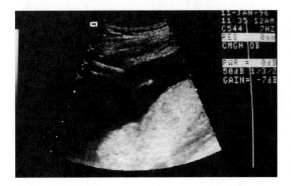

Figure 4-3. Genetic amniocentesis under continuous ultrasound guidance at 16 weeks gestation. Note the needle shadow along the shaft and flare at tip.

obtain cytogenetics, and document ruptured membranes by the instillation of 1–5 mL of indigo carmine dye. If there is ruptured membranes, dye inserted into the amniotic cavity by amniocentesis will usually be noted within 30 minutes on a sterile gauze pad within the vagina and eventually in the maternal urine. Amniocentesis after a stillbirth can assure that cytogentic studies are obtained in an optimal timely sterile fashion. A wide variety of in utero medications have been administered by amniocentesis. In utero amniotic infusion of levothyroid (500 μg) has been administered on a weekly basis to treat hydramnios and fetal goiter resulting from fetal hypothyroidism and also to improve pulmonary maturity.[6,7] See Figure 4-3 for an ultrasound of a genetic amniocentesis at 16 weeks.

Early Amniocentesis

Early amniocentesis for antenatal diagnosis is performed at 14 weeks gestation or less. In 1987, Hanson reported on 541 amniocenteses performed between 11 and 14 weeks gestation with a total fetal loss rate of 4.7%.[8] The technique of early amniocentesis is similar to routine amniocentesis but requires continuous guidance with high-resolution ultrasound and operators skilled with routine amniocentesis. Because of clinical concern about removing too much amniotic fluid early in gestation the common practice is to remove 1 cc of amniotic fluid

per week of gestation for analysis. Early amniocentesis permits screening for fetal anomalies by evaluation of alpha-fetoprotein. Rh immune globulin (300 μg) should be given to unsensitized rhesus negative women after early amniocentesis. The procedure risk and complications due to early amniocentesis are probably slightly higher than routine amniocentesis but roughly equivalent to the risk of chorionic villus sampling.[8]

Chorionic Villus Sampling

Chorionic villus sampling (CVS) is a technique to obtain a small sample (5–40 mg) of placental tissue (chorionic villi). CVS for first trimester genetic diagnosis is generally performed between 9 and 12 weeks gestation and can be performed either transabdominally or transcervically. Chorionic villi can be used for the same indications for prenatal diagnosis as amniocentesis but cannot be used for the diagnosis of neural tube defects, which requires the assessment of amniotic fluid alpha-fetoprotein. CVS has been used for rapid karyotyping (mean 2 days) in the second and third trimesters of pregnancy.[9,10]

CVS is an outpatient procedure and requires no special preparation or post procedure care. The bladder may be filled or emptied to help provide a better position of the uterus, to straighten an anteflexed uterus, or displace bowel from the field with a retroflexed uterus. Prior to transcervical or transabdominal CVS the cervix or abdomen, respectively, is prepped with betadine or other antiseptic solution. Manipulation of the cervix may aid with repositioning a sharply anteflexed or retroflexed uterus. As a general rule it is better to delay a CVS procedure for a few minutes until a uterine contracture noted on ultrasound has resolved. The transcervical technique is performed using a flexible 1.45-mm-outer-diameter polypropylene catheter with a malleable internal stylet (Portex, Ltd.) inserted through the cervix into the placenta under continuous ultrasound guidance. After removal of the stylet the villi are aspirated with a syringe into growth media. See

Figure 4-4 for an ultrasound of a transcervical CVS. A transabdominal approach is used in the Fetal Diagnostic Center at MetroHealth if the placenta is anterior fundal or more easily accessed transabdominally because of cervical fibroids, cervical stenosis, or other technical reasons. The transabdominal approach can be performed freehand with a 20-gauge, 9-cm spinal needle or by a double-needle technique using an 18-gauge needle positioned as a guide to the placenta with a 20-gauge needle then inserted within the 18-gauge needle for repeated passes. No more than two CVS procedures should be performed at one session. Pregnancies with multiple gestations can be sampled with CVS but require a skilled operator and being able to clearly separately sample the placenta of each fetus at the cord insertion site. See Tables 4-5 for a pre-CVS checklist. See Table 4-6 for a transcervical and Table 4-7 for a transabdominal technique for performing CVS. Unsensitized Rh-negative women should receive RhoGAM® after CVS (300 μg). Rh-sensitized patients are at high risk for increased sensitization with CVS and should not have the procedure performed because of the risk of developing severe early fetal hydrops. Total loss rates up through 28 weeks of pregnancy have been reported as 2.5% after transcervical and 2.3% after transabdominal CVS.[11] Complications after CVS may include spotting, fetomaternal hemorrhage, fluid leakage, and chorioamnionitis.

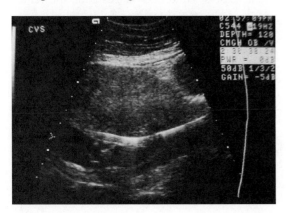

Figure 4-4. Ultrasound showing a transcervical chorionic villus sampling procedure at 12 weeks gestation using a Portex catheter.

Table 4-5. A Pre-Chorionic Villus Sampling (CVS) Checklist

1. Counseling complete
2. Consent signed and in chart
3. Gonorrhea culture of the cervix done (if transcervical CVS)
4. Blood type and Rh known
5. RhoGAM® to be given if unsensitized Rh negative patient (do not perform CVS if Rh sensitized)
6. Fetal ultrasound confirming appropriate gestational age (10–12 weeks)
7. Instructions and follow-up form given to patient

CVS performed by inexperienced operators or prior to 9 weeks gestation may result in increased risk of fetal developmental abnormalities including limb defects.[12,13]

Embryoscopy

Embryoscopy is observing an embryo transcervically or transabdominally through an intact amnion via an endoscope introduced into the extraembryonic coelom. In ongoing pregnancies

Table 4-6. Transcervical Chorionic Villus Sampling Technique in the Fetal Diagnostic Center at MetroHealth Medical Center (Cleveland, OH)

1. Counseling performed and informed consent obtained.
2. Blood type obtained.
3. Ultrasound for: viability, gestational age, and placental location.
4. Speculum placed in vagina, cervix cleansed with betadine, and clamp placed on the anterior lip of the cervix.
5. Uterine sound placed into the cervix under ultrasound guidance and removed.
6. Portex inserted into placental body under continuous ultrasound guidance and stylet removed.
7. 20-cc syringe with 5 cc of growth media attached to syringe.
8. 15 cc of negative pressure applied to syringe with multiple passes and then catheter removed.
9. Attempt to obtain 15 mg of wet-weight villi (confirm under microscope if indicated). If villi insufficient (less than 5 mg) perform one more pass.
10. RhoGAM® given if indicated.
11. Counseling and follow-up scheduled. Ultrasound in 1 week and at 16 weeks. Schedule triple check (AFP, hCG, uE3) at 16–18 weeks.

Table 4-7.   Transabdominal Chorionic Villus Sampling Technique in the Fetal Diagnostic Center at MetroHealth Medical Center (Cleveland, OH)

1. Counseling performed and informed consent obtained.
2. Blood type obtained.
3. Ultrasound for: viability, gestational age, and placental location.
4. Abdomen cleansed with betadine.
5. Ultrasound guidance off field.
6. 20-gauge beveled spinal needle inserted into the placental body (parallel to placental disc) under continuous ultrasound guidance.
7. 20-cc syringe with 5 cc of growth media attached to syringe.
8. 15 cc of negative pressure applied to syringe with multiple passes and then needle removed.
9. Attempt to obtain 15 mg of wet weight villi (confirm under microscope if indicated). If villi insufficient (less than 5 mg), perform one more needle insertion.
10. RhoGAM® given if indicated.
11. Counseling and follow-up scheduled. Ultrasound in 1 week and at 16 weeks. Schedule triple check (AFP, hCG, uE3) at 16–18 weeks.

embryoscopy should be performed after 9 weeks gestation after development of the embryo's eyelids in order to minimize the risk of eye damage due to excessive exposure to light. Transcervical embryoscopy is possible as long as the thickest part of the trophoblast is not in direct contact with the internal cervical os and involves inserting a rigid endoscope (outer diameter 1.7–3.5 mm) through the cervix. The embryo can be seen directly through the endoscope or via video camera and monitor. Antibiotics are given after a transcervical embryoscopy. The risks of bleeding and infection of transcervical embryoscopy are assumed to be similar to the risks of chorionic villus sampling. Transabdominal thin wall 18-gauge embryofetoscopy has been used in the diagnosis of Meckel-Gruber at 11 weeks gestation prior to fusion of the chorion and amnion (12–13 weeks gestation). Embryoscopy permits prenatal diagnosis of face and limb defects as early as 9 weeks gestation but because of its invasive nature has limited clinical application. Embryoscopy may be useful in patients with a high risk of transmitting a severe congenital disorder that

can be identified by morphology or by directly sampling blood and skin. Embryoscopic in utero injection of cells may be a means of early treatment of genetic, metabolic, hematologic, and immune disorders.[14–16]

CORDOCENTESIS

Ultrasound-guided access to the fetal circulation was first described in 1982 by Bang into the fetal body and then in 1983 by Daffos into the umbilical cord.[17,18] Cordocentesis, also known as percutaneous umbilical blood sampling (PUBS) or fetal blood sampling (FBS), has had many indications including: red cell isoimmunization, fetal hemolytic disease, hemoglobinopathies, coagulation defects, platelet abnormalities, evaluation of nonimmune hydrops, fetal acid-base status, rapid karyotype, intrauterine infections (rubella, toxoplasmosis, cytomegalovirus), and fetal drug levels. Cordocentesis involves an initial ultrasound to evaluate the fetus and determine the most appropriate access to the umbilical cord (see Fig. 4-5). The easiest access to the umbilical cord is often at its insertion into the placenta. The umbilical cord can usually be sampled relatively easily between 20 and 26 weeks gestation. Earlier in gestation cordocentesis can be technically difficult and the loss rate higher because of the small size of the fetal umbilical vessels while later in gestation the fetus

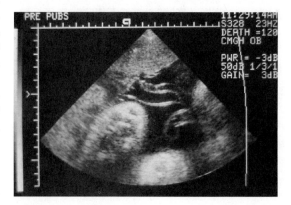

Figure 4-5.   Ultrasound of a cordocentesis procedure. (Needle tip in umbilical vein through an anterior placenta.)

may obstruct ultrasound visualization and access to the cord insertion site. Fetal vascular access sites used at MetroHealth if a cord insertion site is not available include a free-floating loop of umbilical cord, the intrahepatic vein, or a cardiac ventricle.

Using sterile technique the patient is prepped with betadine or other antiseptic, the abdomen draped and local anesthetic (2% lidocaine) infiltrated into the maternal abdomen and subcuticular tissues taking care to avoid entering the maternal abdominal cavity or uterine wall. A 22-gauge single spinal needle is inserted into the umbilical cord using a freehand technique and either a sector or curvilinear 3.5–5 MHz transducer for ultrasound guidance. Blood is aspirated into a 3-cc heparinized syringe and sent for a Coulter counter analysis to document a pure fetal sample. Ferning can demonstrate amniotic fluid contamination and the Kleihauer-Betke maternal cells. Infusion of normal saline or blood can document fetal arterial or venous access. RhoGAM® is administered if indicated after the procedure. Complications after cordocentesis include leakage of blood from the cordocentesis puncture site, cord hematoma, bradycardia, rupture of membranes, and chorioamnionitis. A fetal loss rate of 1.2% has been attributed to diagnostic cordocentesis.[19–22]

Cordocentesis has come to play a major role in the treatment of hemolytic disease of the fetus. Patients with hemolytic disease are followed with monthly titers until a critical titer of 1:16 is reached. Once a critical titer is reached the patient can be managed by amniocentesis to determine the fetal antigenicity and to monitor the amniotic fluid delta OD 450. See the section on amniocentesis in this chapter and Figures 4-1 and 4-2. If the delta OD 450 is at the 80th percentile or Zone 2 of the Liley curve then cordocentesis may be indicated to sample the fetal hematocrit. Ultrasound findings of hydrops, ascites, effusions, hydramnios, hepatomegaly, or cardiomegaly may suggest fetal isoimmunization and aid management. The fetus is transfused if the fetal hematocrit is less than 30. An intravascular dose of vecuronium (0.1 mg/kg estimated fetal weight) can be used to paralyze the

fetus during the transfusion. The paralysis will last 1–2 hours. The transfused blood can be O-negative cytomegalovirus-negative donor blood or fresh maternal blood. Prior to transfusion maternal blood can be washed to remove the antibodies, filtered to remove leukocytes, irradiated to prevent graft versus host reaction and concentrated to a final hematocrit of 75–85% or even higher.

Previous to the use of cordocentesis, fetal transfusions were done by intraperitoneal transfusions (IPT) giving a volume of blood in mL equal to 10 times the result of the gestational age subtracted by 20. However, a major drawback of IPT was that fetuses with hydrops did not absorb blood well given by IPT. Hydrops usually occurs at a hematocrit of 15 or if the fetal hemoglobin level is 7 g/dL below the mean hemoglobin for gestational age. Intravascular transfusions (IVT) can provide accurate direct sampling of the initial hematocrit and final hematocrit and the transfusion of hydropic fetuses. Final goals for hematocrit levels for IVT are 50–65% while for IPT are 35–40%. The initial two transfusions can occur at 2-week intervals and then be spaced out for 3–4 weeks depending on the fetal hematocrit. Clinical experience suggests that with severe disease the fetal hematocrit may initially decrease by 2% per day declining to 1% per day with milder disease or after several transfusions. Combining IPT and IVT may decrease the number and frequency of fetal transfusions. Fetuses with severe hydrops may have better survival if the initial posttransfusion hematocrit is only 20–25% and only brought up to 35% after 48 hours. The final transfusion should be not later than 35 weeks gestation with delivery by 37–38 weeks. The survival rate for hydropic fetuses can be 82% and for nonhydropic fetuses 90%. Up to 50% of infants treated in utero may require "top up" transfusions within the first few weeks of life.

Despite the use of prophylactic immunoglobulin it is unlikely that red cell alloimmunization will ever be totally eliminated. It appears unlikely that fetal survival can be much improved beyond the current techniques of cordocentesis and ultrasound-guided IVT. It is unclear what

the long-term outcome of fetuses will be after
IPT and IVT. Future therapy may involve suppression of the maternal B-lymphocytes that
produce the antibodies resulting in alloimmunization. Alternately, artificial insemination,
prenatal screening, in vitro fertilization, or gene
therapy can prevent alloimmunization.[22,23]

FETOSCOPY

One of the older methods to access the fetus is
fetoscopy which can be used to obtain fetal
blood and skin biopsy samples. The fetoscope
has an outer diameter of 1.7 mm and a sidearm
permitting insertion of a 26- or 27-gauge needle
for fetal sampling. Maternal sedation, local anesthesia, and a small skin insertion is required
prior to uterine insertion of the fetoscope. The
loss rate associated with fetoscopy is operator
dependent and has been estimated at 5–7%. Fetoscopy has largely been replaced by other diagnostic and invasive techniques.[24]

STENT PROCEDURES (SHUNT)

In utero surgery placement of fetal stents has
been performed in the fetal genitourinary system, pleural cavities, and cerebral ventricles.
The value of these procedures in terms of immediate benefit and long-term improvement appears to be limited. Complete parental informed
consent is important as the procedures are invasive, take time to perform, have increased risk
of infection, and are in the realm of experimental clinical care (see Fig. 4-6).

The use of shunt (stent) procedures may be
helpful in fetuses with bladder outlet obstruction
severe enough to compromise renal and pulmonary development but prior to irreversible fetal renal and pulmonary damage. Bladder outlet
obstruction (BOO) due to posterior urethral
valves (PUV) should be suspected on ultrasound
if there is a dilated bladder, hydroureter and hydronephrosis in a male fetus. Often the proximal
urethra will be dilated with PUV and the bladder
wall will be hypertrophied. Renal dysplasia may

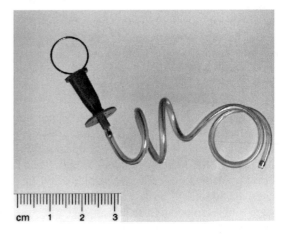

Figure 4-6. Fetal stent. (Courtesy Rocket, Ltd., UK.)

be suspected if there are multiple cysts and hy-
perechogenicity of the renal parenchyma. Oligohydramnios is not an invariable sign of BOO
or PUV and depends on the severity of the obstruction but is a poor prognostic sign. Urinary
ascites from bladder rupture or other causes may
also be seen with BOO. A normal male karyotype should be obtained before contemplating a
shunt procedure or fetal surgery in order to
avoid operations on a genetically abnormal fetus.

Persistent fetal lower urinary obstruction has
a very poor prognosis because of diminished renal function and pulmonary hypoplasia secondary to oligohydramnios. Severely affected fetuses in the third trimester are probably best
treated by delivery and neonatal treatment. The
overall survival rate has been no more than
30%. Early attempts at in utero shunt placement
to provide renal decompression and prevent the
development of pulmonary hypoplasia may not
have been successful because of poor patient selection. Appropriate candidates for in utero surgery for bladder outlet obstruction include fetuses with a normal male karyotype and normal
fetal urine biochemistry parameters. Normal fetal urine would be a sodium (Na) less than 100
mEq/L, chlorine (Cl) less than 90 mEq/L, calcium (Ca) less than 6 mg/dL, urine osmolarity
less than 210 mOsm/L, low beta-2 microglob-
ulin, and a urine output greater than 2 cc/hr.
There is controversy about the predictive value

of fetal urinary electrolytes.[25] A single fetal urine determination by bladdercentesis may be insufficient to declare irreversible damage. After decompression, improvement or the lack of improvement in urine biochemistry may be more representative of the ultimate fetal outcome. Also, some fetuses spontaneously improve after serial bladdercenteses, possibly due to release of intravesicular pressure allowing release of the obstructed posterior urethral valve or relief of bladder neck spasm. Fetuses that do not show improvement of fetal urine biochemistry despite serial decompression have a poor prognosis.[26] The decompression of the fetal bladder by either needle aspiration or intrauterine shunting may be warranted in carefully selected fetuses with bladder outlet obstruction. Fetuses with persistent megacystis whose urine biochemistry's improve after serial decompression represent the group most likely to benefit from invasive fetal therapy. Predicting lung pathology or pulmonary hypoplasia is difficult but increasing the amniotic fluid will improve fetal lung development and maturation. The earlier in pregnancy that the fetus is treated the more likely that normal development will take place.

Stent procedures can be performed under continuous ultrasound guidance with a Rodeck shunt apparatus (Rocket of London, UK) (see Fig. 4-7). After an initial ultrasound to determine the proper approach and maternal sedation, the maternal skin is prepped, the skin anesthetized with 2% lidocaine, and a scalpel blade is used to nick the skin. The shunt loader is inserted into the uterine cavity and then into the fetal cavity to be shunted. After the fluid cavity is sampled to confirm the position and for appropriate studies the central trocar is removed. A plastic double-pigtailed catheter with a central wire stylet is passed down the shunt apparatus. The wire stylet is then removed. A short plunger is used to push the distal portion of the catheter into the fetal cavity. The short plunger is removed and a long plunger inserted to just touch the catheter. The shunt introducer apparatus is then pulled back while holding the long plunger steady, so that the proximal portion of the catheter is placed into the amniotic cavity.

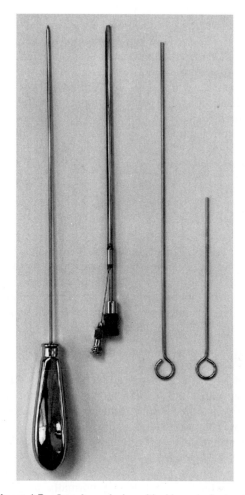

Figure 4-7. Introducer device with side port, short and long plungers for fetal stent placement. (Courtesy Rocket, Ltd., UK.)

Complications after fetal suprapubic stent placement include rupture of membranes, chorioamnionitis, injury to the fetus, obstruction, displacement, and ventral wall defects. See Figures 4-3 and 4-4 showing the shunt placement apparatus and the Rocket catheter.[27]

FETAL SURGERY

Open fetal surgery (in utero or ex utero surgery with replacement of fetus in utero) is a relatively rare technique that may allow the treatment of simple anatomic defects that untreated would usually result in death in utero or shortly after birth. The younger the fetus at the time of surgery the less likely the formation of surgical scars. Conditions that might be alleviated by open fetal surgery include bilateral urinary tract obstruction with oligohydramnios, congenital cystic adenomatoid malformation, congenital diaphragmatic hernia, sacrococcygeal teratoma, complete heart block, and stuck twin. Only a few centers worldwide have the experience and expertise to justify attempting open fetal surgery.

CONCLUSIONS

Maternal-fetal management has extended beyond simply determining the timing and method of delivery to treating or even correcting underlying fetal abnormalities. Steady improvement in antenatal diagnostic and invasive techniques is transforming the fetus into a patient.

State of the Art

In 1995, De Lia reported fetoscopic laser ablation with a 2.9 × 3.85 mm dual-channel fetoscope and neodymium:yttrium-aluminum-garnet laser light of chorioangiopagus vessels in 35 patients with severe previable (6–17 weeks, mean 11.7 weeks) twin-twin transfusion syndrome. De Lia found that 53% of fetuses survived with 96% developing normally at 35.8 weeks. In midpregnancy the difficulty of identifying and laser ablating chorioangiopagus vessels combined with the successful symptomatic therapy of twin-twin transfusion with amniocentesis has made laser therapy controversial. De Lia states that laser surgical interruption of the common vasculature is the only treatment that can halt the twin-twin transfusion and protect the survivor if one fetus dies in utero. De Lia maintains that laser occlusion of chorioangiopagous vessels in monochorionic fetuses provides the most favorable environment for continued development.[28]

Future of Fetal Diagnosis and Therapy

The "holy grail" of prenatal diagnosis, the genetic analysis of fetal cells obtained from the maternal circulation early in gestation, may eventually provide a noninvasive way to screen or diagnose genetic abnormalities in the fetus. In the future it may be possible to identify, separate, and analyze fetal cells in a reproducible fashion.[29]

Eventually gene therapy and fetal stem cell transplantation may permit antenatal treatment of prenatally diagnosed cellular deficiency states. Advances in fetal endoscopic surgery may allow fetal surgery in utero through small puncture sites avoiding the morbidity of a large uterine incision.

REFERENCES

1. Ashmead GG, Krew MA. Amniocentesis (early and late). In Reed GB, Claireaux AE, Cockburn F (eds), *Diseases of the Fetus and Newborn*, 2nd ed. London: Chapman & Hall, 1995, pp. 1083–1087.

2. Elias S, Gerbie AB, Simpson JL. Genetic amniocentesis in term gestation. *Am J Obstet Gynecol* 1980;138:169–174.

3. Evans MI, Drugan A, Koppitch FC, et al. Genetic diagnosis in the first trimester: The norm for the 1990s. *Am J Obstet Gynecol* 1989;160:1332–1339.

4. Garite TJ, Yabusaki KK, Moberg LJ, et al. A new rapid slide agglutination test for amniotic fluid phosphatidylglycerol: Laboratory and clinical correlation. *Am J Obstet Gynecol* 1983;147:681–686.

5. American College of Obstetricians and Gynecologists. Management of isoimmunization in pregnancy. *ACOG Technical Bulletin 148.* Washington, DC: ACOG, 1990.

6. Polk DH. Diagnosis and management of altered fetal thyroid status. *Clin Perinatol* 1994;21:647–662.

7. Romaguera J, Ramirez M, Adamsons K. Intraamniotic thyroxine to accelerate fetal maturation. *Semin Perinatol* 1993;17:260–266

8. Hanson FW, Zorn EM, Tennany FR, et al. Amniocentesis before 15 weeks gestation: Outcome, risks and technical problems. *Am J Obstet Gynecol* 1987;156:1524–1531.

9. American College of Obstetricians and Gynecologists. Chorionic villus sampling. *ACOG Committee Opinion 69.* Washington, DC: ACOG, 1989.

10. Shulman LP, Tharapel AT, Meyers CM, et al. Direct analysis of uncultured cytotrophoblastic cells from second and third trimester placentas: An accurate and rapid method for detection of fetal chromosome abnormalities. *Am J Obstet Gynecol* 1990;163:1606–1609.

11. Jackson L, Zachary JM, Fowler SE, et al. A randomized comparison of transcervical and transabdominal chorionic villus sampling. *N Engl J Med* 1992;327:594–598.

12. Kaplan P, Normandin J, Wilson GN, et al. Malformations and minor anomalies in children whose mothers had prenatal diagnosis: Comparison between CVS and amniocentesis. *Am J Med Genet* 1990;37:366–370.

13. Brambati B. Chorionic villus sampling (early and late). In Reed GB, Claireaux AE, Cockburn F (eds), *Diseases of the Fetus and Newborn,* 2nd ed, London: Chapman & Hall, 1995, pp. 1077–1082.

14. Copel JA, Cullen MT, Grannum PA, Hobbins JC. Invasive fetal assessment in the antepartum period. *Obstet Gynecol Clin North Am* 1990;17: 201–221.

15. Quintero RA, Abuhamad A, Hobbins JC, et al. Transabdominal thin-gauge embryofetoscopy: A technique for early prenatal diagnosis and its use in the diagnosis of a case of Meckel-Gruber syndrome. *Am J Obstet Gynecol* 1993;168: 1552–1557.

16. Dumez Y, Oury JF, Dommergues M, et al. Embryoscopy and first trimester prenatal diagnosis. In Reed GB, Claireaux AE, Cockburn F (eds), *Diseases of the Fetus and Newborn,* 2nd ed. London: Chapman & Hall, 1995, pp. 1065–1070.

17. Bang J, Bock JE, Trolle D. Ultrasound guided fetal intravenous transfusion for severe rhesus haemolytic disease. *British Medical Journal* 1982;284:373–374.

18. Daffos F, Pavlovsky M, Forrestier F. A new procedure for fetal blood sampling in utero: Preliminary results of fifty-three cases. *Am J Obstet Gynecol* 1983;146:985–986.

19. Ludomirski A, Weiner S, Ashmead CG, et al. Percutaneous umbilical fetal blood sampling procedure safety and normal hematological indices. *Am J Perinatol* 1988;5:264–266.

20. Lazebnik N, Hendryx PV, Ashmead GG, et al. Detection of amniotic fluid contamination of fetal blood obtained by cordocentesis. *Am J Obstet Gynecol* 1990:163:78–80.

21. Ashmead GG, Lazebnik N, Ashmead JW, et al. Normal blood gases in fetuses with absence of end-diastolic umbilical artery velocity. *Am J Perinatol* 1993;10:67–70.

22. Johnson P, Maxwell DJ. Cordocentesis (percutaneous umbilical blood sampling and fetal blood sampling). In Reed GB, Claireaux AE, Cockburn F (eds), *Diseases of the Fetus and Newborn,* 2nd ed. London: Chapman & Hall, 1995, pp. 1071–1076.

23. Moise KJ, Ashmead GG. Rhesus alloimmunization. In Reed GB, Claireaux AE, Cockburn F (eds), *Diseases of the Fetus and Newborn,* 2nd ed. Chapman & Hall, London, 1995, pp. 1301–1306.

24. Grannum PA, Copel JA. Invasive fetal procedures. *Radiol Clin North Am* 1990;28:217–226.

25. Elder JS, O'Grady JP, Ashmead G, et al. Evaluation of fetal renal function: Unreliability of fetal urinary electrolytes. *J Urol* August 1990; 144:574–578.

26. Evans MI, Sacks AJ, Johnson MP, et al. Sequential invasive assessment of fetal renal function and the intrauterine treatment of obstructive uropathies. *Obstet Gynecol* 1991;77:545–550.

27. Ashmead GG, Burrows WR. Shunts in closed fetal surgery. In Reed GB, Claireaux AE, Cockburn F (eds), *Diseases of the Fetus and Newborn,* 2nd ed. London: Chapman & Hall, 1995, pp. 1315–1318.

28. De Lia JE, Kulmann RS, Harstad TW, et al. Fetoscopic laser ablation of placental vessels in severe previable twin-twin transfusion syndrome. *Obstet Gynecol* 1995;172:1202–1211.

29. Senyei AE, Wassman ER. Fetal cells in the maternal circulation: Technical considerations for practical application to prenatal diagnosis. *Obstet Gynecol Clin North Am* 1993;20:583–598.

30. Weinstein L. Irregular antibodies causing hemolytic disease of the newborn. *Clin Obstet Gynecol* 1982;25:321–332.

31. Liley AW. Liquor ammi analysis in management of pregnancy complicated by rhesus sterilization. *Am J Obstet Gynecol* 1961;82:1359–1370.

BIBLIOGRAPHY

Harrison MR, Golbus MS, Filly RA (eds). *The Unborn Patient: Prenatal Diagnosis and Treatment*, 2nd ed. Philadelphia: Saunders, 1990.

Reece EA, Goldstein I, Hobbins JC (eds). *Fundamentals of Obstetric and Gynecologic Ultrasound*. Norwalk, CT: Appleton & Lange, 1994.

Reed GB, Claireaux AE, Cockburn F, et al. (eds). *Diseases of the Fetus and Newborn: Pathology, Imaging, Genetics and Management*, 2nd ed., 2 vols. New York: Chapman & Hall Medical, 1995.

Romero R, Pilu G, Jeanty P, et al. *Prenatal Diagnosis of Congenital Anomalies*. Norwalk, CT: Appleton & Lange, 1988.

QUESTIONS
(choose the single best answer)

1. Routine amniocentesis:
   a. Has the same risk as early amniocentesis.
   b. Has a risk of 1% in skilled hands.
   c. Is better than chorionic villus sampling in screening for neural tube defects.
   d. Is better than chorionic villus sampling in screening for genetic abnormalities.
2. Indications for amniocentesis include all except:
   a. Advanced maternal age (35 or greater at delivery).
   b. Parental chromosome abnormality.
   c. Maternal age 25 but prior child with trisomy 21.
   d. Maternal reassurance.
3. Chorionic villus sampling cannot (should not):
   a. Be performed transabdominally.
   b. Diagnose neural tube defects.
   c. Provide preliminary results in under 2 days.
   d. Be used in the third trimester.
4. Cordocentesis transfusions:
   a. Should not be performed after 32 weeks.
   b. Should not be used in combination with intraperitoneal transfusions.
   c. Are only indicated in the treatment of Rh isoimmunization.
   d. May be indicated if the fetal hemoglobin level is 7 g/dL below the mean hemoglobin for gestational age.
5. Stent procedures:
   a. Are of proven immediate and long-term benefit for placement in pleuritic cavities and cerebral ventricles.
   b. Are appropriate in severely affected fetuses with bladder outlet obstruction in the third trimester.
   c. Are most likely to be successful in fetuses with persistent megacystis whose urine biochemistries improve after serial decompression.
   d. Are not indicated in fetuses with urine concentrations of Na less than 100 mEq/L or Cl less than 90 mEq/L.

Part III

MATERNAL-FETAL COMPLICATIONS DURING PREGNANCY

5

Intrauterine Growth Restriction (IUGR)

Sangithan J. Moodley

INTRODUCTION

Fetuses suffering restriction of intrauterine growth constitute one of the primary causes of stillbirth, prematurity, increased neonatal morbidity, and mortality and fetal stress during labor. The diagnosis and subsequent management of pregnancies complicated by intrauterine growth restriction (IUGR) continues to present multiple challenges.[1] Current screening policies only identify 25% of cases,[1] and in the low-risk population this figure may be much lower.

This chapter will define the problem of IUGR, and discuss current concepts in diagnosis and management.

DEFINITIONS

1. *Low birth weight (LBW)*[2]. This term includes all infants weighing less than 2500 g at birth, irrespective of gestational age. Further categorization has recently separated these births as follows: 1000–1499 g (very LBW), 500–999 g (extremely LBW), and <500 g (micropremies). About two thirds of LBW infants are appropriate for the gestational age (preterm), and the remainder are smaller than expected for the

gestational age (small for dates, IUGR, or dysmature).

2. *Small for dates (SGA, SFD)*. These are infants whose weight at birth is below the lower confidence limit of a normal distribution of infants (Figure 5-1). Several important facts must be understood in relating birth weight to gestational age under such circumstances. These include:
   a. The lower confidence limit is arbitrarily assigned and must be defined [3rd, 5th, or 10th percentile or −1 or −2 standard deviation (SD)].
   b. Such charts are frequently constructed from cross-sectional data, include high-risk obstetric patients, and have not been corrected for the multiple variables which influence fetal growth. For example, the Denver Birth weight charts[3] commonly used in the United States, are inclusive of high-risk patients living at an altitude of about 10,000 ft and appear not to be representative of many regions of the country (Figure 5-1).
   c. Constitutionally, normal infants may be distributed below the lower confidence limit. These infants are commonly referred to as SGA infants.

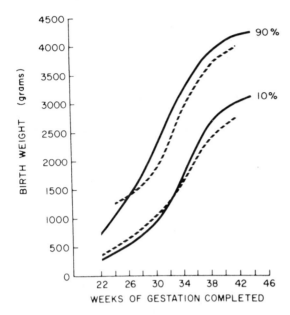

Figure 5-1. Solid line represents births in California 1970–1976. Dotted line represents births in Colorado General Hospital 1948–1960. (Adapted from ref. 20.)

d.   Infants within the normal distribution curve could demonstrate evidence of IUGR (thin infants, frequently referred to as dysmature).[4]

3.   *Intrauterine growth restriction (IUGR).* It is important to separate small infants who have not suffered restraint of growth (SGA) from those showing evidence of undernutrition (IUGR). Up to 40% of infants born SFD show no evidence of undernutrition (IUGR).[4] Neonatal indices such as the ponderal index and crown heel length attempt to separate these two groups. In utero fetal biometry also attempts to separate these types. The heterogeneity of intrauterine growth failure often makes this task difficult.

INCIDENCE

Incidence significantly varies (3–7%)[5,6] in various communities due to some of the factors noted above. Some of these factors include ethnic, racial, social, and economic, geopolitical

factors and the definitions utilized. The clinical recognition of IUGR in pregnancies presenting little or no apparent risk factors is of primary importance. For example, unrecognized IUGR is a frequent accompaniment (20%)[7] of stillbirth.

NORMAL FETAL GROWTH

Fetal growth can be divided into the embryonic (up to $8\frac{1}{2}$ weeks) and subsequent fetal period. Growth is also physiologically divided into an early hyperplastic, midhyperplastic-hypertrophic, and finally a hypertrophic phase[8] (Figure 5-2). From a clinical standpoint, these divisions may be useful in understanding pathological alterations of growth. For example, factors predisposing to an early restraint of growth will probably lead to an overall reduction of cellular hyperplasia [hence deoxyribonucleic acid (DNA)] and reduction in overall size (symmetrical IUGR),[9,10] whereas any influence occurring later will lead to a maximum effect on the size of cells (protein content), and will be especially responsive to metabolic fuels (liver, fat, muscle). The relative sparing of head size and length leads to a thin (undernourished-asymmetric) infant (Figure 5-3).[9,10]

From a clinical standpoint it is important to recognize the heterogeneity of the condition, and to differentiate those infants suffering restriction of growth (IUGR) from those who are constitutionally small (SGA). The pattern of restricted fetal growth is dependent on multiple factors and does not commonly conform to a symmetrical and/or asymmetrical pattern. For example, while maternal undernutrition would more likely lead to a depression of cellular hypertrophy, and hence to asymmetrical IUGR, very severe early undernutrition (such as occurring in droughts and famines) could result in early depression of cellular hyperplasia and later hypertrophy, causing a mixed (heterogeneous) pattern of fetal growth. The combinations of clinical and sonographic information usually establishes the likely etiology(ies) of IUGR.

The term ''growth'' usually implies an in-

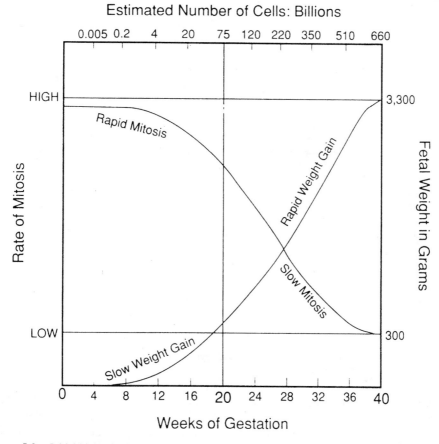

Figure 5-2.   Initial high mitotic activity is not associated with substantial changes in mass (hyperplasia). Later decreased mitotic activity is associated with rapid changes in mass (hypertrophy). (Adapted from refs. 67 and 68.)

crease in body mass (and also encompasses hyperplasia and hypertrophy) while the term ''development'' signifies the process of attainment of physiological function. The intrinsic potential of an organism to grow is dependent upon genetic and subsequently hormonal mechanisms (i.e., is growth promoting). The restraining effect on fetal growth is the environment.

Genetic factors dominate in the first half of pregnancy while hormonal and environmental factors exert their effects later (Table 5-1).

The rate of fetal growth has been studied in abortuses and live births. The cross-sectional data obtained indicate the following pattern:

- 5 g/day at 14–15 weeks
- 10 g/day at 20 weeks
- 30–35 g/day at 32–34 weeks
- 230 g/week at 33–36 weeks
- 0 g/week to decrease at 41–42 weeks

ETIOLOGY OF IUGR

In discussing the etiology of IUGR, it is important to realize that smallness (SGA), in up to 40% of instances, may be constitutional (genetic) in origin. Also, a significant percentage of neonates whose weights are average at birth may be the products of restricted intrauterine growth.

Table 5-2 outlines factors associated with IUGR. This list is by no means complete. The

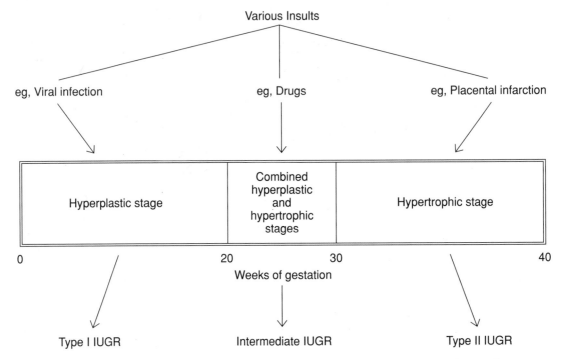

Figure 5-3. Some influences on fetal growth and the types of IUGR that could result. (Adapted from ref. 68.)

factors associated with IUGR can be divided into three broad groups; maternal, uteroplacental, and fetal. These factors may occur in isolation or may act in concert in causing IUGR. For example, fetal aneuploidy is frequently associated with placental abnormalities.

Maternal age at both extremes is associated with IUGR. Socioeconomic status encompasses a multiplicity of risk factors. Afro-Americans have lower-birth-weight infants, even after correction for socioeconomic factors.

Severe maternal undernutrition in wars and famines can predispose to substantial reductions in birth weight. This effect can be enhanced by low preconceptual maternal weight. Dietary supplementation under these circumstances increases birthweight. Marked maternal undernutrition is uncommon in industrialized societies. It usually accompanies maternal disorders such as eating disorders or gastrointestinal disease.

Oxygen deprivation such as associated with high-altitude living or maternal cardiorespiratory disease predisposes a fetus to reduced growth.

Chronic hypertension remains one of the most common problems associated with IUGR and preterm delivery. The antiphospholipid syndrome and connective tissue disease are associated with an increased risk of hypertension, vascular disease, and renal involvement, all of which predispose to IUGR. However, IUGR is also seen with subclinical disease, and is due to the effect of autoantibodies on the microvasculature of the uterus and placenta. These effects are mediated by changes in vascular prostacycline, a potent vasodilator, and thromboxane, a potent vasoconstrictor.

Table 5-1. Contributions of Various Influences on Fetal Growth

Factor	Percentage
Maternal genotype	20%
Fetal genotype	15%
Y chromosome	2%
Maternal environment	31%
Intrauterine environment	31%

Source: Adapted from ref. 68.

Table 5-2. Factors Associated with IUGR

Maternal
  Demographic: age, socioeconomic status, race, ethnic
  Constitutional: genetic, height, weight at birth, maternal
    weight prior to pregnancy
  Inadequate nutrition: dietary calories, oxygen
  Maternal disease: hypertension, autoimmune disease,
    anemia, chronic cardiopulmonary disease, chronic re-
    nal disease, diabetes, with vascular disease
  Addiction: smoking, alcohol, drug use
Uteroplacental
  Placental infarcts
  Placental mosaicism
  Uterine anomalies
  Multiple gestation
Fetal
  Constitutional: genetic, gender, fetal order
  Fetal aneuploidy/inherited syndromes
  Fetal infection
  Fetal anomaly: cardiovascular, single umbilical artery,
    twin-twin transfusion

The impact of toxic substances, such as cigarettes,[11–13] alcohol,[14,15] and drugs[13] on fetal growth are well established.

Primary placental disease may arise from inadequate or poor adaptation of the maternal microcirculation to the fetal villous proliferation and vice versa. Primary placental disease may also arise as a consequence of maternal disease such as connective tissue disease.

With increased utilization of chorionic villus sampling, the association of placental mosaicism and IUGR and perinatal loss has been recognized.[16–18] Kalousek and coworkers[19] have attempted to define three types of mosaicism based on villous cytotrophoblastic and/or mesenchymal cell mosaicism, and have attempted to further define fetal outcome based on these findings. Prognosis appears to be associated with fetal karyotype and the ratio of euploid to aneuploid cells in culture.

Multiple gestation is complicated by IUGR in 20–30% of cases. The onset and degree of growth failure is directly related to the number of fetuses. The decline in fetal weight increases in singleton and twin gestations occurs when the total fetal mass is 3000–3500 g.[20] In twins, the incremental weekly gain peaks between 28 and 32 weeks gestation. The decrease in weight in

twins is due to the inability of the environment to meet fetal needs. Monozygotic twins complicated by significant vascular anastomosis may reveal varying onset and severity of IUGR.

Fetal chromosome abnormality is commonly associated with IUGR. Examples include trisomy 13, 18, and 21, Turner's syndrome (45XO), sex chromosome trisomies (XXX, XYY, XXY), and segmental chromosome imbalances (4p— short arm, 18p, 18q). The latter abnormality usually predisposes to early IUGR. Other inherited syndromes may also be associated.

Fetal infection accounts for only 5% of human IUGR. The best known fetal infections are rubella and cytomegalovirus. Others, such as toxoplasmosis, syphilis, plasmodium, herpes, and varicella have also been reported.

A single umbilical artery can be associated with an increased risk of fetal malformations, aneuploidy, inherited syndromes, and IUGR.

DIAGNOSIS OF IUGR

Several important points need to be emphasized regarding diagnosis of IUGR. These include:

1. Early sound clinical dating serves as an important measure of subsequent growth.
2. One half of all pregnancies complicated by IUGR have no risk factors. Strategies for routine screening of this low-risk group need to be developed.
3. Any clinical and/or laboratory measure of fetal growth has its limitations.
4. More often a combination of clinical and laboratory assessments enhances diagnostic accuracy and outcome.
5. More efforts must be directed at prevention of IUGR.

Clinical

This primarily depends upon measurement of the symphysis-fundal height (SFH). Various charts[21–23] have been used in screening programs with varying degrees of success. Overall, the success with this measure indicates 60–85% sensitivity, 80–90% specificity, and a positive predictive rate of 20–80%. These statistics will vary depending upon the prevalence of IUGR within the population studied. Interestingly, in one of the studies,[23] no significant difference was observed between the SFH measurement (76%) and the fetal abdominal circumference measurement (83%) by ultrasound. This finding validates use of the SFH measurement in present obstetric practice.

The accepted deviations in SFH measurements vary dependent upon the author and/or charts utilized. Ideally, charts should be constructed for specific populations, and must be tested for performance and accuracy. Commonly accepted deviations of SFH measurements for IUGR include values reflecting less than 2 standard deviations (SD) and/or <10th percentile from the mean.

Ultrasound

Ultrasound fetal biometry, combined with placental and amniotic fluid assessment and use of Doppler ultrasound, has enabled more precise evaluation of fetal growth and well-being.

Ultrasound Biometry

Several biometric parameters have been described for the detection of IUGR. Table 5-3[24] compares the performance of these parameters.

From the table it should be apparent that the abdominal circumference measurement remains one of the most sensitive parameters for the detection of IUGR. It should be emphasized that

this sensitivity is maximal at the 34th week ± 1 week and decreases thereafter.

Estimated Fetal Weight

Several formulas for the estimation of fetal weight have been published and subsequently tested for accuracy.[30] One study[31] found accuracy in the estimation of the birth weight to be within 10% of the actual weight in 77.1% of a population of LBW infants (520–1500 g).

The ultrasound estimation of fetal weight and comparison to the normal expected percentiles is useful in the diagnosis of IUGR. Such estimation is, however, limited by the accuracy of fetal weight estimation (Table 5-4).

Biometric Ratios

Several ratios have been recommended for use in the diagnosis and classification of IUGR. Two commonly used ratios include the head circumference/abdominal circumference[32] and the abdominal circumference/femur length.[33] A potential advantage of these ratios is that they are gestational age dependent. However, the predictive value of these ratios is limited (Table 5-4).

It can be observed that the individual ultrasound parameters lack the degree of accuracy for either a screening program and/or diagnosis in cases clinically suspected for IUGR. The problem is accentuated in cases where the clinical dates are not known and/or where the weight of a growth-restricted fetus lies within the normal weight distribution percentile for the gestational age. However, these limitations are

Table 5-3. Specificity, Sensitivity, and Predictive Value of Various Ultrasound Biometric Variables

			Predictive Value	
	Sensitivity	Specificity	Positive	Negative
Biparietal diameter (BPD)[25,26]	45	74.5	23	81.5
Cephalic circumference (HC)	52	80	26	94.3
Cephalic area	60	80	23	95.2
Abdominal circumference (AC)[23,27,28]	83	87.7	43	97.8
Abdominal area	85	88	44	98.1
Femur length (FL)[29]	58	81	23.3	95

Adapted from ref. 69.

Table 5-4. Available Data on Sensitivity, Specificity, and Predictive Values of Various Ultrasound Biometric Parameters in the Prediction of IUGR

Parameter	Sensitivity	Specificity	PPV	NPV
Estimated weight[34]	87	87	78	92
HC/AC ratio[34]	36	90	67	72
FL/AC ratio[33]	60	90	—	—
Ponderal index[35]	77	82	—	—
Total intrauterine volume[36]	60	—	30	—
Amniotic fluid volume[34,37]	84	97	90	95
Thigh circumference[38]	78	—	85	—
Placental grading[39]	62	—	59	—

Abbreviations: AC, abdominal circumference; FL, femur length; HC, head circumference; NPV, negative predictive value; PPV positive predictive value.

overshadowed by the benefits of dynamic ultrasound scanning, including use of Doppler ultrasound, in the evaluation of fetal well-being and timing of delivery. This subject will be more fully discussed in the section "Management of IUGR," below.

Doppler Ultrasound

Disappointing results have been obtained by the use of Doppler ultrasound to either diagnose or predict the type of IUGR, since not all cases of IUGR are associated with placental insufficiency. Doppler has a lower sensitivity and predictive value than biometric data.[40]

Umbilical artery Doppler ultrasound has been shown to be superior to uterine artery Doppler in prediction. Doppler ultrasound may be useful in the clinical management of patients following biometric confirmation. Abnormal waveforms in the IUGR fetus are associated with increased perinatal risk.[41] Absent or reversed umbilical-arterial flow has been shown to have the greatest significance. Recently, attempts have been made to correlate Doppler ultrasound and other tests of fetal well-being with fetal acid-base status, through percutaneous umbilical cord sampling.[42] This study revealed increasing levels of fetal hypoxia/acidosis with worsening umbilical Doppler indices.

Doppler ultrasound abnormalities usually precede abnormalities in other biophysical parameters, and fetal death.

PREVENTION OF IUGR

In reviewing the etiologies of IUGR (Table 5-2), it becomes apparent that certain factors may be accessible to change. Early interventions addressing nutrition and lifestyle changes (smoking, alcohol, drugs) are important. In other cases, (autoantibodies, vascular problems) the problem may be more complex. Some attempts at enhancing nutritional (glucose, O_2) delivery to the fetus have had limited success.

Use of aspirin in prevention of IUGR has recently been shown to be ineffective in large randomized controlled studies.[42a] Magnesium therapy has been demonstrated to have some success (The Szegled Magnesium Study).[43]

MANAGEMENT OF IUGR

Following the diagnosis of IUGR, obstetric management will depend upon several factors. These factors include:

- Evaluation of etiology
- Maternal state
- The degree of IUGR

- Fetal well-being
- Timing and mode of delivery
- Availability of neonatal services
- Counseling regarding prevention

Evaluation of Etiology

This includes a complete history, examination, and specific laboratory testing. Frequently the clinical examination will yield no identifiable risk factors. Diagnostic studies should include detailed ultrasound examination, selective use of karyotype and drug screening, detection of autoantibodies, viral studies, and other targeted screening.

Maternal State

Maternal disease may be associated with and/or may necessitate delivery.

Degree of IUGR

Generally, IUGR of a moderate to severe degree at term ($\geq$37th week) is treated with delivery. This strategy was based upon the recognition of an increased risk of stillbirth in late pregnancy.

For the preterm fetus with IUGR, estimation of fetal size and maturity are important variables in survival. For the very-LBW (<750 g) growth-restricted fetus, measures utilizing maternal hyperoxygenation and glucose infusions may be considered.

Fetal Well-Being

Current recommendations for the evaluation of fetal well-being include serial fetal biometry, use of biophysical testing, and Doppler evaluation. In serial biometry, it is important to realize the standard error of sonographic measurements and utilize these at the approximate intervals (minimum 2 weeks). Arrested fetal growth would constitute an indication for delivery.

Biophysical testing may incorporate any of the current methods [nonstress test (NST), contraction stress test (CST), biophysical profile (BPP)].[44-46] The only caveats include frequency

of testing. The NST, and possibly the BPP, requires twice weekly testing. The CST may provide the earliest indication of fetal compromise. It does, however, carry other disadvantages such as a 25% incidence of equivocal tests, requiring retest in 24 hours. The BPP does have the advantage of combining several modalities in a single test [biometry, BPP, amniotic fluid volume (AVF) assessment].[47-48]

AFV assessment by single pocket size or the amniotic fluid index is very important in IUGR. Twice-weekly assessment of AFV is important, as decreases in AFV can be fairly rapid in onset. Oligohydramnios is an indication for delivery.[49-50]

Doppler assessment of the umbilical circulation and, more recently, the fetal circulation, is a useful adjunct in evaluating the degree of fetal compromise and in timing delivery.[51]

Timing and Mode of Delivery

The timing and mode of delivery will depend upon multiple factors. Reassuring tests of fetal well-being are associated with a low risk of stillbirth. The improved neonatal survival rates currently experienced should not lure clinicians to delivery. Appropriate biophysical testing and assessment of fetal maturity should remain primary factors in timing delivery.

Cesarean section delivery may be necessary for other maternal and/or fetal indications. There is an increased risk of meconium-stained amniotic fluid and abnormal fetal heart rate patterns in labor. Amnioinfusion may be a useful adjunct in management. Cesarean section delivery may be primarily indicated for absent or reversed umbilical arterial diastolic flow because of the high risk of abnormal fetal heart rate patterns and fetal hypoxia.

Availability of Neonatal Services

It is imperative that complete antenatal evaluation assess the available resources for care of the neonate. Transfer of high-risk mothers to appropriate facilities for delivery is important. Me-

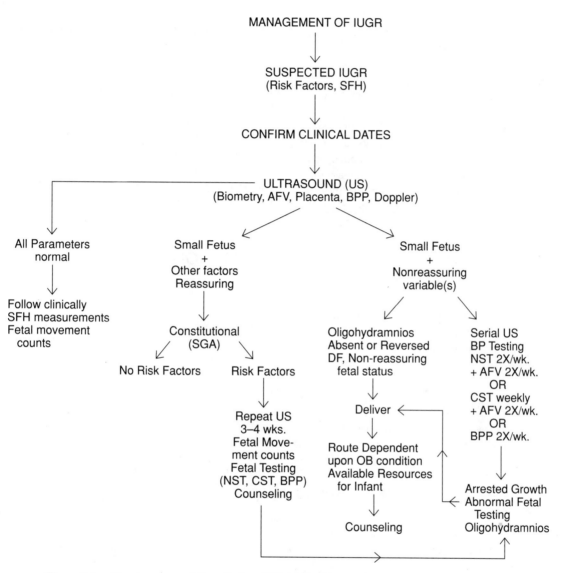

Figure 5-4. Absent or reversed diastolic flow (DF) implies increased impedance to placental flow. AFV = amniotic fluid volume; BPP = biophysical profile; CST = contraction stress test; NST = non-stress test; OB = obstetric; SFH = symphysis-fundal height; SGA = small for gestational age.

conium aspiration, respiratory distress, and hypoglycemia are frequent early complications.

Counseling Regarding Prevention

It is important after evaluation of the intra-partial situation and neonate that the patient be counseled about more specific etiology and future implications. Uterine exploration, neonatal examination, and placental examination may provide valuable insights into etiology.

The scheme outlined in Figure 5-4 summarizes obstetric management.

POSTNEONATAL SEQUELAE OF IUGR

Most studies evaluating outcome in SDF infants do so on the basis of birth weight.[3,5] For reasons cited above, this procedure results in confusing data on long-term outcome. Data sets must attempt to collect longitudinal information on normal newborns, and must also attempt to correct for the numerous factors affecting fetal and neonatal growth.

Birth weight fails to reflect nutritional status at birth.[52] Up to 40% of SFD infants are constitutionally small. The rest show evidence of restraint of intrauterine growth (i.e., they are thin). To facilitate the diagnosis of intrauterine malnutrition at birth, the Rohrer's ponderal index (PI) may be applied. The formula is:

$$I = \frac{Wt(g) \times 100}{[Length\ (cm)]^3}$$

This formula relates body weight to length and is independent of gestational age. Values below the third percentile embody 50% of all babies born as SFD.

Immediate Consequences

Early neonatal complications of IUGR include an increased risk of meconium aspiration, respiratory distress, hypoglycemia, and hyperviscosity due to polycythemia. Hypoglycemia[53] and hyperviscosity[54] can be associated with later problems.

Physical Development

Physical growth is influenced by genetic and environmental factors. While the velocity of growth may be similar in SFD and appropriate for gestational age (AGA) infants, postneonatal growth restriction is identified by many studies.[55,56]

Early (<6 months), rates of growth correlate to later growth and size. Catchup growth occurs primarily in infancy. The degree of growth restriction at birth is no indicator of subsequent size. Between 10 and 46% of infants remain subnormal.[57,58]

LBW AGA infants do better than LBW SGA infants.[59]

Psychomotor Development

Eventual prognosis is related to head circumference at birth[60] and its subsequent growth, and the presence of neurologic abnormality in the newborn period.[61]

The timing, severity, and duration of the insult correlates with neurologic outcome.[62]

Neurologic abnormalities that are described include perceptual problems, diminished IQ, changes in verbal expression, minimal brain dysfunction, and cerebral palsy.[63–66]

CONCLUSION

The identification of IUGR in patients at low risk remains a significant problem. Biochemical markers (elevated serum alpha-fetoprotein) and Doppler evaluation of the fetal-placental-uterine circulation may provide early clues as to the risk of the fetus for IUGR. These techniques are currently investigational.

Unfortunately, in most cases of IUGR specific therapy to prevent IUGR and/or enhance fetal growth is not available. The primary goal of early detection of IUGR is the evaluation of an etiology, and, in the timing of the delivery, the prevention of stillbirth.

Following the diagnosis of IUGR, ultrasound, biometry, amniotic fluid volume assessment, and Doppler velocimetry have proven to be invaluable tools in management. The relationship between the fetal circulation, fetal acid-base balance, and fetal biophysical parameters requires further study. Such inquiries will also permit more accurate noninvasive fetal assessment and will make available further help in the timing of delivery.

REFERENCES

1. Hepburn M, Rosenberg K. An audit of the detection and management of small for gestational age babies. *Br J Obstet Gynaecol* 1986;93:212–216.

2. World Health Organization. Aspects of LBW. *WHO Technical Report* 1961;217:3–16.

3. Lubchenko IO, Hansman C, Dressler M, et al. Intrauterine growth as estimated from liveborn birth weight at 24 to 42 weeks of gestation. *Pediatrics* 1963;32:793–800.

4. Weiner CP, Robinson D. The sonographic diagnosis of intrauterine growth retardation using the postnatal ponderal index and the crown-heel length as standards of diagnosis. *Am J Perinatol* 1989;6:380–383.

5. Battalgia FC, Lubchenko LO. A practical classification of newborn infants by weight and gestational age. *J Pediatr* 1967;71(2):159–163.

6. Gailbraith RS, Karchmar EJ, Pievey WN, et al. The clinical prediction of intrauterine growth retardation. *Am J Obstet Gynecol* 1979;133(3):281–286.

7. Manara LR. Intrapartum fetal morbidity and mortality in I.U.G.R. infants. *J Am Osteopathic Assoc* 1980;80(2):101–104.

8. Winick M. Cellular changes in placental and fetal growth. *Am J Obstet Gynecol* 1971;109(1):166–176.

9. Gruenwald P. Growth of the human fetus. *Am J Obstet Gynecol* 1962;94:1112–1119.

10. Gruenwald P. Chronic fetal distress and placental insufficiency. *Biol Neonate* 1963;5:215.

11. Butler NR, Alberman ED. *Second Report of British Perinatal Problems*. Edinburgh: Churchill-Livingstone, 1969.

12. Goldstein H. Smoking and pregnancy. *Nature* 1973;245:277–283.

13. Naeye RL, Blanc W, Leblanc W, et al. Fetal complications of maternal heroin addiction: Abnormal growth infections, and episodes of stress. *J Pediatr* 1973;83:1055–1061.

14. Ulleland CN. The offspring of alcoholic mothers. *Ann NY Acad Sci* 1972;197:67–69.

15. Palmer RH, Oullette EM, Warner I, et al. Congenital malformations in offspring of chronic alcoholic mothers. *Pediatrics* 1974;53:490–496.

16. Kalousek DK, Howard-Pecbles PN, Olson SB, et al. Conformation of CVS mosaicism in terms of placenta and high frequency of I.U.G.R. associated with confined placental mosaicism. *Prenat Diag* 1991;11:743–750.

17. Verp MS, Unger NL. Placental chromosome abnormalities and I.U.G.R. in proceedings of the 35th annual meeting of the S.G.I. Baltimore, March 17–20, 1988, p. 143.

18. Holzgneve B, Exelor R, Holzgneve W, et al. Nonviable trisomies confined to the placenta leading to poor pregnancy outcome. *Prenat Diagn* 1992;12:(Suppl.) S95.

19. Kalousek DK, Barret I, McGuilliuray BC. Placental mosaicism and intrauterine survival for trisomies 13 and 18. *Am J Hum Genet* 1989;44:338–343.

20. Williams RL, Creasy RK, Cunningham GC, et al. Fetal growth and perinatal viability in California. *Obstet Gynecol* 1982;59(5):624–632.

21. Westin B. Gravidogram and poor intrauterine fetal growth. In Salvadori B, Bacchi-Modena A (eds), *Poor Intrauterine Fetal Growth*. Parma, Italy: Minerva Medica, 1977, pp. 44–47.

22. Effer SB. Management of high risk pregnancy: Report of a combined obstetrical and neonatal intensive care unit. *Can Med Assoc J* 1969;101:389–404.

23. Campbell S, Soothill P. Detection and management of IUGR. A British approach. In Chervenak FA, Isaacson J, Campbell S (eds), *Ultrasound in Obstetrics and Gynecology*. London: Little Brown, 1993, p. 1431.

24. Carrera JM, Mallafre J. Intrauterine growth retardation. In Kurjak A, Chervenak FA (eds), *The Fetus as a Patient*. New York: Parthenon, 1994, pp. 251–287.

25. Seeds JW. Impaired fetal growth: Ultrasonic evaluation and clinical management. *Obstet Gynecol* 1984;63:577–582.

26. Sabbagha R, Hughey M, Depp R. Growth adjusted sonographic age. A simplified method. *Obstet Gynecol* 1978;51:383–386.

27. Campbell S, Wilkin P. Ultrasonic measurement of fetal abdominal circumference in the estimation of fetal weight. *Br J Obstet Gynaecol* 1975;82:689–697.

28. Wittman BK, Robinson HP, Aitchison T, et al. The value of diagnostic ultrasound as a screening test for intrauterine growth retardation. Comparison of 9 parameters. *Am J Obstet Gynecol* 1979;134:30–35.

29. O'Brien G, Queenan JJ. Growth of the ultrasound fetal femur length during normal pregnancy. *Am J Obstet Gynecol* 1981;141:833–837.

30. Deter RL, Hadlock FP, Harrist RB, et al. Evaluation of 3 methods of obtaining fetal weight estimates using dynamic image ultrasound. *J Clin Ultrasound* 1981;9(8):421–425.

31. Warsof SL, Gohari P, Berkowitz RL, et al. The estimation of fetal weight by computer-assisted analysis. *Am J Obstet Gynecol* 1977;128(8):881–892.

32. Campbell S, Thoms A. Ultrasound measurement of the fetal head to abdomen circumference ratio in the assessment of growth retardation. *Br J Obstet Gynaecol* 1977;84(3):165–174.

33. Hadlock FP, Deter RL, Harrist RB, et al. A date independent predictor of intrauterine growth retardation: FL/AC ratio. *Am J Roentogenol* 1983;141:979–984.

34. Divon MY, Guidetti DA, Brauerman JJ, et al. Intrauterine growth retardation—a prospective study of the diagnostic value of realtime sonography combined with umbilical artery flow velocimetry. *Obstet Gynecol* 1988;72(4):611–614.

35. Vintzileos AM, Lodeiro JG, Feinstein SJ, et al. Value of fetal ponderal index in predicting fetal growth retardation. *Obstet Gynecol* 1986;67(4):584–588.

36. Giersson RT, Patel NB, Christie AD. Intrauterine volume, fetal abdominal area and BPD measurements with ultrasound in the prediction of small for dates babies in a high-risk obstetric population. *Br J Obstet Gynaecol* 1985;92:936–940.

37. Chamberlain PF, Manning FA, Morrison I, et al. Ultrasound evaluation of AF, Volume 1. The relationship of marginal and decreased AF volumes to perinatal outcomes. *Am J Obstet Gynecol* 1984;150(3):245–249.

38. Hill LM, Guzick D, Thomas ML, et al. Thigh circumference in the detection of IUGR. *Am J Perinatol* 1989;6(3):349–352.

39. Kazzi GM, Gross TL, Sokol RJ, et al. Detection of IUGR. A new use of placental sonographic grading. *Am J Obstet Gynecol* 1983;145:733–737.

40. Ng A, Trudinger B. The application of umbilical artery studies to complicated pregnancies. In Malcolm Pearce J (ed), *Doppler US in Perinatal Medicine*. Oxford: Oxford University Press, 1992, pp. 142–158.

41. Lowery CL, Henso B, Wan I, et al. A comparison between umbilical velocimetry and standard antepartum surveillance in hospitalized high-risk patients. *Am J Obstet Gynecol* 1990;162:710–714.

42. Pardi G, Cetin I, Marconi AM, et al. Diagnostic value of blood sampling in fetuses with growth retardation. *N Engl J Med* 1993;328:601–602.

42a. CLASP (Collaborative Low Dose Aspirin Study in Pregnancy). Collaborative Group. *Lancet* 1994;343:619–629.

43. Kovacs L, Bodis L, Szabo J. Magnesium Substitution Wahrend der Schwangerschaft "Szededer Magnesium Studie." In Weidinger H (ed), *Magnesium in der Frauenheil Kunde*. Munich: Munchner Wissenschaftsliche Publikationen, 1985, p. 110.

44. Eden R, Seifert L, Kodack L, et al. A modified biophysical profile for antenatal surveillance. *Obstet Gynecol* 1988;71:365–369.

45. Freeman R, Anderson G, Dorchester W. A prospective multi-institutional study of antepartum fetal heart rate monitoring I. The risk of perinatal morbidity and mortality according to antepartum heart rate test results. *Am J Obstet Gynecol* 1982;143(7):771–777.

46. Freeman R, Anderson G, Dorchester W. A prospective multi-institutional study of antepartum fetal heart rate monitoring II. Contraction stress test versus non-stress test for primary fetal surveillance. *Am J Obstet Gynecol* 1982;143(7):278–281.

47. Manning F, Morrison I, Lange I, et al. Fetal assessment based on fetal biophysical scoring: Experience in 12,620 high-risk pregnancies. 1. Perinatal mortality by frequency and etiology. *Am J Obstet Gynecol* 1985;151(3):343–350.

48. Manning F, Morrison I, Lange I, et al. Fetal biophysical profile score and the non-stress test. A comparable trial. *Obstet Gynecol* 1984;64(3):326–331.

49. Chamberlain PF, Manning FA, Morrison I, et al. Ultrasound evaluation of amniotic fluid. The relationship of marginal and decreased amniotic fluid volumes to perinatal outcome. *Am J Obstet Gynecol* 1984;150:245–249.

50. Rutherford S, Smith C, Phelan J, et al. Four quadrant assessment of amniotic fluid volume. *J Reprod Med* 1987;32:587–589.

51. Neilson JP. Doppler ultrasound study of umbilical artery waveforms in high risk pregnancy. In Chalmers I (ed), *Oxford Database of Perinatal Trials*. New York: Oxford University Press, Version 1.3. Disk issue 7, 1992, Record 3889.

52. Wacether FJ, Remaekers, LHJ. Neonatal morbidity in SGA infants in relationship to their nutritional status at birth. *Acta Paediatr Scand* 1983;72(3):437–440.

53. Koivisto MM, Blanco-Sequeiros M, Krause U. Neonatal symptomatic and asymptomatic hypoglycemia: A follow-up study of 151 infants. *Dev Med Child Neurol* 1972;14(5):603–614.

54. Black VD, Lubchendo LO, Luckey DW, et al. Developmental and neurological sequelae of neonatal hyperviscosity syndrome. *Pediatrics* 1982;69(4):426–431.

55. Fitzhardinge PM, Steven EM. The SFD infant. 1. Later growth patterns. *Pediatrics* 1972;49(5):671–681.

56. Westwood M, Kramer MS, Munz D, et al. Growth and development of full-term nonasphyxiated small-for-gestational-age newborns: Follow-up through adolescence. *Pediatrics* 1983;71(3):376–382.

57. Dunsted M, Moar V, Scott A. Growth in the first four years II. Diversity within small for dates and large for dates babies. *Early Hum Dev* 1982;7(1):29–39.

58. Hack M, Merkatz IR, McGarth SK, et al. Catch up growth in very LBW infants. *Am J Dis Child* 1984;138(4):370–375.

59. Lubchenko LO. Assessment of gestational age and development at birth. *Pediatr Clin North Am* 1970;17(1):125–145.

60. Davies H, Kirman BH. Microcephaly. *Arch Dis Child* 1962;37:623.

61. Nelson KB, Ellenberg JH. Neonatal signs as a predictor of cerebral palsy. *Pediatrics* 1979; 64(2):225–232.

62. Beargie RA, Vernon LJ, Green JW. Growth and development of SFD newborns. *Pediatr Clin North Am* 1970;17(1):159–167.

63. Rubin PA, Rosenblatt C, Balou B. Psychological and educational sequelae of prematurity. *Pediatrics* 1973;52(3):352–363.

64. Villar J, Smeriglio V, Martorell R, et al. Heterogeneous growth and mental development of intrauterine growth retarded infants during the 1st three years of life. *Pediatrics* 1984;74(5):783–791.

65. Eaves LC, Nuttal JC, Klonoff H, et al. Development and psychological test scores in children of low birth weight. *Pediatrics* 1970;45(5):886–887.

66. Commey JO, Fitzhardinge PM. Handicap in the preterm small for gestational age infants. *J Pediatr* 1979;94(5):779–786.

67. Vorherr H. Factors influencing fetal growth. *Am J Obstet Gynecol* 1982;142:577.

68. Reece EA, Hobbins JC, Mahoney MJ, et al. (eds). *Medicine of the Fetus and Mother*. Philadelphia: Lippincott, 1992, p. 673.

69. Kuriak A, Chervenak FA (eds). *The Fetus as a Patient*. New York: Parthenon, 1994, p. 262.

QUESTIONS
(choose the most appropriate answers to the following questions)

1. Current clinical screening policies allow for what percentage of detection of IUGR?
   a. 100%.
   b. 50%.
   c. 25%.
   d. 5%.

2. Late (32–34 weeks) screening with ultrasound is superior to clinical (SFH) methods in the detection of IUGR.
   a. True.
   b. False.

3. Maternal exercise is known to increase the risk for IUGR.
   a. True.
   b. False.

4. Early (<24 weeks) IUGR is usually due to poor nutrition.
   a. True.
   b. False.

5. The following may be associated with IUGR, except:
   a. Chronic hypertension.
   b. Maternal exercise.
   c. Living at high altitudes.
   d. Fetal malformations.

6. The following conditions in IUGR pregnancies are usually indications for delivery, except:
   a. Oligohydramnios.
   b. Positive contraction stress test (CST).
   c. Abnormal umbilical Doppler velocimetry.

6

Antepartum and Intrapartum Fetal Infection

Michael A. Krew
Prabhcharan Gill

INTRODUCTION

Maternal infection frequently confronts the perinatologist. Viral or parasitic infection may complicate 5–15% of pregnancies but cause congenital defects in only 1–2% of exposed fetuses. Group B streptococcal (GBS) vaginal colonization is present in up to 40% of screened women but 1% of exposed neonates develop early-onset GBS sepsis.[1] TORCH is an acronym that has traditionally stood for Toxoplasmosis, Other (including syphilis), Rubella, Cytomegalovirus (CMV), and Herpes simplex virus (HSV) but which of late has become synonymous with these and many other agents responsible for perinatal infection. This chapter will provide an overview of the fetal effects of maternal infection as summarized in Table 6-1.

The perinatologist will most likely be involved in the diagnosis of intrauterine infection in the following settings: (1) prenatal ultrasound findings associated with intrauterine infection are noted such as nonimmune hydrops, fetal calcifications, echogenic bowel, or severe early growth retardation; (2) maternal counseling is requested after infection or exposure to agents such as varicella, parvovirus B19, or rubella that affect the fetus; (3) routine maternal screening

by history, serology, or culture may indicate or identify agents known to cause intrauterine infection such as human immunodeficiency virus (HIV) or syphilis or reveals agents that are transmitted to the neonate in the peripartum period such as GBS or genital herpes.

Diagnosis of infection after fetal anomalies have been detected will provide parents information about recurrence risk, may allow the option of pregnancy termination, and will occasionally prevent further fetal damage with initiation of treatment. Preventive strategies hold more promise but screening programs need to be carried out with well-established methods in order to avoid unnecessary parental anxiety and potential fetal harm arising out of unnecessary invasive testing or ill-advised termination of pregnancy.

TOXOPLASMOSIS

Toxoplasma gondi is an intracellular protozoan parasite which can infect many birds and mammals but for which the cat is the only known definitive host. Transmission to humans occurs by ingestion of oocyst-contaminated food or water or consumption of undercooked meat or eggs of infected animals. Infection also occurs

Table 6-1. Summary of Antepartum and Intrapartum Fetal Infection

Agent	Diagnosis		Treatment	
	Maternal	Fetal	Maternal	Fetal
Toxoplasmosis	Serology	Amniotic fluid PCR		Spiramycin, pyrimethamine, sulfadiazine
Syphilis	Dark-field microscopy, serology	Ultrasound?	Penicillin (desensitize if allergic)	Penicillin (desensitize if allergic)
Rubella	Clinical serology	Ultrasound?	Vaccinate postpartum if seronegative	None
CMV	Serology	Amniotic fluid culture, ultrasound	None	None
Genital herpes	Culture of lesions		?Acyclovir	Delivery by C-section when maternal lesions present
Parvovirus B19	Serology	MSAFP, ultrasound	None	Intrauterine transfusion
Varicella zoster	Clinical	Ultrasound?	Acyclovir for varicella pneumonia	Neonatal IgG and vaccination as indicated
HIV	Serology	Invasive procedures could increase risk of fetal infection	AZT and PCP prophylaxis as needed	AZT
Group B streptococcus	Selective medium rectovaginal cultures at 36 weeks		Only needed antepartum for UTI	Penicillin during labor
Listeria monocytogenes	Blood cultures	Amniotic fluid culture	Ampicillin	Ampicillin and gentamycin
Plasmodium falciparum	Blood smear	Placental pathology	Chloroquine unless CDC recommends alternative	Chloroquine unless CDC recommends alternative
Mycobacterium tuberculosis	Chest x ray and culture sputum		Isoniazid and ethambutol and rifampin unless CDC recommends alternative	Isoniazid prophylaxis or full treatment as indicated
Boriellia burgdorferi	Clinical, serology	Ultrasound?	Penicillin or erythromycin	Penicillin or erythromycin

Abbreviations: AZT, zidovudine; CDC, Centers for Disease Control; C-section, cesarean section; IgG, immunoglobulin G; MSAFP, maternal serum alpha-fetoprotein; PCP, pneumocystis carinii pneumonia; UTI, urinary tract infection.

transplacentally. Adult infection is generally asymptomatic or produces only mild nonspecific symptoms. The classic triad of congenital infection is hydrocephalus, intracranial calcifications, and chorioretinitis. Effects may also include hydrops and fetal demise. Congenital infection may have mild or no symptoms at birth but may progress to neurologic injury, blindness, or death unless treated.

Maternal infection prior to pregnancy almost never results in fetal infection. An important exception to this rule is the immunocompromised HIV patient in whom reactivation of old infection has been reported to cause severe fetal infection. In general, the earlier in pregnancy toxoplasmosis is acquired, the more severe the effects of fetal infection. The likelihood of fetal infection; however, increases with gestational age.[2] When maternal infection is suspected, serial serology may be confirmatory but specific immunoglobulin M (IgM) toxoplasma antibodies may persist for years though usually not in high titer. The presence of specific immunoglobulin A (IgA) and immunoglobulin E (IgE) is more suggestive of recent infection. Maternal infection does not always result in fetal infection. Polymerase chain reaction (PCR) analysis of amniotic fluid for toxoplasma deoxyribonucleic acid (DNA) is replacing umbilical blood sampling for the diagnosis of fetal infection.[3]

If fetal infection is confirmed, the severity cannot be predicted in all cases. The sonographic findings of ventriculomegaly, central nervous system (CNS) and hepatic calcifications, thickened placenta, or hydrops suggest a poor outcome but the absence of these signs does not exclude significant sequelae including massive cerebral necrosis.[4] When acute maternal infection is suspected, use of the macrolide antibiotic spiramycin will reduce the risk of fetal infection but alone is not effective against established fetal infection. If PCR or umbilical blood testing confirms fetal infection then a combination of pyrimethamine and sulfadiazine with leucovorin appears to significantly improve newborn outcome. Other antibiotics including clindamycin, azithromycin, clarithromycin, atovaquone, and trimethoprin sulfamethoxazole are being evaluated in adult infection but experience for use for fetuses and newborns is lacking.[5]

Unlike the current policy in France, screening for toxoplasmosis infection during pregnancy is not organized and is somewhat controversial in the United States. It is carried out by some practitioners. It is important to use a laboratory experienced with the diagnosis of toxoplasmosis when evaluating a positive screening test. In our practice we have found the Research Institute of the Palo Alto (CA) Medical Foundation to be a useful resource. It is not controversial to advise pregnant women to avoid eating raw or undercooked meat, avoid cat feces, and practice good hand washing after contact with raw meat or garden soil.

SYPHILIS

The incidence of congenital syphilis increased by over 10-fold from 1983 to 1991 (110 cases per 100,000 live births). Reasons for this rise include the trading of sex for crack cocaine, increasing numbers of women with no or little prenatal care, and revised reporting guidelines introduced in 1989. By 1994 the incidence had fallen 50% from its peak but still represents a major public health problem.[6] Fetal infection can result in hydrops, fetal death, growth retardation, a neonate with early congenital syphilis, or an asymptomatic neonate that if untreated will go on to develop late congenital disease. Early congenital infection may be characterized by mucocutaneous rash, hepatospenomegaly, snuffles (rhinitis), or hydrops. Late disease may result in Hutchinson's triad (notched central incisors, interstitial keratitis of the eye, and eighth nerve deafness), bone deformities ("saber shins" and "saddle nose"), as well as neurosyphilis. Maternal primary syphilis is much more likely to result in fetal infection than secondary or latent syphilis. Fetal infection with spirochetes has been demonstrated as early as 6 weeks gestation but fetal manifestations do not become apparent until 16–18 weeks when the fetus is capable of mounting an immune response.

All pregnant women should undergo screening for syphilis in early pregnancy. Women with high-risk behavior or who live in a community with a high prevalence should undergo screening again in the late third trimester and again at delivery. Diagnosis of infection is made by a positive screening nontreponemal test, Venereal Disease Research Laboratory (VDRL) or rapid plasma reagin (RPR) tests, confirmed by a treponema-specific test which include the *Treponema pallidum* immobilization (TPI), fluorescent treponemal antibody absorption (FTA-ABS) or microhemagglutination test (MHA-TP). A lesion suspected of being a chancre should have fluid expressed for examination under a dark-field microscope or more conveniently a direct fluorescent antibody *T. pallidum* (DFA-TP) test of a fixed smear or the lesion can be performed. Serology may be negative in early primary syphilis but will be positive by 4 weeks. A false-positive nontreponemal test will always be of low titer. Treatment of syphilis in pregnancy is with penicillin as outlined by the CDC for non-pregnant patients of a given stage.[7] HIV testing should be carried out on all patients diagnosed with syphilis.

Special considerations exist for the pregnant patient. Penicillin is the only antibiotic demonstrated to be effective in treating the fetus for syphilis. Pregnant women who are penicillin allergic should undergo a desensitization protocol in the hospital as referenced.[8] A treated pregnant woman should be monitored with a monthly VDRL or RPR to demonstrate adequate treatment by at least a fourfold fall in titer. A rising titer requires retreatment. Any patient with positive serology should be treated unless previous treatment and appropriate decline of antibody titers have been unequivocally documented. Women treated after fetal viability are at risk of premature labor or fetal distress if treatment causes a Jarisch-Herxheimer reaction. They should be cautioned to report contractions or decreased fetal movement. Stillbirth has also been reported and so antenatal testing for fetal well-being can be considered; however, treatment should not be delayed.

RUBELLA

Congenital rubella syndrome (CRS) is the result of maternal infection during the first 20 weeks of pregnancy. The risk of severe fetal damage is as high as 90% with maternal infection in the first trimester and rapidly decreases with advancing gestational age. Manifestations include intrauterine growth retardation, congenital heart disease, cataracts, deafness, microcephaly, and mental retardation. Effects may not all be apparent at birth. Since the introduction of a live attenuated rubella vaccine in 1969, maternal infection and CRS have been rare and until recently appeared to be on the verge of elimination. Cluster outbreaks still occur and appear to be a result of inadequate vaccination rates of socioeconomically disadvantaged and immigrant populations.[9]

When suspected, paired maternal acute and convalescent serology can confirm infection. Presence of rubella IgM usually indicates recent infection. Because of the relative rarity of infection it is important to obtain testing from an experienced reference laboratory. Amniocentesis and umbilical blood sampling do not appear to be useful in determining the extent of fetal infection although manifestations of CRS may be detectable by sonography at an advanced gestational age. Postexposure use of immune globulin does not appear to be useful.

Vaccination with rubella vaccine within 3 months of conception or during pregnancy is contraindicated as it is a live virus which in theory could cause CRS. In actual practice no case of CRS has been reported due to the vaccine despite more than one thousand reported periconceptual vaccinations. Thus the risk should be considered very low when counseling a pregnant patient who has been inadvertently vaccinated.[10]

CYTOMEGALOVIRUS

Cytomegalovirus (CMV) virus is a DNA herpesvirus. Up to 60% of all pregnant women can be expected to have serologic evidence of a prior infection depending on the socioeconomic status of the population, and approximately 3% will be actively shedding the virus in cervical secretions. CMV is the most common congenital viral infection in the United States with an estimated 0.2–2.2% of all live infants acquiring the virus perinatally.[11] Only 1 of 10 such infants will have clinically obvious neonatal disease and the remaining infants will be asymptomatic. Any particular maternal episode of CMV infection may be a primary infection or a reactivation of a prior infection. Approximately half of all the infected infants occur as a result of reactivation of maternal disease. Early severe neonatal disease is associated with primary CMV maternal infections when the overall risk for an infected infant may be as high as 40%, whereas reactivation maternal illness places the infant at an 8% risk for milder long-term sequelae, principally deafness.[12,13] Currently there is no effective strategy that can minimize this risk. Women of childbearing age who work in day care settings, neonatal, and dialysis units can be exposed to CMV, however, they should be counseled about the relatively low risk of fetal exposure to CMV.[14] Whereas negative serology excludes fetal infection, a positive maternal serology is clinically less helpful, although evidence of primary infection increases the risks for early neonatal disease. Paired-interval (3 weeks) IgG serology showing a fourfold rise suggests an active maternal infection but it does not distinguish between primary versus reactivation of a prior infection. From the perspective of acquiring intrauterine fetal infection, the occurrence of any maternal disease opens the possibility of congenital infection. Unfortunately no test can exclude fetal infection although some findings such as amniotic fluid positive for CMV (detection by virus culture or PCR, DNA-based test) raise a strong possibility of fetal CMV infection. Furthermore, the tests are uninformative with regard to predicting the severity of neonatal disease should it occur. No maternal-fetal treatment is known to alter the clinical course of the illness. Ultrasound findings of fetal CMV infection are nonspecific and include intrauterine fetal growth restriction, intracerebral calcifications, cerebral ventriculomegaly, microcephaly, hepatic calcifications, and fetal hydrops. In summary, CMV fetal infection can cause significant short- and long-term neonatal morbidity but its prenatal diagnosis with certainty remains elusive.

HERPES SIMPLEX VIRUS

Transplacental congenital infection with herpes simplex virus (HSV) is probably a rare event but has been documented in a few cases.[15] Adult HSV-1 infections are usually found in the oral region and HSV-2 is usually a genital infection although either type can cause infection at either site. Neonatal infection is usually acquired by delivery through an infected cervix or by ascending infection though ruptured membranes. Neonates with disseminated HSV have up to a 50% mortality and 50% of survivors have serious sequelae including seizures, mental retardation, and blindness. If an active primary genital infection is present at the time of delivery the risk of infection may be up to 40% but the risk with recurrent infection may be less than 5%. Maternal antibodies are probably not completely protective. More than half of mothers giving birth to an infected infant have asymptomatic infections and 10% of neonatal infections occur after cesarean delivery with intact membranes.

Routine surveillance cultures of women with a genital HSV infection history are no longer recommended. Amniocentesis and umbilical blood sampling do not appear to have a role. Cultures should be done only to confirm the diagnosis when a suspected HSV lesion is present. Vaginal delivery is considered safe if no lesions or prodromal symptoms are present at the start of labor. HSV culture of asymptomatic women allowed to have a vaginal delivery can be considered. Cesarean section should be route of delivery if active lesions are present and membranes have ruptured regardless of the duration of rupture.[17] The role of the antiviral agent acyclovir is uncertain and it is not routinely used to suppress recurrent lesions near term. As fetal risk from the drug is probably small it should not be withheld for severe maternal disease.[18]

Management of preterm rupture of membranes complicated by HSV genital lesions requires the balancing of the risks of prematurity versus those of intrauterine HSV infection. One reported series of 18 such patients presenting at less than 32 weeks gestation managed expectantly resulted in none of the 18 infants developing neonatal HSV.[19] Antepartum use of acyclovir should be considered in this setting.

PARVOVIRUS B19

Human parvovirus B19 causes erythema infectiosum (fifth disease) which in otherwise healthy children results in a mild illness characterized by a mild constitutional illness followed by a "slapped cheek" rash. An erythematous maculopapular rash then appears on the trunk and extremities. The child is not contagious after the rash appears. In adults the most common symptoms include a reticular trunk rash and arthropathy, especially in the hands. Asymptomatic infection is frequent and 30–60% of young adults show immunity. Infection of a patient with a preexisting chronic hemolytic anemia can lead to aplastic crisis.

Infection acquired during pregnancy may be transmitted to the fetus and cause fetal hydrops and demise. The hydrops is most likely due to bone marrow failure and anemia but direct myocardial toxicity has been proposed as a mechanism. Despite early reports to the contrary the risk of adverse pregnancy outcome after a pregnant woman is exposed to parvovirus B19 is probably small (1–3%).[20] The virus does not appear to increase the risk of anomalies. If maternal exposure is suspected, testing for parvovirus B19 IgG and IgM should be offered. Presence of IgG indicates immunity and therefore no further follow-up is needed. A positive IgM indicates acute infection.[21]

If acute maternal infection is suspected then serial ultrasound evaluations for fetal hydrops are indicated. Maternal serum alpha-fetoprotein levels may increase prior to the onset of hydrops. Intrauterine blood transfusion has been reported as a method of fetal salvage when hydrops is present but spontaneous resolution has been reported.[22,23] Parvovirus B19 infection should be considered in the workup of nonimmune fetal hydrops.

VARICELLA

Varicella-Zoster virus (VZV) can cause varicella (chickenpox) or Herpes zoster (shingles). The maternal incubation period is 11–21 days and the rash usually lasts 7–10 days. Whereas an isolated episode of shingles carries no risk to the fetus, maternal varicella carries substantial maternal and fetal risks. In the United States, the seroconversion rate is as high as 95%, however, the serologic antenatal testing to describe maternal vulnerability may be helpful in timely institution of preventive measures as well as prompting postpartum vaccination. Maternal complications are more apt to occur in adults, with varicella pneumonia occurring in 14% of the infected gravida. The risk for fetal embryopathy has been estimated at 2% when the maternal varicella occurs before 20 weeks gestation.[24] The miscarriage rates are unaltered but the overall prematurity risk is increased. Fetal embryopathy has a very broad spectrum and includes denuded skin, cutaneous scars, rudimentary digits, limb hypoplasia, muscle atrophy, microcephaly, intracranial calcifications, cortical atrophy, cataracts, chorioretinitis, microphthalmia, and psychomotor retardation. The ultrasound-detectable abnormalities appear approximately 5–19 weeks after the onset of the rash and include deformities of the hands and feet, hepatic calcifications, hydrocephalous, fetal hydrops, along with polyhydramnios which is the most common manifestation.[25] Infants with varicella embryopathy are not infectious at birth but may develop herpes zoster later in life.

Reliable detection of fetal disease is presently not possible, although innovative approaches have been reported in case reports. Worthy of note is the lack of diagnostic value of chorionic villus biopsy as positive varicella-zoster virus (VZV). DNA detection using PCR does not reliably denote fetal infection.[26] Suspicion of fetal infection may be strengthened by recovering the virus from the amniotic fluid or by the presence of VZV-specific IgM in fetal blood. Maternal administration of immunoglobulin or acyclovir has not been shown to minimize the risk for fetal infection or alter its course. Neonatal disease can occur when maternal varicella occurs in the peripartum period (within 5 days prior to delivery and 2 days postpartum), and this vulnerability is based on the risk of acquiring the virus without the benefit of sufficient transplacental acquisition of maternal immunoglobulins. These infants should receive varicella immunoglobulin and be isolated from their mothers until maternal lesions have crusted. Varicella is one of the most contagious agents in humans.

HUMAN IMMUNODEFICIENCY VIRUS

Human immunodeficiency virus (HIV) infection is the fourth leading cause of death in women of reproductive age and carries a substantial risk for vertical transmission of the virus.[27] The virus does not cause anomalies or miscarriages and the manifestations of the fetal illness begin after birth once transplacentally acquired natural immunity deteriorates. Detection of maternal infection is accomplished by the universal offering of HIV testing. Mothers that have HIV infection need to receive appropriate vaccinations and rigorous baseline screens for infections. In the interest of optimizing maternal health, those that have CD4 counts below 500 μ/L are considered for antiretroviral agent treatment and those with CD counts of below 200 μ/L are at exaggerated risk for *Pneumocystis carinii* pneumonia and should receive prophylaxis in addition to the antiretroviral treatment. Neither maternal viral load, antibody titers, nor viral phenotype appears to affect the risk of fetal transmission.[28]

The use of zidovudine (AZT) for all HIV-infected women during pregnancy has been demonstrated to substantially reduce (from 25.5 to 8.3%) the perinatal transmission risk.[29] At 14 weeks of gestation all HIV-infected women should therefore be offered zidovudine (oral 100 mg five times a day) and during labor a loading dose (2 mg/kg/hr) is followed by a maintenance dose (1 mg/kg/hr) until delivery; infants also receive oral AZT syrup (2 mg/kg four times a day) for 6 weeks.[30] The mother needs to understand that the efficacy has been only shown in those women who started the treatment before 34 weeks. Close maternal surveillance with complete blood count (CBC) (every 2 weeks, twice;

and then monthly), transaminases (each month), and creatinine (each month) is necessary to detect adverse drug reactions. Intrapartum fetal infection can be minimized by avoidance of invasive monitoring and personnel precautions must be exercised. Breast feeding is not recommended and a pediatric HIV specialist should be involved.

GROUP B STREPTOCOCCUS

GBS perinatal infection remains a clinical challenge as it has emerged as the major infectious cause of neonatal morbidity and mortality and a significant cause of chorioamnionitis, endomyometritis, urinary tract infection, and wound infection. Neonatal infection has a bimodal distribution of incidence with 60–80% of cases, early onset, occurring within 24 hours of birth. Late-onset disease occurs after the first week of life. Early-onset disease is most likely due to vertical transmission during labor and its incidence is increased in cases with prematurity, prolonged rupture of membranes, maternal fever, or a history of a previously infected neonate.[31]

Selective media cultures are sensitive for GBS but slow. Currently available rapid detection techniques are fast but relatively insensitive. Maternal cultures obtained remote from term do not have adequate predictive value of maternal anovaginal carriage at term. Intrapartum treatment of GBS-colonized women with antibiotics will greatly decrease the risk of their newborns acquiring early onset disease.[32] Several strategies have been developed to determine who should receive intrapartum antibiotics. Decision analysis suggests that intrapartum antibiotics given to all women in premature labor and to all in whom anovaginal carriage has been determined by culture within 1 month of term may prevent 86% of early-onset GBS disease but expose 27% of laboring women and their fetuses to antibiotics. Universal intrapartum antibiotic administration would prevent 94% of cases. Antibiotic use based on risk factors alone would prevent 69% of cases by treating 18% of deliveries.[33]

A consensus conference which included representatives of the CDC, The American College of Obstetricians and Gynecologists, and the American Academy of Pediatrics has endorsed anogenital culture with selective media at 35–37 weeks gestation and intrapartum antibiotics of all GBS carriers.[34] If culture status is not known at the time of labor antibiotics should be given if either prematurity, maternal fever or prolonged membrane rupture is present. Treatment of GBS carriers prior to labor is not recommended; however, women with GBS bacteriuria are usually heavily colonized and should be treated at the time of diagnosis and again in labor. A patient with a previous neonate with GBS disease should receive antibiotics regardless of culture status. Treatment based on risk factors alone was also declared to be an acceptable strategy.

Because of its narrow spectrum, the preferred antibiotic for intrapartum prophylaxis is intravenous penicillin G with an initial dose of 5 million units followed by 2.5 million units every 4 hours until delivery. Ampicillin is also acceptable. Clindamycin or erythromycin can be used for the penicillin-allergic patient. A fast, sensitive intrapartum screening test for GBS carriage is not as yet available but should one be developed the prevention of early-onset GBS disease will be greatly simplified.

LISTERIA MONOCYTOGENES

Listeria monocytogenes is a small, aerobic, non-spore-forming, gram-positive rod that is β-hemolytic on blood agar. It has been recognized as a cause of human disease since 1929 and 50% of reported cases are currently maternal or neonatal. Maternal listeria infection may result in abortion, preterm labor, and fetal infection and the neonatal mortality has been reported from 7% to more than 50%. The median incubation period is 31 days and the prodromal symptoms include fever, myalgias, nausea, vomiting, and diarrhea. It is a food-borne pathogen and occurs sporadically or in epidemics. Maternal consumption of contaminated soft cheese and other dairy products is a known cause of epidemics. Maternal listeriosis is suspected when a pregnant woman presents with flulike syndrome characterized by chills, back pain, and fever which can mimic pyelonephritis; however, most maternal illness are asymptomatic. Blood, rectovaginal, and amniotic fluid cultures and Gram stain should be performed. Intravenous administration of ampicillin and gentamycin is essential for infection diagnosed in pregnancy since it may prevent fetal infection. Penicillin-allergic patients can be treated with trimethoprim/sulfamethoxazole or erythromycin.[35] Transplacental treatment of fetal infection with intravenous ampicillin has been reported.[36] Congenital listeriosis should be considered as a diagnosis for a depressed preterm infant born after a labor complicated by fetal distress and meconium- or brown-stained amniotic fluid.

OTHER PATHOGENS

Perinatal infections have not been shown to occur with maternal infection with polio, rabies, and influenza. Malaria caused by the genus *Plasmodium* can cause congenital illness. The incidence of congenital malaria is estimated at 0.39% and as high as 10% in those that are nonimmune.[37] When traveling to endemic areas, consideration to malaria prophylaxis must be given. Coxsackie B maternal infections have also been reported to cause fetal infection, but the risks for such occurrences are unknown.[38]

Active *Myobacterium tuberculosis* infection during pregnancy, especially if there is evidence for hematogenous spread [military tuberculosis (TB), meningitis, osteomyelitis], carries risk for fetal infection. The neonate will have fever, respiratory distress, and possibly hepatomegaly and other nonspecific manifestations of fetal infection. In the absence of congenital tuberculosis, and in the scenario of active treated disease in the mother, prophylactic isoniazid treatment of the neonate is recommended until evidence of seroconversion. Consideration can also be given to administration of isoniazid-resistant bacillus Calmette-Guérin (BCG) vaccination.

Lyme disease is caused by *Borellia burgdorferi*, a spirochete acquired from bites from a tick that inhabits wooded areas.[39] The initial distinctive bulls-eye skin lesion occurs in most patients and if untreated will progress to cardiac and joint disease. The fetus can be affected from transplacental infection which can lead to fetal anomalies and fetal death. The frequency of fetal infection is unknown. It is recommended that maternal treatment with penicillin or erythromycin be instituted on the basis of a clinical diagnosis as definitive serologic diagnosis may be both elusive and may lead to delay in treatment.

REFERENCES

1. American College of Obstetricians and Gynecologists. *Group B Streptococcal Infections in Pregnancy.* ACOG Technical Bulletin 170. Washington, DC: ACOG, 1992.

2. Daffos F, Forestier F, Capella-Pavlovsky M, et al. Prenatal management of 746 pregnancies at risk of congenital toxoplasmosis. *N Engl J Med* 1988;318:271–275.

3. Freij BJ, Sever JL. What do we know about toxoplasmosis? *Contemporary OB/GYN* 1996; 41:41–69.

4. Hohlfeld P, MacAllese J, Capella-Pavlovski Y, et al. Fetal toxoplasmosis: Ultrasonographic signs. *Ultrasound Obstet Gynecol* 1991;1:241–244.

5. Remington JS, McLeod R, Desmonts G. Toxoplasmosis. In Remington JS, Klein JO (eds), *Infectious Diseases of the Fetus and Newborn Infant,* 4th ed. Philadelphia: Saunders, 1995, pp. 140–267.

6. Centers for Disease Control. Summary of notifiable diseases, United States. *MMWR* 1995; 43:56–59.

7. Centers for Disease Control. Sexually transmitted diseases treatment guidelines. *MMWR* 1995; 42:39–46.

8. Wendel GD, Stark BJ, Jamison RB, et al. Penicillin allergy and desensitization in serious infections during pregnancy. *N Engl J Med* 1985; 315:1229–1232.

9. Lee SH, Ewert D, Frederick P, et al. Resurgence of congenital rubella syndrome in the 1990s. *JAMA* 1992;267:2616–2620.

10. Briggs GG, Freeman RD, Yaffe SJ. *Drugs in Pregnancy and Lactation,* 4th ed. Baltimore: Williams & Wilkins; 1994, pp. 863–866.

11. American College of Obstetricians and Gynecologists. *Perinatal Viral and Parasitic Infections.* ACOG Technical Bulletin 177. Washington, DC: ACOG, 1993.

12. Fowler KB, Stagno S, Pass RF, et al. The outcome of congenital cytomegalovirus infection in relation to maternal antibody status. *N Engl J Med* 1992;326:663–667.

13. Stagno S, Pas RF, Cloud G, et al. Primary cytomegalovirus infection in pregnancy: Incidence, transmission to fetus, and clinical outcome. *JAMA* 1986;256:1904–1908.

14. American Academy of Pediatrics, American College of Obstetricians and Gynecologists. *Guidelines for Perinatal Care,* 3rd Ed. Elk Grove Village, IL: AAP; Washington, DC: ACOG, 1992, pp. 145–146.

15. Hutto C, Arvin A, Jacobs R, et al. Intrauterine herpes simplex virus infections. *Journal Pediatrics* 1987;110:97–101.

16. Gibbs RS, Sweet RI. Maternal and fetal infections. In Creasy RK, Resnik R (eds), *Maternal-Fetal Medicine, Practice and Principles,* 3rd ed. Philadelphia: Saunders 1994, pp. 639–703.

17. American College of Obstetrics and Gynecology. *Perinatal Herpes Simplex Virus Infection.* ACOG Technical Bulletin 122. Washington, DC: ACOG, 1988.

18. Briggs GG, Freeman RK, Yaffe SJ. *Drugs in Pregnancy and Lactation,* 4th ed. Baltimore: Williams & Wilkins; 1994, pp. 10–16.

19. Majors CA, Towers CV, Lewis DF, et al. Expectant management of patients with both preterm premature rupture of the membranes and genital herpes. Abstract 16. Society of Perinatal Obstetricians. *Am J Obstet Gynecol* 1991;164: 248.

20. Gratacos E, Torres P, Vidal J, et al. The incidence of human parvovirus B19 infection during pregnancy and its impact on perinatal outcome. *J Infect Dis* 1995;171:1360–1363.

21. Centers for Disease Control. Risks associated with human parvovirus B19 infection. *MMWR* 1989;38:81–88.

22. Pryde PG, Nugent CE, Pridjian G, et al. Spontaneous resolution of nonimmune hydrops fetalis secondary to human parvovirus B19 infection. *Obstet Gynecol* 1992;79:859–861.

23. Humphrey W, Magoon M, O'Shaughnessy R. Severe nonimmune hydrops secondary to parvovirus B19 infection. Spontaneous reversal in utero and survival of a term infant. *Obstet Gynecol* 1991;78:900–902.

24. Patuszak AL, Levy M, Schick B, et al. Outcome after maternal varicella infection in the first 20 weeks of pregnancy. *N Engl J Med* 1994;330:901–905.

25. Pretorius DH, Hayman I, Jones KL, et al. Sonographic evaluation of pregnancies with maternal varicella infection. *J Ultrasound Med* 1992;11:459–463.

26. Isada NB, Paar DP, Johnson MP, et al. In utero diagnosis of congenital varicella zoster virus infection by chorionic villus sampling and polymerase chain reaction. *Am J Obstet Gynecol* 1991;165:1727–1730.

27. American College of Obstetricians and Gynecologists. *Human Immunodeficiency Virus Infection*. ACOG Technical Bulletin Number 169, 1992.

28. Husson RN, Lan Y, Kojima E, et al. Vertical transmission of human immunodeficiency virus type 1: Autologous neutralizing antibody titer, virus load and virus phenotype. *J Pediatr* 1995; 126:865–871.

29. Sperling RS, Stratton P, O'Sullivan MJ, et al. Survey of Zidovudine use in pregnant women with human immunodeficiency virus infection. *N Engl J Med* 1992;326:857–861.

30. American College of Obstetricians and Gynecologists. *Zidovudine for the Prevention of Vertical Transmission of Human Immunodeficiency Virus*. Committee Opinion Number 148, 1994.

31. Baker CJ, Edwards MS. In Remington JS, Klein JO (eds), *Infectious Diseases of the Fetus and Newborn Infant*, 4th ed. Philadelphia: Saunders, 1995, pp. 980–1054.

32. Pylipow M, Gaddis M, Kinney JS. Selective intrapartum prophylaxis for group B streptococcus colonization: Management and outcome of newborns. *Pediatrics* 1994;93:631–635.

33. Rouse DJ, Goldenberg RL, Cliver SP, et al. Strategies for the prevention of early-onset group B streptococcal sepsis: A decision analysis. *Obstet Gynecol* 1994;83:483–494.

34. Centers for Disease Control. Prevention of perinatal group B streptococcal disease: A public health perspective. *MMWR* 1996;45(RR7):1–24.

35. Yonekra MI, Mead PB. Listeria infections in pregnancy. In Mead PB, Hager WD (eds), *Infection Protocols for Obstetrics and Gynecology*. Montvale, NJ: Medical Economics Publishing, 1992, pp. 62–65.

36. Kalstone C. Successful antepartum treatment of listeriosis. *Am J Obstet Gynecol* 1991;164:57–58.

37. Quinn TC, Jacobs RF, Mertz GJ, et al. Congenital malaria: A report of four cases and a review. *J Pediatr* 1982;10:229–232.

38. Gibbs RS, Sweet RL. Maternal and fetal infections. In Creasy RK, Resnik R (eds), *Maternal-Fetal Medicine, Practice and Principles*, 3rd ed. Philadelphia: Saunders 1994, pp. 639–703.

39. Markowitz LE, Steere AAC, Bench JL, et al. Lyme disease during pregnancy. *JAMA* 1986; 255:3394–3396.

BIBLIOGRAPHY

Duff P, Blanco J (eds). Perinatal infectious diseases. *Semin Perinatol* 1993;17:367–451.

Remington JS, Klein JO (eds). *Infectious Diseases of the Fetus and Newborn Infant*. 4th ed. Philadelphia: Saunders, 1995.

QUESTIONS

1. Which of the following statements is correct regarding cytomegalovirus infection in pregnancy:
   a. It is the most common congenital viral infection in the United States.
   b. Maternal primary and reactivation infection are both just as likely to cause severe neonatal disease.
   c. Universal serologic testing during pregnancy is recommended.
   d. Cytomegalovirus immunoglobulin is recommended for all exposed infants.

2. What is the risk for fetal embryopathy in maternal varicella occurring before 20 weeks gestation?
   a. Less than 1%.
   b. 40%.
   c. 2%.
   d. 10%.

3. Vertical transmission may be prevented in maternal *Listeria monocytogenes* infection diagnosed in pregnancy by the following treatment?
   a. Ampicillin and gentamycin.
   b. Zidovudine.
   c. Spiramycin.
   d. Acyclovir.

4. Fetal infection has been shown to occur with maternal infection with which of the following?
   a. Polio.
   b. Rabies.
   c. Influenza.
   d. Coxsackie B.

5. Which of the following is a correct statement regarding maternal administration of zidovudine to reduce perinatal transmission of HIV?
   a. Antenatal zidovudine is recommended only when maternal CD4 count is <200 μ/L.
   b. Antenatal zidovudine is recommended only when maternal CD4 count is <500 μ/L.
   c. Oral administration should begin at 14 weeks gestation regardless of maternal CD4 counts and should be administered intravenously through labor.
   d. Maternal treatment with zidovudine need not be followed by treatment of the neonate.

6. What is the recommended treatment of the penicillin allergic pregnant patient with syphilis?
   a. Azithromycin.
   b. Tetracycline.
   c. Erythromycin.
   d. Penicillin after desensitization.

7. Which of the following cases is likely to be associated with significant fetal effects?
   a. Asymptomatic pregnant woman with positive toxoplasmosis IgM.
   b. Asymptomatic mother with positive CMV IgM.
   c. Positive rubella IgM at 12 weeks gestation.
   d. Rubella vaccination 1 week prior to conception.

8. Risk factors for early-onset neonatal group B streptococcus infection include all but which of the following:
   a. Breast feeding.
   b. Prematurity.
   c. Maternal fever in labor.
   d. Prolonged membrane rupture.

7

Prematurity

Patricia L. Collins

INTRODUCTION

Definition

Preterm birth is the delivery of a fetus prior to 37 completed weeks of gestation.[1,2] Creasy[1] also suggests that the definition include a lower limit of 20 weeks since most obstetricians consider the delivery of a fetus less than 20 weeks to be an abortion. *Preterm labor* is the onset of uterine contractions associated with cervical change (effacement and/or dilation) prior to 37 weeks of gestation.[1,2] Because birth weight is inherently linked to gestational age, some literature includes low-birth-weight (<2500 g) infants or small for gestational age (<10th centile) infants in the definition of prematurity. However, if the weight definition is used, some infants that are at term but growth restricted will be labeled premature, thus complicating the study of preterm labor. Additionally, the etiology of the growth disorder may be obscured which can have consequences for future pregnancies.

Incidence

The incidence of premature delivery is about 10% of all births. Despite the advances in med-icine, the incidence of preterm birth has not changed in the last 40 years.[2] This is because there is still a poor understanding of the basic biology and physiology underlying the process of normal parturition. Excluding neonatal deaths due to congenital anomalies, prematurity accounts for 60–80% of all neonatal deaths and is a major cause of morbidity in the survivors (e.g., cerebral palsy, chronic lung disease, seizures, etc.).

Epidemiology

The risk factors for premature labor and birth identified by epidemiologic studies include poor socioeconomic status, nonwhite, less education (age appropriate), unmarried, maternal age less than 18 years, poor prenatal care, and low prepregnancy weight. There remains a racial discrepancy in preterm delivery and in infant mortality in the United States. The preterm birth rate for black women is at least double that of white women. Correspondingly, infant mortality related to preterm birth is about 18% for black infants compared to 8.7% for white infants.[3] If one uses statistical methods to separate marital status, adequacy of prenatal care and educational level, teenage mothers ≤17 years of age still have a higher incidence of prematurity (relative risk, 1.9)[4] Maternal age of ≥40 years also increases the risk for prematurity.

ETIOLOGY

Infectious Etiology

Infectious etiology can account for about 30% of preterm labor and births. Identified organisms that are associated with preterm labor and delivery are shown in Table 7-1.[2,5-8] The current hypothesis is that bacteria ascend from the vagina to the cervix. At this point, the bacteria or bacterial products set up a cascade of inflammatory mediators such as interleukin-1 (IL-1), IL-6, and tumor necrosis factor (TNF). There is recruitment of white cells with their mediators which may release enzymes capable of degrading the matrix of the cervix and weakening fetal membranes leading to rupture. This series of events seems to be able to bypass the normal mechanisms that maintain cervical integrity and uterine quiescence. In addition to local vaginal infections, maternal systemic infections such as pyelonephritis, pneumonia, septicemia, appendicitis, etc. can also predispose a woman to deliver prematurely.

A test for fetal fibronectin will soon be available. Fetal fibronectin may be a marker for degradation of the extracellular matrix at the chorion-decidual junction. Some advocate the use of this test to predict preterm labor.[9] However, one should exercise caution in the interpretation of this test since this molecule is found in amniotic fluid and many other intrauterine tissues.

Table 7-1. Microorganisms Associated with Preterm Labor and Delivery

Group B streptococcus (GBS)
Neisseria gonorrhoeae
Chlamydia trachomatis
Trichomonas vaginalis
Bacterial vaginosis (BV) (*Gardnerella vaginalis* plus bacteroides species)
Mycoplasma hominis
Ureaplasma urealyticum
Treponema pallidum

The basic biology of the normal function of fetal fibronectin is still unclear.

Even though there is an association of infection with prematurity, there are inconsistent results in the recovery of organisms from amniotic fluid after amniocentesis or in the pathologic examination of the placenta for organisms. In patients suspected of having an infectious etiology for their preterm labor, 0–30% have a positive amniotic fluid culture.[5] There is histologic evidence of chorioamnionitis in 19–74% of placentas from preterm deliveries and yet 18–49% are culture-negative and 15–45% of infected membranes show no signs of inflammation.[5]

If overt infection or subclinical infection is responsible for about one third of preterm labor, the use of antibiotics to treat the infection should prevent premature labor and premature birth.[5,6,10] The clearest data on the use of antibiotics to prevent prematurity are those on the treatment of bacterial vaginosis (BV) identified in women during the second trimester. Studies are emerging to suggest that pregnant women should be screened for BV at about 20 weeks of gestation and treated if BV is present.[7,8,11,12] Studies on the use of antibiotics as an adjunctive therapy to tocolytic agents are much less consistent in showing efficacy for latency (time from onset of preterm labor to delivery), frequency of preterm delivery, frequency of preterm, premature rupture of membranes, or differences in mean birth weight. The use of antibiotics alone, without tocolytics, is ineffective.[13]

Preterm, Premature Rupture of the Membrane (PPROM)

PPROM is the rupture of fetal membranes prior to term gestation (less than 37 completed weeks) and prior to the onset of labor. PPROM is associated with about 30% of preterm deliveries and therefore has an important impact on perinatal morbidity and mortality. Once PPROM occurs, 60–80% of patients will be in labor within 48 hours. The etiology and pathophysiology of PPROM are still not well understood.[14] Ascending bacterial infection is thought to play a role in PPROM although amniotic fluid cultures are positive in only about 30% of patients.[15] Other risk factors for PPROM include maternal cigarette smoking, incompetent cervix, vaginal bleeding, and antenatal diagnostic procedures such as amniocentesis or chorionic villus sampling. One of the highest risks for PPROM is a prior pregnancy with PPROM with a recurrence risk of about 20%.

Indicated Preterm Delivery

There are some maternal or fetal conditions in which preterm delivery is indicated or in which preterm labor, if it occurs, should not be stopped. Table 7-2 lists some of these conditions. When continuation of the pregnancy is deemed life-threatening to the mother or to the fetus, preterm delivery is indicated. Examples of some of these conditions include severe preeclampsia or eclampsia, some maternal cardiovascular conditions, or end-stage diabetes. Chorioamnionitis is an indication for delivery independent of gestational age. Some examples of fetal anomalies which may predispose to preterm labor and in which tocolysis would be contraindicated include anencephaly, renal agenesis with oligohydramnios, or chromosomal anomalies such as trisomy 18 or 13.

Other

Table 7-3 lists several other risk factors associated with preterm labor. One of the highest risks for preterm labor and delivery in the current pregnancy is a history of prior preterm labor and/or delivery. The recurrence risk for one prior preterm birth is 17–34% and it almost

Table 7-2. Indicated Preterm Delivery

Maternal Conditions	Fetal Conditions
Severe preeclampsia	Fetal distress
Placental abruption with maternal or fetal compromise	Chorioamnionitis or evidence of fetal infection
Cervix dilated ≥5 cm	Intrauterine fetal demise
Life-threatening complications of pregnancy	Fetal anomaly incompatible with life

Table 7-3. Risk Factors for Preterm Labor

Prior preterm delivery
Multiple gestation
Incompetent cervix
Cervical surgery
Uterine anomalies
Cocaine abuse
Tobacco use
Standing or walking at work >4 hours

doubles with two or more prior preterm births.[1] Multiple gestations account for about 10% of preterm births.[2] Whether this is the result of overdistension of the uterus or because of other intrinsic factors specific to multiple gestations is unknown. The term ''cervical incompetence'' refers to painless cervical dilation in the midtrimester without preterm labor resulting in pregnancy loss. Diagnosis of this condition is usually by history, a workup between pregnancies, or more recently, an ultrasound measurement of cervical length less than 2.5 cm or funneling of the internal os.[16] Prior conization of the cervix or other cervical trauma such as repeated second-trimester pregnancy terminations may also predispose to preterm labor. First-trimester pregnancy terminations are not risk factors for subsequent preterm births. Preterm births are also more common when uterine anomalies such as unicornuate uterus, uterus didelphus, bicornuate uterus, or septated uterus are present. Cocaine use is associated with preterm birth at a variable incidence (20–50%) depending on the population studied.[1] Several studies have assessed the risks for prematurity associated with hazards in the workplace. Although there are discrepancies in this literature, one fairly consistent finding is that long periods of standing (>4 hr/day) carries a relative risk for premature labor of about 2.0.[17–20]

DIAGNOSIS

History

A history for risk factors should be elicited from the patient. Several risk scoring systems have been developed to identify women at risk for preterm labor. However, these scoring systems have sensitivities of 40–60% and positive predictive values of only 15–30%.[21–23] The symptoms of preterm labor may include: uterine contractions, uterine "tightening" which may or may not be associated with pain, menstrual-like cramps, pelvic pressure, low back pain, diarrhea, or symptoms of urinary tract infection. A history for fever, chills, nausea, vomiting, or other systemic symptoms of illness should be obtained. It is also important to determine if the patient has symptoms consistent with rupture of the membranes. She may complain of a gush of vaginal fluid or a small, steady stream of vaginal fluid. Any change in vaginal discharge, the amount and duration of any vaginal bleeding and the time of last intercourse should also be recorded. Fetal activity or any decrease in fetal activity is also important.

Physical Examination

Note whether the patient is febrile or has tachycardia and whether the fetus has tachycardia (fetal heart rate ≥ 160 bpm) which could be indicative of infection. A general physical examination should be performed. On abdominal examination, one should palpate the uterus to assess lie and presentation of the fetus and to assess for uterine tenderness which may be a sign of chorioamnionitis or abruption. One can palpate for uterine contractions and record strength and frequency of contractions. Tocodynamometry can also be used to record frequency of uterine contractions. A fetal heart rate monitoring strip should be obtained to assess fetal status.

A sterile speculum examination should be done. If there is a suspicion of PPROM, check for pooling of amniotic fluid, test the pool of fluid for a pH change with nitrazine paper, and prepare a microscope slide of the pool to look for ferning, all evidence of rupture of the membranes. If PPROM is present, visualize the cervix and avoid digital cervical examinations. Look for any vaginal or cervical discharge and prepare slides for a wet preparation to assess for

yeast, *Trichomonas viginalis* and "clue cells" (evidence for BV). Obtain cultures of the cervix for *Neisseria gonorrhea*, Chlamydia, and vaginal and rectal cultures for Group B streptococcus (GBS). If there is no vaginal bleeding and the fetal membranes are intact, then examine the cervix, recording dilation, effacement, consistency, position of the cervix, and station of the presenting part. In the presence of vaginal bleeding, one should assess placental location to rule out a placenta previa before performing a cervical examination.

Laboratory

The blood work which should routinely be obtained includes; a complete blood count (CBC) with differential, a urinalysis and urine culture, and the vaginal/cervical cultures mentioned above. If the suspicion is high for chorioamnionitis, an amniocentesis should be performed for Gram stain, cell count, glucose, protein, and for culture of the amniotic fluid. If available, an ultrasound can be performed to corroborate the gestational age, to document the fetal lie and presentation, placental location, and the amniotic fluid status.

Diagnosis

The diagnosis of preterm labor is made when there are regular uterine contractions (one criterion often used is more than four uterine contractions per hour) with any of the following: documented cervical change, effacement of the cervix of 80% or more or cervical dilation of 2 cm or more. The diagnosis of PPROM is made when there is preterm, documented rupture of the fetal membrane which occurs before the onset of labor.

TREATMENT

If premature contractions are present but without cervical change or rupture of the membranes, one may try conservative measures to stop the contractions. This may include decreased activity, pelvic rest, IV isotonic fluid bolus of 500 mL (no more than 1 L because of the risk of pulmonary edema if tocolytics are needed) or a subcutaneous injection of 0.25 mg of terbutaline. If conservative measures seem to be successful, then the patient must still be observed for a period of time (usually several hours) to ensure that the contractions have stopped and that there is no cervical change.

If the diagnosis of PPROM is made, then management depends on whether or not infection is present and the gestational age of the fetus. If there is chorioamnionitis, delivery is indicated independent of gestational age. If no infection is present and the gestational age is between 34 and 37 weeks, an attempt should be made to obtain amniotic fluid for fetal lung maturity studies. The fluid can be obtained from a vaginal pool or from an amniocentesis. If the fetus is mature, then it can be delivered. If the fetus is younger or the lung studies show immaturity, expectant management is warranted with fetal monitoring (nonstress test or biophysical profile) and monitoring for maternal infection.

If the diagnosis of premature labor with intact fetal membranes is made, treatment with tocolytic agents should be considered to prevent preterm delivery. The administration, dosage, monitoring, side effects, and antidotes for the most commonly used tocolytics are outlined in Table 7-4. There are some absolute contraindications to tocolysis. If continuation of the pregnancy is deemed life threatening to the mother or to the fetus, then tocolytics should not be used (Table 7-2).

Tocolytic Agents

Magnesium Sulfate

Magnesium sulfate is known to inhibit uterine contractions in both in vitro and in vivo studies[1,25] and is the first-line tocolytic in many centers. There is a direct tocolytic effect on uterine muscle, probably because it antagonizes calcium at the cellular level. After the initial loading dose (4–6 g) of magnesium sulfate, a maintenance dose of 2 g/h is used. If the con-

tractions persist, then the dose can be increased by 0.5–1.0 g/hr, titrating to the clinical response of decreased uterine contractions and to maternal side effects. The serum level at which most women respond is 4–8 mg/dL ("therapeutic range"). Magnesium sulfate has systemic effects as well as local uterine effects (see Table 7-4). Deep tendon reflexes are lost at serum levels of magnesium of ≥ 9.0 mg/dL and respiratory depression/arrest can occur at serum levels of $\geq 12-14$ mg/dL. The most serious side effects include pulmonary edema and respiratory depression/arrest. Once the premature labor has abated, the magnesium sulfate should be continued for another 12–72 hours. At the end of therapy, the magnesium sulfate can be discontinued or weaned by 0.5–1.0 g/hr, monitoring for any increase in uterine contractions or further cervical change. An absolute contraindication to the use of magnesium sulfate is myasthenia gravis.

The fetus will have serum levels of magnesium which are equivalent to maternal levels. Fetal heart rate tracings will often show a decrease in long-term variability during the magnesium sulfate therapy. Therefore, it is important to have a reassuring fetal monitor strip before initiation of therapy. If tocolysis is unsuccessful and premature delivery ensues, side effects in the newborn may include hypotonia, drowsiness, respiratory depression, and hypocalcemia.

There has been some interest in the use of oral magnesium as a tocolytic for maintenance therapy after IV therapy is completed. However, data suggest that oral magnesium sulfate is no more effective in preventing preterm delivery than plecebo or oral terbutaline.[26,27]

Ritodrine

Ritodrine is a β_2-adrenergic agonist which exerts its action by increasing intracellular cellular adenosine monophosphate (cAMP). cAMP phosphorylates myosin light chain kinase, causing inhibition of its kinase activity. This decreases myosin and actin interactions, resulting in inhibition of uterine contractions. The best available data on efficacy suggests that intra-

Table 7-4. Tocolytic Agents

Tocolytic Agent	Mix	Loading Dose	Maintenance Dose	Clinical Monitoring	Elimination	Side Effects	Antidote
Magnesium sulfate	Remove 100 cc from a 500-ml D5 ½ NS and add 50 g (100 cc) MgSO$_4$ (10% solution) for load. For maintenance, 40 g MgSO$_4$ in 1 L	4–6 g MgSO$_4$ IV by infusion pump over 10–30 minutes	2–4 g/hr MgSO$_4$ by IV infusion pump	Respirations Mental status Deep tendon reflexes Cardiac arrhythmias Urine output Mg^{2+} levels q 6 hours	Renal	Flushing Headache Lethargy Drowsiness Hypotonia Respiratory depression Urinary retention Hypocalcemia Pulmonary edema	1 g calcium gluconate IV slow push over 5 minutes
Ritodrine	150 mg ritodrine in 500 cc of D5 ½ NS (10 cc/hr ≡ 50 µg/min)	Start at 100 µg/min (20 cc/hr) by IV infusion pump	Increase by 50 µg/min every 20–30 minutes up to 350 µg/min maximum by IV infusion pump	EKG prior to and during therapy Maternal and fetal heart rate Blood pressure Serum K$^+$, glucose I & O	Excreted unaltered by kidney May also be conjugated with renal excretion	Nausea Tachycardia (maternal and fetal) Anxiety Hyperglycemia Hypotension Hypokalemia Cardiac arrhythmia S-T segment changes Myocardial ischemia	
Nifedipine	Oral	10 mg PO or bite and swallow q15–20 minutes up to 4 doses	10–20 mg q4–6 hours	Blood pressure during load q5 minutes then q15 minutes for 1 hour after load Blood pressure before each additional dose until stable	Liver metabolism, 70–80% renal excretion of inactive metalbolites	Dyspnea Flushing Headache Nausea Hypotension	
Indomethacin	Oral	100 mg rectal suppository	25–50 mg oral q6 hours	Do not use ≥32 weeks gestation Limit therapy to ≤48 hrs Avoid in asthmatics Check hematocrit platelets, liver, and renal function	Metabolized in liver, 10% renal excretion (unchanged)	Renal failure GI bleed Thrombocytopenia Prolonged bleeding time Fetal effects (see text)	

Abbreviations: EKG, electrocardiogram; GI, gastrointestinal; I & O, input and output; IV, intravenous; NS, normal saline.

venous ritodrine therapy will delay preterm delivery for at least 48 hours but improvement in perinatal mortality and rate of preterm delivery have not been proven.[28,29] The starting and maintenance doses are shown in Table 7-4. Ritodrine has an initial half-life of 6 minutes and a second-phase half-life of 2.5 hours. There are significant metabolic and cardiovascular side effects associated with the use of the β-adrenergic tocolytic agents. Therefore, β-mimetics should not be used in women with cardiovascular disease and only with careful monitoring in women with diabetes. The most significant cardiovascular side effects include pulmonary edema, cardiac arrhythmias, and cardiac ischemia. β-Adrenergic tocolytic agents can cause lipolysis and an increase in glucagon secretion resulting in gluconeogenesis and glycogenolysis. With the rise and utilization of the increased serum glucose, serum potassium shifts intracellularly causing a transient hypokalemia. Another property of this class of tocolytics is tachyphylaxis, that is, the same dose of medication has declining efficacy, probably because of down-regulation of the β$_2$-adrenergic receptor. Ritodrine has also been used as an oral tocolytic after IV therapy at doses of 10–20 mg every 4 hours.

Terbutaline

Terbutaline is another β$_2$-adrenergic agonist. Terbutaline is much more potent than ritodrine and therefore dosages for these two drugs are different. Terbutaline is most often used as a 0.25-mg subcutaneous bolus injection or as an oral tocolytic after IV therapy at doses of 2.5–5 mg every 4–6 hours. Terbutaline has also been used in a continuous subcutaneous infusion pump.[30]

Although both ritodrine and terbutaline are commonly used as oral maintenance therapy after IV tocolysis, the data to support this practice is poor. A recent metaanalysis of four randomized trials failed to show any efficacy to oral therapy.[31]

The β$_2$-adrenergic agonists readily cross the placenta and can cause significant tachycardia in the fetus. In animal models, increases in fetal cardiac output, fetal hypoxemia and elevated fetal blood glucose have been demonstrated.

Nifedipine

Nifedipine blocks calcium L-channels, thus reducing intracellular calcium and inhibiting uterine contractions. Data on efficacy suggests that nifedipine is as effective as ritodrine with fewer side effects.[32] Nifedipine has rapid oral absorption. Onset of action is about 5–15 minutes with a half-life of about 2–3 hours and a duration of action of about 6 hours. The most significant side effect of nifedipine is maternal hypotension. Blood pressure should be monitored carefully during the loading and maintenance doses (Table 7-4).

In animal studies, questions were raised about the fetal safety of nifedipine because of the potential for decreased uteroplacental perfusion with maternal hypotension. There are several studies on the effects of nifedipine on the human fetus and none have shown any deleterious effects, including no evidence for fetal acidosis or hypoxia.[32]

Indomethacin

Indomethacin is a nonsteroidal antiinflammatory drug that irreversibly inhibits cyclooxygenase, causing reduction in prostaglandins and inhibition of uterine contractions. Indomethacin is well absorbed orally and rectally with a serum peak at about 1–2 hours and a half-life of about 2 hours. The studies on efficacy suffer from small numbers, lack of a control group, and from being unblinded. Information that is available suggests that indomethacin is as effective as other tocolytic drugs in delaying delivery for 48 hours.[33] Indomethacin can cause renal failure, interstitial nephritis, gastrointestinal (GI) bleeds, prolongation of bleeding time, and thrombocytopenia. Indomethacin should not be used in women with drug-induced asthma, in patients with renal or hepatic disease, or in women with a history of peptic ulcer disease or bleeding disorders.

The side effects in the fetus can be profound. Indomethacin readily crosses the placenta. The half-life in the term fetus is about 15 hours and is longer in the preterm infant. Indomethacin can cause renal failure in the fetus and neonate.

This condition may manifest as oligohydramnios in utero. These side effects are probably minimized if duration of therapy is less than 48 hours. The ductus arteriosus becomes sensitive to prostaglandins at about 32 weeks and therefore indomethacin, which may cause constriction of the ductus arteriosus in utero, should not be used at this time of gestation. Increased complications of sepsis, intracranial hemorrhage, renal failure, and necrotizing enterocolitis are reported in premature infants.[33]

Atosiban

Atosiban is one of a group of new tocolytic agents that are oxytocin antagonists, competing with oxytocin at the myometrial oxytocin receptor thus reducing uterine contractions. Phase III trials are in progress and this drug may be available soon.

Antenatal Corticosteroids

In women who deliver prematurely, the antecedent use of corticosteroids is proven to reduce the incidence of neonatal respiratory distress syndrome, intraventricular hemorrhage, and necrotizing enterocolitis. The National Institutes of Health Consensus Development Conference on the Effect of Corticosteroids for Fetal Maturation on Perinatal Outcomes recently recommended that antenatal corticosteroid therapy is indicated for women at risk of premature delivery between 24 and 34 weeks of gestation.[34] The dosages are either 12 mg of betamethasone intramuscularly (IM) given 24 hours apart or four doses of 6 mg of dexamethasone IM 12 hours apart. The effects of the steroids on fetal maturation begin about 24 hours after the initial treatment and the benefits last for about 1 week. The use of glucocorticoids may alter carbohydrate metabolism, and therefore maternal serum glucose levels should be monitored. In some institutions, in women who are at high risk of preterm delivery, corticosteroids are repeated on a weekly basis. There is little data to support this practice and this is an area that the National Institutes of Health (NIH) panel targeted for further research.

In preterm pregnancies complicated by PPROM, the data is less clear on the benefits of antenatal steroids. There is already a high risk for infection for both mother and fetus which could possibly be worsened with corticosteroids. The NIH consensus panel recommended antenatal steroids in PPROM at less than 30–32 weeks gestation in the absence of clinical chorioamnionitis. The American College of Obstetrics and Gynecology's Committee on Obstetric Practice agreed with most of the recommendations of the panel except for treatment of women with PPROM and said that further research is needed to evaluate this question.[35]

Group B Streptococcus (GBS) Prophylaxis

Because of the high risk of neonatal morbidity and mortality associated with GBS, women with preterm labor should be screened with a vaginal and rectal culture for GBS. GBS-positive women should be treated with a 5- to 7-day course of antibiotics, usually ampicillin. If tocolysis is successful and these patients progress to term, they should be rescreened for GBS.

Social Issues

Women diagnosed with preterm labor should stop working and are often placed on bedrest or reduced activity, placed on pelvic rest (sexual abstinence), and encouraged to stay well hydrated. Prospective, randomized data to support these widely practiced therapies is not convincing. Trials of in-hospital bedrest in twin gestations failed to show a benefit.[1]

Home Uterine Activity Monitoring (HUAM)

Some advocate the use of HUAM to detect premature uterine contractions in women at high risk for preterm delivery. Women who have preterm delivery will often have a higher frequency of uterine contractions earlier in gestation compared to women who initiate labor at term. The patient is taught to use a tocodynamometer at home and the information on contractions and

Table 7-5. Neonatal Outcomes

	501–750 g (n = 329)	751–1000 g (n = 423)	1001–1250 g (n = 498)	1251–1500 g (n = 554)	501–1500 g (n = 1804)
Deaths	201 (61.1%)	98 (23.2%)	51 (10.2%)	39 (7.0%)	389 (21.6%)
Survivors	128 (38.9%)	325 (76.8%)	447 (89.8%)	515 (93.0%)	1415 (78.4%)
Survived without morbidity	60 (46.9%)	213 (65.5%)	354 (79.2%)	470 (91.3%)	1097 (77.5%)
Survived with morbidity	68 (53.1%)	112 (34.5%)	93 (20.8%)	45 (8.7%)	318 (22.5%)
CLD	32 (25.0%)	38 (11.7%)	30 (6.7%)	12 (2.3%)	112 (7.9%)
IVH	14 (10.9%)	34 (10.5%)	24 (5.4%)	10 (1.9%)	82 (5.8%)
NEC	5 (3.9%)	18 (5.5%)	31 (6.9%)	18 (3.5%)	72 (5.1%)
CLD, IVH	8 (6.3%)	14 (4.3%)	3 (0.7%)	2 (0.4%)	27 (1.9%)
CLD, IVH	3 (2.3%)	3 (0.9%)	1 (0.2%)	3 (0.6%)	10 (0.7%)
NEC, IVH	4 (3.1%)	3 (0.9%)	3 (0.7%)	—	10 (0.7%)
CLD, IVH, NEC	2 (1.6%)	2 (0.6%)	1 (0.2%)	—	5 (0.4%)

Source: from Hack M, et al. Very-low-birth-weight outcomes of the National Institute of Child Health and Human Development Neonatal Network, November 1989 to October 1990. *Am J Obstet Gynecol* 1995;172:475–464.

Abbreviations: CLD, choronic lung disease defined as oxygen requirement at 36 weeks corrected age; IVH, grade III–IV intraventricular hemorrhage; NEC, necrotizing enterocolitis (Bell's classification stage ≥ II).

fetal heart rate is transmitted over the telephone to a central agency where the information is reviewed. There is controversy over whether the efficacy of this system of monitoring is the daily nursing contact with the patient or it is the monitoring device itself.[36,37] The evidence is less than convincing for routine use of HUAM in most patients. HUAM in selective patients, such as in twin gestations,[38] may be beneficial.

PRETERM DELIVERY

Once the decision is made to proceed with a preterm delivery, consideration should be given for maternal transport to a facility capable of neonatal resuscitation and care of the premature neonate. The likely outcome for the infant including mortality and morbidity should be discussed with the parents. Morbidity and mortality by birthweight is shown in Table 7-5.

Intrapartum continuous fetal heart rate monitoring should be done for the premature infant. The mode of delivery is important for the premature infant. If the fetus is vertex presentation and the mother and fetus are stable, a spontaneous vaginal delivery should be attempted. Some advocate the routine use of outlet forceps to protect the premature fetal head, however,

data to support this practice are meager.[1] If the fetus is breech presentation, delivery by cesarean section is probably less morbid for the infant than assisted breech delivery at estimated birthweights of 650–2000 g.[1] Mode of delivery in very-low-birth infants (<650 g, usually 23–25 weeks) is more controversial and some evidence suggests that the route of delivery does not significantly influence neonatal outcome.[39] Often a classical cesarean section is required for the delivery of very-low-birth-weight infants, which has higher morbidity for the woman and also has significant consequences for future pregnancies (risk of uterine rupture and requirement of repeat cesarean section).

REFERENCES

1. Creasy RK. Premature labor and delivery. In Creasy RK, Resnick R (eds), *Maternal Fetal Medicine*, 3rd ed. Philadelphia: Saunders, 1994, pp. 494–520.

2. American College of Obstetricians and Gynecologists. Preterm Labor. *ACOG Technical Bulletin 206*. Washington, DC: ACOG, 1995.

3. Infant Mortality—United States, 1992. *MMWR Weekly Report* 1994;43:905–909.

4. Fraser AM, Brockert JE, Ward RH. Association of young maternal age with adverse reproductive outcomes. *N Engl J Med* 1995;332:1113–1117.

5. Gibbs RS, Romero R, Hillier SL, et al. A review of premature birth and subclinical infection. *Am J Obstet Gynecol* 1992;166:1515–1528.

6. Lewis R, Mercer BM. Adjunctive care of preterm labor—the use of antibiotics. *Clin Obstet Gynecol* 1995;38:755–770.

7. Hauth JC, Goldenberg RL, Andrews WW, et al. Reduced incidence of preterm delivery with metronidazole and erythromycin in women with bacterial vaginosis. *N Engl J Med* 1995;333:1732–1736.

8. Hillier SL, Nugent RP, Eschenbach DA, et al. Association between bacterial vaginosis and preterm delivery of a low-birth-weight infant. *N Engl J Med* 1995;333:1737–1742.

9. Lockwood CJ, Senyei AE, Dische R, et al. Fetal fibronectin in cervical and vaginal secretions as a predictor of preterm delivery. *N Engl J Med* 1991;325:669–674.

10. Kirschbaum T. Antibiotics in the treatment of preterm labor. *Am J Obstet Gynecol* 1993;168:1239–1246.

11. McGregor JA, French JI, Parker R, et al. Prevention of premature birth by screening and treatment for common genital tract infections: Results of a prospective controlled evaluation. *Am J Obstet Gynecol* 1995;176:157–167.

12. Morales WJ, Schorr S, Albritton J. Effect of metronidazole in patients with preterm birth in preceding pregnancy and bacterial vaginosis: a plecebo-controlled, double-blind study. *Am J Obstet Gynecol* 1994;171:345–349.

13. Cox SM, Bohman VR, Sherman ML, et al. Randomized investigation of antimicrobials for the prevention of preterm birth. *Am J Obstet Gynecol* 1996;174:206–210.

14. Allen SR. Epidemiology of premature rupture of the fetal membranes. *Clin Obstet Gynecol* 1991;34:685–693.

15. Romero R, Chidini A, Mazor M, et al. Microbial invasion of the amniotic cavity in premature rupture of membranes. *Clin Obstet Gynecol* 1991;34:769–778.

16. Gomez R, Galasso M, Romero R, et al. Ultrasonographic examination of the uterine cervix is better than cervical digital examination as a predictor of the likelihood of premature delivery in patients with preterm labor and intact membranes. *Am J Obstet Gynecol* 1994;171:956–964.

17. Luke B, Mamelle N, Keith L, et al. The association between occupational factors and preterm birth: A United States nurses' study. *Am J Obstet Gynecol* 1995;173:849–862.

18. Teitelman AM, Welch LS, Hellenbrand KG, et al. Effect of maternal work activity on preterm birth and low birth weight. *Am J Epidemiol* 1990;131:104–113.

19. Klebanoff MA, Shiono PH, Carey JC. The effect of physical activity during pregnancy on preterm delivery and birth weight. *Am J Obstet Gynecol* 1990;163:1450–1456.

20. Henriksen TB, Hedegaard M, Secher NJ, et al. Standing at work and preterm delivery. *Br J Obstet and Gynaecol* 1995;102:198–206.

21. Creasy RK, Gummer BA, Liggins GC. A system for predicting spontaneous preterm birth. *Obstet Gynecol* 1980;55:692–695.

22. Main DM, Richardson D, Gabbe S, et al. Prospective evaluation of a risk scoring system for predicting preterm births in indigent inner city women. *Obstet Gynecol* 1987;69:61–66.

23. Holbrook RH, Laros RK, Creasy RK. Evaluation of a risk-scoring system for prediction of preterm labor. *Am J Perinatol* 1989;6:62–68.

25. Gordon MC, Iams JD. Magnesium sulfate. *Clin Obstet Gynecol* 1995;38:706–712.

26. Ricci J, Hariharan S, Helfgott A, et al. Oral tocolysis with magnesium chloride: A randomized controlled prospective clinical trial. *Am J Obstet Gynecol* 1991;165:603–609.

27. Ridgeway L, Moise K, Wright J, et al. A prospective randomized comparison of oral terbutaline and magnesium oxide for the maintenance of tocolysis. *Am J Obstet Gynecol* 1990;163:879–882.

28. Canadian Preterm Labor Investigators Group. Treatment of preterm labor with the β-adrenergic agonist ritodrine. *N Engl J Med* 1992;327:308–312.

29. King JF, Grant A, Keirse MJNC, et al. Betamimetics in preterm labour: An overview of the randomized controlled trials. *Br J Obstet Gynaecol* 1988;95:211–222.

30. Lam F, Gill P, Smith M, et al. Use of the subcutaneous terbutaline pump for long-term tocolysis. *Obstet Gynecol* 1988;72:810–813.

31. Macones GA, Berlin M, Berlin J. Efficacy of oral beta-agonist maintenance therapy in preterm labor: A metaanalysis. *Obstet Gynecol* 1995;85:313–317.

32. Ray D, Dyson D. Calcium channel blockers. *Clin Obstet Gynecol* 1995;38:713–721.

33. Gordon MC, Samuels P. Indomethacin. *Clin Obstet and Gynecol* 1995;38:697–705.

34. Effect of Corticosteroids for Fetal Maturation on Perinatal Outcomes. *NIH Consensus Statement* 1994;12(2):1–24.

35. American College of Obstetricians and Gynecologists. Antenatal corticosteroid therapy for fetal maturation. *ACOG Committee Opinion. ACOG Technical Bulletin 147.* Washington, DC: ACOG, 1994.

36. Rhoads GG, McNellis DC, Kessel SS. Home monitoring of uterine contractility. Summary of a workshop sponsored by the National Institute of Child Health and Human Development and the Bureau of Maternal and Child Health and Resources Development, Bethesda, Maryland, March 29 and 30, 1989. *Am J Obstet Gynecol* 1991;165:2–6.

37. American College of Obstetricians and Gynecologists. Home uterine activity monitoring. *ACOG Committee Opinion. ACOG Technical Bulletin 115.* Washington, DC: ACOG, 1992.

38. Dyson DC, Crites YM, Ray DA, et al. Armstrong MA. Prevention of preterm birth in high-risk patients: the role of education and provider contact versus home uterine monitoring. *Am J Obstet Gynecol* 1991;164:756–762.

39. Cibils LA, Karrison T, Brown L. Factors influencing neonatal outcomes in the very-low-birth-weight fetus (<1500gms) with a breech presentation. *Am J Obstet Gynecol* 1994;171:35–42.

BIBLIOGRAPHY

Creasy RK. Premature labor and delivery. In Creasy RK, Resnick R (eds), *Maternal Fetal Medicine*, 3rd ed. Philadelphia: Saunders, 1994, pp. 494–520.

Effect of corticosteroids for fetal maturation on perinatal outcomes. *NIH Consensus Statement* 1994; 12(2):1–24.

Premature rupture of the membranes. In Duff P (ed). *Clin Obstet Gynecol* 1991;34:683–795.

Preterm labor. In Iams JD (ed). *Clin Obstet Gynecol* 1995;38:673–810.

QUESTIONS

1. Risk factors for preterm delivery include all of the following except:
   a. Prior preterm delivery.
   b. Prior classical cesarean delivery.
   c. Cocaine use.
   d. Maternal age ≤17 years.
2. Which of the following is an indication for a preterm delivery:
   a. Eclampsia.
   b. Maternal pyelonephritis.
   c. Fetal gastroschisis.
   d. Fetal trisomy 21.
3. Which of the following is true of PPROM:
   a. Give antenatal steroids with PPROM at 33–34 weeks.
   b. Treat with tocolytics and antibiotics if gestational age ≤30 weeks.
   c. It is associated with ascending vaginal/cervical infection.
   d. A positive fetal fibronectin test is predictive of PPROM.
4. Which of the following tocolytics can cause premature closure of the ductus arteriosus:
   a. Nifedipine.
   b. Magnesium sulfate.
   c. Ritodrine.
   d. Indomethacin.

8

Hypertensive Disorders in Pregnancy

Michael T. Gyves

INTRODUCTION

One of the most common medical complications of pregnancy is hypertension, either antedating the pregnancy or arising as a result of a pathologic alteration of the normal physiologic adjustment of pregnancy itself. Not only is hypertension a common complication, it is also a very serious one, with potential for harm to both the mother and her offspring. Careful attention to detail and prompt intervention can usually effect a resolution of the problem and a favorable outcome for both mother and baby.

DEFINITION

Accurate diagnosis and appropriate management is dependent upon precise definition of terms and the appropriate application of those definitions to the clinical situation.

Hypertension

Elevated blood pressure or hypertension can be defined as a systolic blood pressure of 140 mm Hg or greater or a diastolic blood pressure of 90 mm Hg or greater on two occasions at least 6 hours apart. It has also been defined as an increase above baseline pressure of 30 mm Hg systolic or 15 mm Hg diastolic. This definition is often misleading since it may be difficult to establish a true baseline blood pressure due to normal fluctuations and different measurements by different observers. Women with low baseline blood pressure may exhibit such a rise but have no manifestation of a pathologic process, although this is not always true. The standards for increase in pressure are most applicable for the definition of pregnancy aggravated hypertension ("see Pregnancy Aggravated Hypertension," below).

Proteinuria

It is quite common to detect trace or 1+ proteinuria in a random sample during pregnancy. Significant proteinuria is a 24-hour excretion of 300 mg or more or a concentration of at least 1 g/L in two random samples obtained at least 6 hours apart.

Edema

Dependent edema is normal in pregnancy and is not an indication for alarm. Generalized edema, involving the hands and face, may be a sign of preeclampsia. Without an increase in blood pressure, however, it is not diagnostic, and its presence is not required for the diagnosis of preeclampsia.

Pregnancy-Induced Hypertension (PIH)

This is hypertension, as defined above, presenting after 20 weeks gestation. The exception to the rule is that pregnancy-induced hypertension (PIH) may occur as early as the first trimester with a hydatidiform mole.

Chronic Hypertension

Chronic hypertension is a term applied in the obstetrical setting to hypertension of any cause not induced by pregnancy. It includes essential hypertension and that due to renal, endocrine and neurologic disorders. Chronic hypertension is thus any persistent hypertension that antedates the pregnancy, occurs before 20 weeks gestation (except with mole), or persists beyond six weeks postpartum.

Pregnancy-Aggravated Hypertension

When the requisite blood pressure rise for PIH of 30 mmHg systolic or 15 mm Hg diastolic occurs in a woman with chronic hypertension it is called pregnancy aggravated-hypertension. This definition may be modified by the presence of edema and/or seizures, as will be discussed below in ''Classification of Hypertensive Disorders.''

CLASSIFICATION OF HYPERTENSIVE DISORDERS

A classification of the hypertensive disorders which may be encountered during pregnancy should allow for the distinction between hypertension caused by pregnancy and that which is independent of pregnancy, and it should also indicate that the two forms of hypertension can coexist. A modification of the classification pro-

Table 8-1. Classification of Hypertensive Disorders in Pregnancy

1. Pregnancy-induced hypertension (PIH)
   a. Without proteinuria or edema
   b. Preeclampsia (PIH with proteinuria or generalized edema)
      (1) Mild
      (2) Severe
   c. Eclampsia
2. Chronic hypertension
3. Pregnancy-aggravated hypertension (chronic hypertension made worse by pregnancy)
   a. Without proteinuria or generalized edema
   b. With proteinuria or generalized edema
      (1) Superimposed preeclampsia
      (2) Superimposed eclampsia

posed in the Technical Bulletin of the American College of Obstetricians and Gynecologists (ACOG)[1] provides us with a useful working model of a spectrum of hypertensive disorders of increasing severity (Table 8-1).

Preeclampsia may be classified as severe on the basis of one or more of a number of clinical signs or laboratory abnormalities, as listed in Table 8-2. Severe preeclampsia is clearly of much greater significance than mild preeclampsia in terms of risk to mother and fetus.

The diagnosis of eclampsia is based on the occurrence of one or more seizures in a woman who does not have a known seizure disorder. Eclampsia is listed as a distinct entity because it is clearly distinguishable from the other forms of PIH, but in terms of pathophysiology and sig-

Table 8-2. Criteria for Severe Preeclampsia

Blood pressure: systolic $\geq$ 160 mm Hg; diastolic $\geq$ 110 mm Hg
Proteinuria: $\geq$5 g in 24 hours or persistent 3+ or 4+ in random samples
Oliguria: <500 mL urine output in 24 hours
Cerebral/visual disturbances: blurred vision, scotomata, persistent headache, altered consciousness
Pulmonary edema or cyanosis
Epigastric or right upper quadrant pain
Impaired liver function—elevated liver enzymes
Thrombocytopenia
Hemolysis
Intrauterine growth restriction

nificance it may not truly be different from severe preeclampsia.

The diagnosis of pregnancy-aggravated hypertension is based on the previously defined
blood pressure rise of 30 mm Hg systolic or 15
mm Hg diastolic.

EPIDEMIOLOGY

Significance of Hypertension in Pregnancy

Hypertensive disorders constitute a major
cause of both maternal and perinatal mortality
and morbidity in the United States. About one
in six maternal deaths[2] can be directly attributed
to hypertension complicating pregnancy, and
hypertension is also responsible for prolonged
hospitalization and operative deliveries with
their attendant morbidity in numerous pregnancies. With respect to fetal outcome, pregnancies
complicated by hypertension are at high risk for
stillbirth, intrauterine growth restriction (IUGR),
preterm delivery with its short- and long-term
morbidity, and neonatal death.[3]

Incidence

Roughly 1% of pregnancies are complicated
by preexisting hypertension, although the prevalence may be higher among racial groups who
have a predisposition toward essential hypertension. Elevation of blood pressure may be caused
by the pregnancy itself (PIH) in 5–7% of pregnant women.

Predisposing Factors

PIH in its purest form is a disease of nulliparous women. There are a number of predisposing factors besides nulliparity that put a woman
at increased risk for developing PIH (Table
8-3). Young adolescents and women over age
35 are at increased risk. Special mention should
be made of maternal family history. Chesley
noted that if a woman had eclampsia her daughter would have a 26% chance of developing
PIH.[4,5] PIH is clearly more common in multi-

Table 8-3. Factors that Predispose to the Development of Pregnancy-Induced Hypertension

Nulliparity
Lower socioeconomic class
Extremes of reproductive age
Maternal family history
Multifetal gestation
Large placental mass
Chronic vascular disease
Chronic renal disease

fetal gestation with the risk increasing with fetal
number. This may be related to placental mass
rather than fetal number since PIH is also more
common in pregnancies with a large placental mass from other causes such as hydrops,
diabetes and hydatidiform mole. Underlying
vascular disease of any kind such as chronic
hypertension or collagen vascular disease increases the risk for PIH. Up to 20% of women
with chronic hypertension will develop superimposed PIH. Renal disease, with or without hypertension, also raises the risk of developing
PIH.

When a multipara develops PIH, one of the
conditions mentioned above is almost always
present as an underlying or precipitating factor.

PATHOPHYSIOLOGY

To best understand the adverse effects of hypertensive disorders on pregnancy and to be
able to treat them rationally, we must have a
working knowledge of the physiologic derange-
ments responsible for the clinical manifestations.

Chronic Hypertension

When hypertension precedes pregnancy, the
increased peripheral vascular resistance and vascular tone persist into pregnancy. The normal
physiologic adjustment to pregnancy involves
an increase in plasma volume of 50% and an
increase in cardiac output of the same magnitude. This change is dependent upon a decrease
in vascular tone and such a decrease in vascular

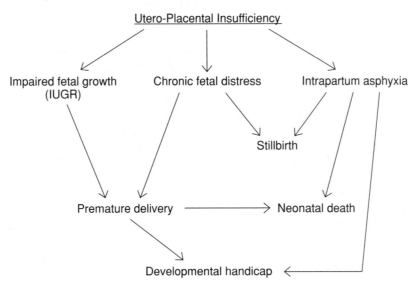

Figure 8-1. Chronic hypertension.

tone may be blunted or absent with chronic hypertension. Thus the normal increase in plasma volume and cardiac output do not occur. The most dramatic consequence of this can be seen in impaired fetal growth which reflects the inadequate uterine blood flow resulting from the deranged physiologic adaptation.

Chronic hypertension, therefore, may cause uteroplacental insufficiency with a spectrum of associated problems for the fetus and newborn (Figure 8-1). These problems include the obvious IUGR and antepartum stillbirth. Fetal distress in labor is more common and may result in intrapartum stillbirth, neonatal death, or long-term disability. Preterm delivery may be necessitated by IUGR and chronic fetal distress or may be spontaneous, and it carries with it all the morbidity and mortality of prematurity.

Soffronoff et al.[6] and Sibai et al.[7] demonstrated a direct correlation between plasma volume deficit and poor fetal outcome manifest as IUGR and intrauterine fetal demise. In the study of Soffronoff et al. the greatest plasma volume deficiency was seen in the women with the most severe hypertension.

Pregnancy-Induced Hypertension

The classic teaching has been that pregnancy-induced hypertension involves increased peripheral vascular resistance and decreased cardiac output, but recent studies indicate that this is not always true.

In the classic model, the basic pathophysiology of PIH is vascular spasm which results in increased resistance to blood flow and hypertension. In normal pregnancy, there is decreased vascular tone, decreased systemic vascular resistance, and a decreased sensitivity to the effects of presser agents. This decreased sensitivity or resistance to pressor agents is lost in PIH. Gant and coworkers,[8] in a longitudinal study, demonstrated that women who remained normotensive throughout pregnancy were resistant to angiotensin II as early as 7–8 weeks gestation and they maintained a high resistance to the pressor effect of infused angiotensin II until term, with maximal resistance to angiotensin II at 28 weeks gestation. In contrast, women who developed preeclampsia were resistant to the pressor effect of infused angiotensin II in early pregnancy, but after 18 weeks gestation this resistance declined and was ultimately lost. A significant difference between the pressor dose of angiotensin II for the two groups appeared by 23–26 weeks gestation.

Vascular spasm causes damage to the vascular endothelium with resultant loss of intravascular fluid into the extravascular space (edema) and hemoconcentration. The combination of arteriolar spasm and hemoconcentration compromises tissue perfusion and can cause organ damage.

Increased systemic vascular resistance due to vascular spasm is not, however, universal or it may be a very late development in PIH. Easterling, et al.[9] studied hemodynamics longitudinally in women who remained normotensive and in women who developed preeclampsia. Those who developed preeclampsia had higher cardiac output throughout pregnancy and did not have elevated peripheral resistance. In that study, some women had late onset of increased peripheral resistance and low cardiac output. The investigators suggested that the combination of high cardiac output and low peripheral resistance is a precursor to PIH. In another publication, Easterling and Benedetti[10] presented the hypothesis that "preeclampsia is a hyperdynamic condition in which the characteristic hypertension and proteinuria are mediated by renal hyperperfusion." They also suggested that instead of arteriolar spasm there may be arteriolar relaxation, exposing capillaries to hyperperfusion and systemic pressures with resultant damage to capillary endothelium, capillary leaks, edema, and end organ damage. Platelets adhere at sites of endothelial damage, release thromboxane (see "The HELLP Syndrome," below), and late onset of vascular spasm results.

When PIH progresses to severe preeclampsia observations of hemodynamics are more consistent. Cotton et al.[11] showed that most women with severe PIH have high systemic vascular resistance, a normal cardiac index and hyperdynamic left ventricular function. A not uncommon complication of severe preeclampsia is pulmonary edema which appears to be the result of altered capillary permeability, decreased colloid osmotic pressure, increased left ventricular filling pressure,[12] and left ventricular decompensation due to a rapid rise in blood pressure.[11]

In the kidney, the classic lesion is glomerular endotheliosis, which is swelling of the glomerular capillary endothelium with resultant narrowing of the capillary lumen and reduced glomerular filtration. This is accompanied by proteinuria with reduction of plasma protein, decreased plasma oncotic pressure, and potentiation of the loss of intravascular volume.

There are also characteristic lesions in the vasculature of the placental bed in preeclampsia. During development of the placenta, cytotrophoblast grows into and replaces the muscularis of the spiral arteries as far as the inner third of the myometrium. This results in dilatation of the distal portion of the spiral arteries and limits their ability to respond to pressors. Brosens[13] showed that in preeclampsia the replacement of muscularis by trophoblast is limited to the decidual portion of the spiral arteries in the placental bed. Thus, the terminal dilatation of the spiral arteries is limited to the decidua, while in the myometrium the spiral arteries retain the muscularis and the ability to respond to pressors. This deficiency in invasion of spiral arteries by trophoblast may result in uteroplacental insufficiency.

HELLP Syndrome

The detrimental effects of severe preeclampsia on various organs have long been recognized, but in 1982, Weinstein[14] brought particular attention to the manifestations of these effects in a syndrome he called HELLP. This syndrome consists of Hemolysis, Elevated Liver enzymes, and Low Platelet count. Each component of the syndrome is a sign of severe vasospasm with endothelial damage and platelet aggregation. When the process is diffused there is sufficient platelet consumption to produce thrombocytopenia. Microthrombi of platelets and fibrin in the microcirculation cause physical damage to the red cells with resultant hemolysis (microangropathic hemolytic anemia). In the liver, the vasospasm and microthrombi cause microinfarcts and periportal hemorrhagic necrosis which result in elevation of liver enzymes. These areas of hemorrhagic necrosis may progress to the development of a subcapsular hematoma. Of particular importance was Weinstein's observation that one or more components of the HELLP syndrome may be present without severe hypertension. Failure to recognize this could lead to mistakenly diagnosing the observed abnormalities as a nonobstetrical condition, resulting in a hazardous delay in appropriate treatment.

ETIOLOGY OF PREGNANCY-INDUCED HYPERTENSION

Although we can demonstrate specific biochemical and physiologic abnormalities in pregnancy-induced hypertension, the precise etiology remains to be identified. The etiology of PIH should be consistent with the following observations about the condition.

1. In its purest form, PIH is a condition of nulliparous women.
2. It is more likely to occur in late pregnancy.
3. The risk of developing PIH is increased by underlying vascular disease, renal disease, and trophoblastic excess (large placental mass).
4. PIH typically resolves after delivery, but may have its onset shortly after delivery.

It may very well be that PIH represents the common manifestation of a variety of pathologic processes.

History

Numerous theories have been proposed for the etiology of PIH most of which have some plausibility but do not withstand thorough scrutiny. Such theories have attributed PIH to uterine ischemia, a coagulopathy, endocrine abnormalities, elevated plasma levels of pressors, dietary deficiencies, fetal metabolic products, placental products, autointoxication (hence the outmoded term "toxemia"), and numerous other causes. In many of these theories the suspected etiologic factors which were observed were, in fact, the results of PIH.

Current Theories

There are currently two theories that dominate thinking about the etiology of PIH. The first theory relates to an immunological mechanism that triggers a hypertensive reaction and the second theory attributes hypertension to an imbalance in prostaglandins.

The immunologic theory for the etiology of preeclampsia is based on the fact that the fetus and placenta have a genetic makeup which is half paternal in origin. They are thus partially antigenically different from the maternal host. It might be expected that the pregnant woman would mount a graft rejection reaction, but in most pregnancies this does not occur. There are a number of factors that protect the fetus from immunologic rejection, one of which is thought to be a blocking (humoral) antibody which appears early in pregnancy and binds with antigenic sites on the placenta to mask them and prevent a cellular immune response, which is the mechanism of graft rejection.

Scott and Beer[15] reviewed the evidence and noted that preeclampsia could develop in those women whose immunologic homeostasis is overwhelmed by the antigenic stimulus of the trophoblast. Inadequate production of blocking antibody permits an effector lymphocyte response to the trophoblast with incidental maternal renal damage. To support this they cited a number of studies that demonstrated common antigens in placenta and kidney and the deposition of immunoglobulin in glomeruli of patients with preeclampsia.

This theory is consistent with the observation that PIH is more common with an increased mass of trophoblast, since the antigenic load may exceed the ability to produce sufficient blocking antibody. It also explains the protection afforded by a prior completed pregnancy and the partial protection afforded by a spontaneous abortion, each of which provides exposure to trophoblast and initiates the production of blocking antibody. The intermediate risk for PIH seen in a multipara with a new partner could be explained on the basis of exposure to a new foreign antigen.

The prostaglandin theory for the etiology of PIH focuses on an abnormal ratio of prostacyclin to thromboxane. Prostacyclin, which is produced in vascular endothelium, is a vasodilator and an inhibitor of platelet aggregation. Thromboxane, produced in platelets, promotes platelet aggregation and vasoconstriction. Walsh[16] has observed that, compared to normal placentas, those from preeclamptic pregnancies had a higher production of thromboxane and a lower production of prostacyclin. He concluded that this might affect uteroplacental blood flow and contribute to uteroplacental insufficiency.

Everett et al.[17] demonstrated that prostaglandin synthetase inhibitors given to normal pregnancy women decreased their resistance to the pressor effect of infused angiotensin II. They assumed that the normal resistance to angiotensin II was mediated by prostaglandins.

On the other hand, Sanchez-Ramos et al.[18] showed that low-dose aspirin (80 mg daily) increased the normal refractoriness to the pressor effect of angiotensin II in the third trimester of pregnancy and Spitz et al.[19] showed that pregnant women who were sensitive to angiotensin II became resistant to the pressor effect after treatment with low-dose aspirin. Spitz et al.[19] measured metabolites or prostacyclin and thromboxane and showed that both were reduced by aspirin, but thromboxane was reduced more, resulting in a more favorable prostacyclin/thromboxane ratio.

High doses of prostaglandin synthetase inhibitors will block production of both prostacyclin and thromboxane. Thus, Everett demonstrated a loss of resistance to the pressor effect of angiotensin II infusion because prostacyclin was reduced. Low doses of aspirin will irreversibly inhibit cyclooxygenase, which is involved in the production of both prostacyclin and thromboxane, but the endothelium can continuously regenerate cyclooxygenase and maintain the synthesis of prostacyclin while platelets cannot

regenerate cyclooxygenase. Thus, low-dose aspirin has more of an inhibitory effect on thromboxane synthesis,[20] promotes a favorable ratio of prostacyclin to thromboxane and maintains or restores the resistance to pressors.

These studies support the theory that PIH is the result of an abnormal ratio of prostacyclin to thromboxane. They do not, however, explain what causes the abnormal ratio.

CLINICAL PRESENTATION AND DIAGNOSIS

As with hypertension in general, PIH is usually asymptomatic. When symptoms do develop they are likely to be associated with severe preeclampsia.

Presenting Signs and Symptoms

With early PIH or mild preeclampsia it is unlikely that the woman will complain of anything more than "swelling." As noted above, some edema is normal in pregnancy, and the edema of preeclampsia is generalized, involving hands and face. Most patient complaints related to edema are not indicative of preeclampsia since hypertension is necessary for the diagnosis. Proteinuria on the spot urine check will change the diagnosis from PIH to preeclampsia. The asymptomatic nature of PIH and the increasing risk of occurrence in later gestation provide the rationale for more frequent prenatal visits as term approaches to assess blood pressure, urine, and weight gain (as a sign of edema).

When a woman has the objective signs of preeclampsia (hypertension and proteinuria) she may have a number of symptoms that signal the progression to severe preeclampsia. These symptoms include headache, altered consciousness, visual disturbances (blurred vision, scotomata), epigastric pain, right upper quadrant abdominal pain, and nausea. Many of these symptoms are common in normal pregnancies and, in the absence of hypertension, do not indicate preeclampsia. As Weinstein[14] noted, how-

Table 8-4. Initial Laboratory Studies in Preeclampsia

Spot urine for protein
Hct/Hgb
Uric acid
Aspartate aminotransferase (AST)
Peripheral blood smear
Platelet count

Abbreviations: Hgb, hemoglobin; Hct, hematrocrit.

ever, severe hypertension may be absent in severe preeclampsia, so appropriate attention must be paid to the above symptoms, especially in late pregnancy. All too often the severe preeclampsia presenting with epigastric or right upper quadrant pain plus nausea and vomiting is mistakenly diagnosed as gallbladder disease.

Laboratory Studies

Very few laboratory studies are necessary for the diagnosis of preeclampsia and for the distinction between mild and severe preeclampsia (Table 8-4). Proteinuria can be documented by spot checks. A 24-hour urine collection will not be very helpful unless spot checks are consistently greater than 1+, since the major purpose of a 24-hour urine collection is to determine whether or not 5 g of protein is excreted. Serum uric acid should be measured since elevated serum uric acid, due to decreased renal clearance, is the first laboratory abnormality to appear after proteinuria. Hematocrit or hemoglobin concentration may be a useful indicator of hemoconcentration. A peripheral blood smear, platelet count, and aspartate aminotransferase (AST) are indicated to screen for severe preeclampsia (HELLP). Although disseminated intravascular coagulation may develop in rare cases of severe preeclampsia, the initial process is platelet consumption, so a full coagulation profile is not necessary in the initial screen.

CLINICAL MANAGEMENT

Management of the woman with PIH will vary depending upon the severity of her disease, the gestational age of the pregnancy, and obstetrical considerations regarding the mode of delivery.

Definitive Treatment

The only true cure for PIH is delivery. Generally speaking, when the fetus is mature it should be delivered. With mild PIH or preeclampsia and a cervix which is unfavorable for induction of labor, delivery may be delayed until the cervix is more favorable. There must, however, be close surveillance of both fetus and mother. Available cervical ripening agents make it difficult to justify a delay of more than 1 or 2 days.

Most authorities agree that with severe preeclampsia beyond 34 weeks gestation, delivery should be effected as soon as possible. There is no place for the use of antihypertensive agents to treat severe preeclampsia beyond 34 weeks gestation except for control of blood pressure during labor.

Early versus Late Onset

The earlier preeclampsia appears the more likely it is to be severe and fulminant in its course. Despite this, conservative or expectant management of severe preeclampsia prior to 34 weeks may be justified in some cases to allow fetal maturation. Odendaal et al.[21] and Sibai et al.[22] showed that before 34 weeks, severe preeclampsia, based on blood pressure criteria only, could be managed expectantly in a perinatal center. Treatment included the use of corticosteroids to induce fetal pulmonary maturation, antihypertensives, and close maternal and fetal surveillance. One to two weeks time was gained in their studies and was associated with better neonatal outcomes. Prior to 24 weeks gestation, however, Sibai et al.[23] showed dismal results with expectant management. The risks to mother and fetus with such early onset of severe preeclampsia dictate immediate delivery. Expectant management must be abandoned and delivery effected when there is evidence of either maternal or fetal deterioration. The former includes uncontrolled severe hypertension, oliguria, persistent severe headache, visual symptoms, epigastric or right upper quadrant pain, vaginal bleeding, preterm labor, rupture of membranes, or signs of the HELLP syndrome. Fetal indications for delivery are severe oligo-hydramnios, repetitive variable or late fetal heart rate decelerations, and an abnormal bio-physical profile.[21,22]

Medical Therapy

Although it is not appropriate to treat PIH with antihypertensive agents except prior to 34 weeks gestation, early and continuing therapy of chronic hypertension is appropriate if the dia-stolic pressure is 100 mm Hg or greater. It is usually appropriate to continue the antihyperten-sive therapy that a woman was taking at the time of conception, the exception being angio-tensin-converting enzyme (ACE) inhibitors which may cause fetal anomalies, renal failure in the newborn, and fetal or neonatal death. ACE inhibitors must, therefore, be discontinued as soon as possible.

The most widely used antihypertensive agent in pregnancy is alpha-methyldopa and this is the preferred drug for starting therapy in pregnancy, since it is not known to put the fetus at risk. Beta blocking agents, specifically labetalol and aten-alol, may be used as primary therapy or in com-bination with alpha-methyldopa. There is some evidence of increased risk for IUGR with beta blockers, but the risks of untreated or uncon-trolled hypertension outweigh the risk of IUGR. Treatment with diuretics is discouraged because of a potential reduction in plasma volume, but diuretic therapy may be used if absolutely nec-essary to control blood pressure and may be con-tinued if in use at the time of conception.

In severe preeclampsia, antihypertensive therapy is appropriate to extend the very pre-term pregnancy or to control blood pressure while effecting delivery if the pressure is con-sistently 160/110 mm Hg or greater. For pro-longing the preterm pregnancy, the agents of choice are beta blockers and calcium channel blockers. To control blood pressure acutely dur-ing labor and delivery, the recommended agents are hydralazine, labetalol, and calcium channel blockers. Hydrazine and labetalol may be given as continuous infusions or as intermittent bolus doses. Bolus therapy is hydralazine 5–10 mg IV every 20 minutes or labetalol 20 mg IV every 10 minutes as needed.

Management of Labor and Delivery

Vaginal delivery should be the goal for the woman with PIH, but cesarean section will often be necessary because of an urgent need for de-livery. Control of blood pressure during labor is discussed in "Medical Therapy," above. It is generally recommended to institute seizure pro-phylaxis during labor, with magnesium sulfate being the drug of choice. A magnesium sulfate infusion is started with a loading dose of 4 g over 20 minutes followed by a continuous in-fusion of 2–3 g per hour. Urine output should be monitored closely since magnesium sulfate is eliminated via the kidneys and oliguria in-creases the risk of toxicity (apnea, cardiac ar-rest). A loss of deep tendon reflexes and slowed respirations will precede severe toxicity. If there is any question about whether or not toxicity is developing, a serum magnesium level can be measured. The therapeutic range is 4–7 mEq/L. Deep tendon reflexes disappear at 8–10 mEq/L and respiratory arrest may occur at 12 mEq/L. Toxicity can be reversed with calcium gluconate 1 g IV.

Magnesium sulfate is also the treatment of choice for eclamptic seizures. For a seizure the loading dose is 4–6 g IV over 20 minutes, fol-lowed by a continuous infusion of 2–3 g per hour. Although some prefer the use of phenytoin sodium for prophylaxis and/or treatment of eclamptic seizures, an extensive record of clin-ical experience and recent studies[24,25] hold mag-nesium sulfate to be superior.

Invasive hemodynamic monitoring is rarely necessary for management intrapartum or post-partum. Those conditions that warrant pulmo-nary artery catheterization include hypertension which is extremely difficult to control, persistent oliguria despite a careful (500 ml) fluid chal-lenge, and pulmonary edema.[26,27]

PROGNOSIS

Short Term

Pure PIH should resolve shortly after delivery. With earlier onset or more severe hypertension, complete resolution may be delayed, but blood pressure should be normal by 6 weeks after delivery. Unless the blood pressure remains at 160/110 mm Hg or greater, there is no need for antihypertensive therapy after delivery. The risk of eclamptic seizures continues for 24–48 hours after delivery, so seizure prophylaxis is generally continued for at least 24 hours after delivery. Beyond 48 hours postpartum, the risk of a seizure is very low.

Future Pregnancies

A woman who has mild preeclampsia has little risk of PIH in a future pregnancy. The risk of recurrent PIH is increased if a woman has had severe preeclampsia or eclampsia, especially if the onset was early.[28] Chronic hypertension with pregnancy-aggravated hypertension and hypertension persisting beyond 6 weeks postdelivery also increase the risk of PIH in future pregnancies.

Antiphospholipid antibodies (lupus anticoagulant and anticardiolipin antibody) are known to predispose to early onset of severe preeclampsia. It is therefore wise to screen for these antibodies in any woman with PIH developing before 34 weeks gestation. A positive screen for antiphospholipid antibodies indicates a high risk for recurrence of PIH.

Long Term

PIH that is not related to underlying vascular or renal disease does not put a woman at increased risk for the later development of hypertension. If, however, there is known renal or vascular disease it is not purely "pregnancy-induced" hypertension and there is an increased risk for developing hypertension later in life. Early onset of PIH, its occurrence in a multipara, and persistence at 6 weeks postdelivery

also increase the risk for later hypertension.[28,29] These features suggest that it is not "pure" PIH.

PROPHYLAXIS

In view of the previously stated association between prostacyclin and thromboxane and their presumed roles in PIH, we might assure that we could prevent PIH by inducing or maintaining an appropriate ratio of prostacyclin to thromboxane. Low doses of aspirin will inhibit thromboxane production more than prostacyclin and might be an effective prophylaxis. Several studies[30-32] have demonstrated a significant reduction in the incidence of PIH and preeclampsia in both normal nulliparous women and women at high risk for PIH using low doses of aspirin (60–100 mg daily). One of these studies,[31] however, noted a small increase in the risk of abruptio placentae with aspirin prophylaxis. Another large collaborative study[33] showed a decrease in the incidence of preeclampsia with low-dose aspirin which was not statistically significant.

Calcium supplementation of 2 g daily has also been shown to reduce the incidence of PIH in nulliparous women.[34] The mechanism of this effect is not clear and the reduction is small but significant. More investigation must be done on the use of calcium for prevention of PIH.

At this time, there is no prophylaxis that can be recommended for use in all women. There are enough data, however, to justify the use of low-dose aspirin in women who are known to be at high risk for the early onset of severe preeclampsia. In this group, the benefit outweighs the small risk of abruptio placentae.

REFERENCES

1. American College of Obstetricians and Gynecologists. Management of Preeclampsia. ACOG Technical Bulletin 91. Washington, DC: ACOG, 1986.
2. Rochat RW, Koonin LM, Atrash HK, et al. The Maternal Mortality Collaborative: Maternal mortality in the United States: Report from the

maternal mortality collaborative. *Obstet Gynecol* 1988;72:91–97.

3. Lin C-C, Lindheimer MD, River P, et al. Fetal outcome in hypertensive disorders of pregnancy. *Am J Obstet Gynecol* 1982;142:255–260.

4. Chesley LC, Cooper DW. Genetics of hypertension in pregnancy: Possible single gene control of pre-eclampsia and eclampsia in the descendants of eclamptic women. *B J Obstet Gynaecol* 1986;93:898–908.

5. Chesley LC, Cosgrove RA, Annitto JE. Pregnancies in the sisters and daughters of eclamptic women. *Obstet Gynecol* 1962;20:39–46.

6. Soffronoff EC, Kaufmann BM, Connaughton JF. Intravascular volume determinations and fetal outcome in hypertensive diseases of pregnancy. *Am J Obstet Gynecol* 1977;127:4–9.

7. Sibai BM, Abdella TN, Anderson GD, et al. Plasma volume determination in pregnancies complicated by chronic hypertension and intrauterine fetal demise. *Obstet Gynecol* 1982;60:174–178.

8. Gant NF, Daley GL, Chand S, et al. A study of angiotensin II pressor response throughout primigravid pregnancy. *J Clin Invest* 1973;52:2682–2689.

9. Easterling TR, Benedetti TJ, Schmucker BC, et al. Maternal hemodynamics in normal and preeclamptic pregnancies: A longitudinal study. *Obstet Gynecol* 1990;76:1061–1069.

10. Easterling TR, Benedetti TJ. Preeclampsia: A hyperdynamic disease model. *Am J Obstet Gynecol* 1989;160:1447–1453.

11. Cotton DB, Lee W, Huhta JC, et al. Hemodynamic profile of severe pregnancy-induced hypertension. *Am J Obstet Gynecol* 1988;158:523–529.

12. Benedetti TJ, Kates R, Williams V. Hemodynamic observations in severe preeclampsia complicated by pulmonary edema. *Am J Obstet Gynecol* 1985;152:330–334.

13. Robertson WB, Brosens I, Dixon G. Uteroplacental vascular pathology. *Eur J Obstet Gynecol Reprod Biol* 1975;5:47–65.

14. Weinstein L. Syndrome of hemolysis, elevated liver enzymes, and low platelet count: a severe consequence of hypertension in pregnancy. *Am J Obstet Gynecol* 1982;142:159–167.

15. Scott JR, Beer AA. Immunologic aspects of pre-eclampsia. *Am J Obstet Gynecol* 1976;125:418–427.

16. Walsh SW. Preeclampsia: An imbalance in placental prostacyclin and thromboxane production. *Am J Obstet Gynecol* 1985;152:335–340.

17. Everett RB, Worley RJ, MacDonald PC, Gant NF. Effect of prostglandin synthetase inhibitors on pressor response to angiotensin II in human pregnancy. *J Clin Endocrinol Metab* 1978;46:1007–1010.

18. Sanchez-Ramos L, O'Sullivan MJ, Garrido-Calderone J. Effect of low-dose aspirin on angiotensin II pressor response in human pregnancy. *Am J Obstet Gynecol* 1987;156:193–194.

19. Spitz B, Magness RR, Cox SM, et al. Low-dose aspirin. I. Effect of angiotensin II pressor responses and blood prostaglandin concentrations in pregnant women sensitive to angiotensin II. *Am J Obstet Gynecol* 1988;159:1035–1043.

20. Vane JR, Anggard EE, Botting RM. Regulatory functions of the vascular endothelium. *N Engl J Med* 1990;323:27–36.

21. Odendaal HJ, Pattinson RC, Bam R, et al. Aggressive or expectant management for patients with severe preeclampsia between 28–34 weeks' gestation: A randomized controlled trial. *Obstet Gynecol* 1990;76:1070–1075.

22. Sibai BM, Mercer BM, Schiff E, Friedman SA. Aggressive versus expectant management of severe preeclampsia at 28 to 32 weeks' gestation: A randomized controlled trial. *Am J Obstet Gynecol* 1994;171:818–822.

23. Sibai BM, Akl S, Fairlie F, et al. A protocol for managing severe preeclampsia in the second trimester. *Am J Obstet Gynecol* 1990;163:733–738.

24. Dommisse J. Phenytoin sodium and magnesium sulphate in the management of eclampsia. *Br J Obstet Gynaecol* 1990;97:104–109.

25. Lucas MJ, Leveno KJ, Cunningham FG. A comparison of magnesium sulfate with phenytoin for the prevention of eclampsia. *N Engl J Med* 1995;333:201–205.

26. Clark SL, Cotton DB. Clinical indications for pulmonary artery catheterization in the patient with severe preeclampsia. *Am J Obstet Gynecol* 1988;158:453–458.

27. Clark SL, Greenspoon JS, Aldahl D, et al. Severe preeclampsia with persistent oliguria: man-

agement of hemodynamic subsets. *Am J Obstet Gynecol* 1986;154:490–494.

28. Sibai BM, El-Nazer A, Gonazalez-Ruiz A. Severe preeclampsia-eclampsia in young primigravid women: Subsequent pregnancy outcome and remote prognosis. *Am J Obstet Gynecol* 1986;155:1011–1016.

29. Chesley LC, Annitto JE, Cosgrove RA. The remote prognosis of eclamptic women. *Am J Obstet Gynecol* 1976;124:446–459.

30. Schiff E, Peleg E, Goldenberg M, et al. The use of aspirin to prevent pregnancy-induced hypertension and lower the ratio of thromboxane A_2 to prostacyclin in relatively high risk pregnancies. *N Engl J Med* 1989;321:351–356.

31. Sibai BM, Caritis SN, Thom E, et al. Prevention of preclampsia with low-dose aspirin in healthy, nulliparous pregnant women. *N Engl J Med* 1993;329:1213–1218.

32. Hauth JC, Goldenberg RL, Parker CR, et al. Low-dose aspirin therapy to prevent preeclampsia. *Am J Obstet Gynecol* 1993;168:1083–1093.

33. CLASP Collaborative Group. CLASP: A randomised trial of low-dose aspirin for the prevention and treatment of pre-eclampsia among 9364 pregnant women. *Lancet* 1994;343:619–629.

34. Belizan JM, Villar J, Gonazalez L, et al. Calcium supplementation to prevent hypertensive disorders of pregnancy. *N Engl J Med* 1991; 325:1399–1405.

BIBLIOGRAPHY

American College of Obstetricians and Gynecologists, *Hypertension in Pregnancy*. ACOG Technical Bulletin 219. Washington, DC: ACOG, 1996.

National High Blood Pressure Education Program Working Group Report on High Blood Pressure in Pregnancy. *Am J Obstet Gynecol* 1990;163:1689–1712.

QUESTIONS
(choose the best single answer)

1. A rising hematocrit in preeclampsia reflects:
   a. Disseminated intravascular coagulation.
   b. Accelerated erythropoiesis.
   c. Hepatic failure.
   d. Decreased plasma volume.
2. Which of the following laboratory findings would be typical of severe preeclampsia:
   a. Low serum uric acid.
   b. Low platelet count.
   c. Low serum creatinine.
   d. Low 24 hour urine protein.
3. Hypertension in pregnancy may result in which of the following:
   a. Postterm delivery.
   b. Intrauterine growth restriction (IUGR).
   c. Hydatidiform mole.
   d. Fetal anomalies.
4. The basic pathophysiology in preeclampsia is:
   a. Increased vascular reactivity to pressors.
   b. Renal failure.
   c. Disseminated intravascular coagulation.
   d. Cardiac failure.
5. Intrapartum management directed at prevention of seizures in the preeclamptic patient should include:
   a. Pulmonary artery catheterization.
   b. Antihypertensive therapy with beta-blocking agents.
   c. Therapy with magnesium sulfate.
   d. Diurectic therapy.

SELECT THE ONE INCORRECT ANSWER

6. Appropriate antihypertensive therapy for the pregnant woman with longstanding hypertension may include all of the following except:
   a. Diuretics.
   b. Angiotensin-converting enzyme inhibitors.
   c. Beta-blocking agents.
   d. Alpha-methyldopa.
7. The risk that a woman will develop pregnancy-induced hypertension is increased by each of the following except:
   a. Multiple gestation.
   b. Maternal family history of eclampsia.
   c. Coexistent seizure disorder.
   d. Antiphospholipid antibody.
8. Severe preeclampsia may present with each of the following except:
   a. Pulmonary edema.
   b. Oliguria.
   c. Epigastric pain.
   d. Polyhydramnios.

9

Pregnancy in the Woman with Diabetes Mellitus

Carol A. Lindsay

Diabetes mellitus (DM) continues to be a challenging problem facing the obstetrician/gynecologist. Pregnancy represents a diabetogenic state. The incidence of diabetes mellitus (DM) in women of childbearing age is 0.4–1.5%. The incidence of gestational diabetes is 1–4%.

CLASSIFICATION OF DIABETES MELLITUS IN PREGNANCY

There are two classes of diabetes encountered in the pregnant woman. First there is gestational diabetes (GDM) in which glucose intolerance evolves during the index pregnancy and may resolve at the conclusion of the pregnancy (White's classes A1 and A2). The second group consists of those which have been diagnosed with DM prior to the onset of pregnancy Type I (insulin-dependent) and Type II (non-insulin-dependent) DM or White's classes B through R). A modification of White's classification of diabetes in pregnancy is listed in Table 9-1.[1]

GESTATIONAL DIABETES MELLITUS

Risk Factors

Risk factors for the development of GDM include a strong family history of Type II DM, a previous pregnancy with an unexplained fetal demise, a congenitally malformed infant or a fetus with macrosomia, or the index pregnancy complicated by obesity, hypertension, persistent glycosuria, maternal age >25 years, fasting glucose >140 mg/dL, or random glucose >200 mg/dL.[2] The American Diabetes Association recommends screening all patients for gestational diabetes at 24–28 weeks gestation regardless of the presence of risk factors because as many as 50% of patients identified as having GDM will not have an identifiable risk factor. If strong risk factors exist, however, many practitioners will screen patients at the initial visit and again at the usual 24–28 weeks if the initial screen was negative.

Diagnosis of Gestational Diabetes Mellitus

The diagnosis of GDM is determined by the 100-g, 3-hour oral glucose tolerance test. First the patient is given a screening test which consists of a 50-g glucose oral load followed by a plasma glucose determination 1 hour later. Values greater than 130–140 mg/dL constitute a positive screening test. Each individual center must choose its cutoff for a positive screening test. Higher values (i.e., 140 mg/dL) decrease the sensitivity but increase the specificity for de-

Table 9-1. White's Classfication of Diabetes in Pregnancy

A1	Gestational diabetes treated with diet only
A2	Gestational diabetes treated with insulin
B	>20 years of age at onset or less than 10 years duration
C	10–19 years of age at onset of 10–19 years duration
D	<10 years old at onset or greater than or equal to 20 years duration, or background retinopathy or chronic hypertension
F	Any age at onset or duration with nephropathy (proteinuria greater than 300 mg/dL)
R	Any age at onset or duration with proliferative retinopathy or vitreous hemorrhage
H	Any age of onset or duration with arteriosclerotic heart disease
T	Any duration or age of onset with prior renal transplant

tecting diabetes. This means that a few patients who have GDM will be missed but a larger percentage of those people with a positive screening test will actually have the disease. Conversely, a lower value such as 130 mg/dL will increase the number of diabetic women that are identified (increased sensitivity) but there will be more false-positives (decreased specificity). A positive screening test is followed by a 100-g oral glucose tolerance test. The patient should be fasting for 8–10 hours prior to this test. The diagnostic criteria for GDM are listed in Table 9-2.[3] Two or more abnormal values are considered diagnostic.[4] A glucose value greater than 200 mg/dL on the screening test is also generally considered diagnostic for GDM.

Pathophysiology

The pathogenesis of GDM is not clearly understood. Pancreatic insulin secretion has been shown to be delayed and blunted in women with GDM. There is also impaired peripheral glucose

Table 9-2. Normal Values for the 3-Hour, 100-g Glucose Tolerance Test, mg/dl

FBS < 105	1 < 190	2 < 165	3 < 145

Abbreviations: FBS, fasting blood sugar.

utilization that is associated with increased peripheral and hepatic insulin resistance.[5,6]

Antenatal Management

The antenatal management of the woman with GDM is aimed at maintaining euglycemia. This has been shown to decrease the perinatal morbidity and mortality associated with impaired glucose tolerance.[7]

In addition to those procedures recommended as part of routine prenatal care, attention should be addressed to both glucose control and the detection and prevention of complications. At each visit a capillary blood glucose value is obtained with relation to the last meal noted. Urine is also checked for ketones. Capillary blood sugars obtained by the patient are evaluated and appropriate adjustments in insulin or diet are made. These visits also allow for an assessment of fetal growth and well-being. This can also be an opportunity for interaction with the diabetic nurse educator (a registered nurse specializing in the care of women with diabetes) and with the nutritionist and social worker as needed if these services are available. The diabetic nurse educator can reinforce the information the physician has explained to the patient about her disease. In addition, he or she can teach the patient home capillary glucose monitoring and insulin administration and monitor the patient's ability to correctly perform these tasks. The nutritionist is instrumental in explaining the dietary recommendations to the patient and can also determine individual caloric requirements based on activity and desired weight gain. The nutritionist can help make adjustments in diet for the special needs of an individual patient.

Improved results have been obtained with home capillary blood glucose monitoring in terms of neonatal complications and fetal macrosomia. At our institution we commonly use three times a week self monitoring blood glucose (SMBG) for women with gestational diabetes not requiring insulin and daily monitoring in all patients requiring insulin.

All patients are taught how to perform home self-monitoring of fingerstick capillary blood glucose. These are read with either a glucose reflectance meter if available or visually with oxidase reagent strips.

In the patient with A1 GDM, SMBG monitoring is done three times a week. Each of these days the patient checks a fasting blood sugar. One day the patient also does all preprandial (ac) SMBG. The other two days the patient checks 2-hour postprandial (pc) glucose levels. These values are evaluated on a regular basis to determine the patient's need for insulin or diet adjustment. Normal values are fasting and preprandial less than 100 mg/dL and postprandial glucose less than 120 mg/dL. In addition to home monitoring, a capillary glucose determination is made at each clinic visit with a notation made as to when the determination was made with relation to the time of the last meal. The purpose of this is twofold. This allows one to compare the glucose levels the patient reports to that obtained by the clinic personnel. This allows one to detect defective meters or oxidative strips and it helps identify those patients that are having difficulty performing capillary blood sugar monitoring or interpreting oxidative strips. It also allows one to detect patients who are noncompliant with home glucose monitoring.

Those patients requiring insulin therapy use a more intensive glucose monitoring program (see Figure 9-1). Patients check capillary blood sugars seven times daily: fasting, preprandial, 2-hour postprandial, and at bedtime (hs). Some patients also check at 3 am to rule out nocturnal hypoglycemia. These patients also have glucose determinations at each office visit. In addition hemoglobin A1c (HbA1c), blood urea nitrogen (BUN), serum creatinine, and urine culture and antibiotic sensitivity determinations are performed on all patients starting insulin.

In addition to glucose monitoring patients perform daily urinary ketone determinations again by oxidative reagent strips to identify inadequate diet or insulin.

Patients requiring insulin therapy require close follow-up, often necessitating telephone calls at home during the week in order to check on patient progress and to make insulin adjustments as necessary.

The above scheme is the one practiced at our institution. In other centers the glucose monitoring of GDM varies from only once-weekly preprandial and postprandial glucose to eight times daily including fasting, preprandial, postprandial, bedtime, and between 2 and 4 am.

The mainstay of therapy in GDM is diet. Patients with a diagnosis of gestational diabetes are placed on a diet consisting of approximately half complex carbohydrates with the remainder divided between protein and fat. Diet alone is successful in maintaining euglycemia in approximately 50–80% of women with GDM. The goal of dietary therapy is to prevent hyperglycemic episodes and starvation ketosis. Weight

| Date | Breakfast ac/pc | Lunch ac/pc | Dinner ac/pc | Bedtime hs | Urine ketones | Insulin dose | | | Notes* |
						time	NPH	Reg	

*Notes includes alterations in diet, symptoms of hypoglycemia or hyperglycemia, illnesses, insulin reactions or anything that makes the day unusual for the patient.

Figure 9-1. Example of daily capillary glucose determinations. ac, preprandial; hs, bedtime (hours of sleep); pc, postprandial.

gain of 20–25 lb is recommended in gestation. However, specific recommendations for weight gain in the individual patient must be based on pregravid weight. Lean women should gain approximately 35 lb, average-size women should gain 25 lb, obese women should gain 15 lb, and very obese women should gain 10 lb.

The recommended daily caloric requirements average 30–35 kcal/kg ideal body weight. Lean patients should have higher caloric requirements (35–40 kcal/kg/day). Patients in the normal weight ranges should have approximately 30 kcal/kg/day. Obese patients should have 15–25 kcal/kg/day.[3] The distribution of calories should be 40–50% carbohydrate, 20–30% protein, and 25–40% fat. Simple sugars should be avoided. Patients should avoid unsweetened fruit juices, carbonated beverages, and concentrated sweets.[8] A liberal exercise program should be encouraged which could involve continuing with her current exercise regimen or in the patient not currently exercising beginning a program of postprandial walking.[9] If fasting ketonuria is detected an increase in bedtime caloric intake is instituted.

When to start insulin therapy in the patient with GDM is a difficult management decision. We attempt to maintain euglycemia in all patients with diabetes defined as preprandial glucose values less than 100 mg/dL and 2-hour postprandial glucose values less than 120 mg/dL. When a patient with GDM exhibits persistent values in excess of those previously described, they are started on insulin. If a patient has borderline SMBG values, we include other factors in decision making. For example one may be more inclined to start insulin therapy in presence of fetal macrosomia or a patient who is relatively early in gestation, in whom it is anticipated that insulin resistance will increase.

Most patients can be managed on a multidose insulin regimen ranging from one to four or more doses each day. A typical regimen consists of a combination of short (regular) and intermediate (neutral protamine Hagedorn or NPH) acting humulin insulin in the morning, with short-acting insulin, at dinner and intermediate-acting insulin at bedtime. A few patients who

are difficult to control or who have irregular schedules may be best managed with very long-acting insulin (ultralente) to give the patient a basal level of insulin with short-acting insulin at meals.

Insulin doses are adjusted throughout gestation to maintain euglycemia. Insulin requirements tend to increase in the woman with GDM throughout pregnancy but may decrease in the latter half of the third trimester.

Some clinicians use a set regimen of insulin while others use empiric doses to maintain euglycemia. An alternative dosing regimen is 0.3–0.4 units/kg ideal body weight of NPH at nighttime in a lean patient and 0.5–0.7 units of NPH/kg ideal body weight in obese patients. Once a patient is started on insulin close follow-up must be arranged. The patient may be started as an inpatient for education and to allow for rapid detection of hypoglycemia. Alternatively, in the compliant patient, many can be taught insulin administration as an outpatient. However, a physician or a nurse knowledgeable in the management of diabetes and insulin should maintain frequent contact with the patient. The patient should have 24-hour access to someone who can answer questions. Patients are also given glucagon for use in case of severe hypoglycemia and unresponsiveness. Her family members are instructed in its use. Glucagon is a hormone which has glycogenolytic and gluconeogenic actions which can be administered into the buccal mucosa. This facilitates the rapid increase in serum glucose concentrations. It should also be noted that the normal hypoglycemic response may be blunted in pregnancy due to the tighter glycemic control of the patient or the pregnancy itself.

The laboratory evaluation of the woman with GDM includes a clean void urine culture obtained each trimester because these patients are at increased risk of developing pyelonephritis secondary to asymptomatic bacteriuria.

The fetus of the woman with DM is at risk for many complications. Disturbances in fetal growth are not uncommon. In the past intrauterine fetal demise was a serious concern, but with the current ability of antenatal monitoring this is an infrequent complication.

In the third trimester fundal height is used as a screen for fetal growth abnormalities. Fundal height should correlate in centimeters with gestational age. If it differs by more than 3 cm an ultrasound is obtained to estimate fetal weight so as to detect macrosomia, polyhydramnios, or occasionally intrauterine growth restriction. Once macrosomia is detected an ultrasound close to the time of delivery (around 36 weeks) is helpful to plan the route of delivery. If the estimated fetal weight is greater than 4000–4500 g in the diabetic patient elective cesarean section must be considered due to the increased risk of shoulder dystocia.[10] The macrosomic infants of diabetic mothers tend to have truncal obesity leading to a higher likelihood of shoulder dystocia.

In our institution all patients with GDM have weekly antenatal monitoring with nonstress testing beginning at 36 weeks until delivery. Once a patient has been started on insulin, the patient is monitored with nonstress tests twice weekly starting at 32 weeks. If other complications develop more intensive monitoring may be necessary including biophysical profiles, contraction stress tests, or oxytocin challenge tests.

Labor and Delivery in the Woman with GDM

The timing of delivery of the woman with GDM is controversial. Other factors to be considered include the management of plasma glucose levels during labor and fetal monitoring.

In our institution, the patient with A1 GDM who is well controlled on diet and who does not develop any other complications, is delivered by term. If complications develop such as pre-eclampsia, poor glycemic control, fetal macrosomia, or intrauterine growth restriction (IUGR), delivery may be considered earlier. If a patient is electively delivered before 39 completed gestational weeks, an amniocentesis is performed to ensure fetal lung maturity. Lung maturity is determined by the lecithin/sphingomyelin ratio or a positive phosphatidyl glycerol. The value of a mature lecithin/sphingomyelin ratio varies from institution to institution. Some centers are allowing well-controlled gestational diabetics to advance to 42 weeks before an induction of labor is instituted.[11]

The night before the patient is scheduled for induction she is instructed to take her usual insulin dose and to remain NPO after midnight. She comes to labor and delivery in the morning when an infusion of 5% dextrose in 0.45 normal saline ($D_5$1/2NS) (at 125 cc/hr) or 10% dextrose in 0.45 normal saline (D_{10}1/2NS) (at 60 cc/hr) is started. Glucose levels are monitored at 1- to 2-hour intervals. The goal is to maintain glucose levels less than 100 mg/dL. If this is not achieved a continuous intravenous infusion of insulin is started (Table 9-3). Most women with GDM A1 or A2, however do not require insulin therapy during induction of labor.

If a woman with GDM on insulin presents in spontaneous labor, consideration must be given to the patient's last dose of insulin. The patient should be given an intravenous infusion of a glucose-containing solution with frequent monitoring of blood glucose levels to prevent the development of hypoglycemia. Continuous electronic fetal monitoring is mandatory in all patients with GDM.

Table 9-3. Calculation of Intravenous Insulin Infusion

$$\text{Insulin infusion rate} = \frac{\text{Total daily insulin requirements (U)} \times \text{hourly caloric intake (kcal)}}{\text{Total daily caloric intake (kcal)}}$$

Total daily insulin requirement = Total regular + 2/3 total NPH

$$\text{Hourly caloric intake} = \frac{\text{Grams of glucose in IV fluids*}}{\text{Volume of fluid (cc)}} \times \frac{4 \text{ kcal}}{g} \times \text{rate (cc/hr)}$$

*D_{10} contains 100 g of glucose per liter of fluid and D_5 contains 50 g/L.

At the time of delivery special concerns must be addressed. One must anticipate the possible complications of the diabetic woman at the time of delivery. These women are at increased risks for delivering an infant with a shoulder dystocia due to truncal obesity.[12] This woman should be delivered in an area with facilities to address this problem should it arise including the immediate capability for cesarean section. The neonate is also at risk for the development of hypoglycemia, hypocalcemia, hyperbilirubinemia, and hypomagnesemia after birth. Hypoglycemia results from increased fetal insulin. Maternal glucose is transported across the placenta to the fetus by facilitated diffusion. Endogenous or exogenous maternal insulin most probably does not cross the placenta. The fetus makes insulin to counteract the increase levels of glucose. Once delivery occurs, the maternal supply of glucose is abruptly interrupted but the high levels of fetal insulin remain. This along with the relative inability of the fetus for gluconeogenesis leads to neonatal hypoglycemia. The degree of neonatal hypoglycemia is related to glucose levels during labor. Early feeding and sometimes intravenous glucose infusions may be necessary to combat this hypoglycemia. Insulin also acts as a growth hormone in the fetus contributing to the development of macrosomia.[13] Insulin promotes deposition of glycogen in the fetal liver, increasing its size (contributing to truncal obesity and shoulder dystocia). Insulin also promotes increased fat deposition as excess glucose not converted to glycogen is converted to fat.

The Postpartum Period

Postpartum we recommend that the patient continue on the prescribed diet. In those patients treated with insulin, glucose levels are monitored every 4–6 hours while the patient is hospitalized. Frequently insulin requirement drops after delivery and the patient with gestational diabetes will require no insulin at all.[14]

The preferred methods of contraception are barrier methods or sterilization if the patient has completed her childbearing. Low-dose oral con-

Table 9-4. Values for the 75-g Glucose Tolerance Test

	Normal	Impaired Glucose Tolerance	DM
Fasting blood sugar	<115 mg/dl	<140 mg/dl	>140 mg/dl
30, 60, and 90 minutes	All <200	1 value >200	1 value >200
120 minutes	<140	140–199	>200

Source: from ref. 3. Reprinted with permission.

traceptives can be used in women with GDM. Among the oral contraceptives, the newer progestational agents (i.e., Desogesterol) have less of an effect on lipid metabolism and should probably be recommended if available.

Approximately 20–50% of woman with GDM will develop overt DM or impaired glucose tolerance in their lifetime. At the 6-week postpartum visit a 75-g, 2-hour glucose tolerance test is performed on all women with GDM to detect overt diabetes or impaired glucose tolerance.[15] Normal values are listed in Table 9-4. Long-term recommendations to decrease the incidence of Type II DM include a diet high in complex carbohydrates and low in fat, weight loss in the obese patient, and exercise.

DIABETES THAT PREDATES THE PREGNANCY

Type I DM is characterized by an absolute deficiency of endogenous insulin, whereas type II DM is characterized by increased insulin resistance and relative insulin insufficiency. Type I generally presents as White's classes B through R, whereas Type II diabetes generally presents as classes A1, A2, or B in the pregnant woman.

Preconceptual Counseling

Since impaired glycemic control predates the pregnancy in these patients preconceptual counseling is key for optimal prevention of maternal and fetal complications.[16] First the physician should perform a baseline evaluation to assess the extent of the woman's disease. This session provides an opportunity to search for vascular involvement in these patients. A 24-hour urine collection for total protein and creatinine clearance, BUN, and serum creatinine are obtained to evaluate the patient for nephropathy. The patient should also undergo an evaluation for hypertension and ischemic heart disease. A retinal examination should be done to diagnose proliferative retinopathy with therapy preferably initiated prior to pregnancy. Other helpful consultations that are obtained include the nutritionist for optimal dietary management and the nephrologist if abnormal renal function exists. Preconceptual counseling should be aimed at maintaining euglycemia at the time of conception and early gestation. Euglycemia is defined as it is during pregnancy in these patients (fasting and preprandial blood glucose <100 mg/dL and postprandial blood glucose <120 mg/dL). The goal is to maintain normalization or near-normalization of glucose to the level seen in nondiabetic individuals. This can be assessed by normalization of glycosylated hemoglobin. Miller et al. report malformation rates increasing based on increasing HbA1c levels.[17] HbA1c is the major glycosylated hemoglobin that is measured in many laboratories as a substitute for glycosylated hemoglobin. Hypoglycemic and hyperglycemic episodes should also be minimized.

Patients on oral hypoglycemics should be switched to insulin. The maintenance of euglycemia prior to conception and in early gestation has been shown to decrease the rates of anomalies and decrease the rate of spontaneous abortions to near that of the general population.

Imperative in the discussion with the patient prior to pregnancy is a discussion of the effects pregnancy will have on her disease and the effect her disease will have on the pregnancy. In general, pregnancy is not believed to worsen the course of diabetes with a few exceptions: proliferative retinopathy may worsen and in the women with marginal renal function, creatinine clearance may worsen.[18] Creatinine clearance, however, is generally felt to return to prepregnancy values postpartum provided the pregravid

serum creatinine is less than 1.5 mg/dL. Glycemic control is made more difficult by the diabetogenic effect of pregnancy often requiring increasing insulin doses in the second and third trimesters or starting insulin in someone previously controlled by diet or oral hypoglycemics. Insulin requirements may decrease in the first trimester. Diabetic ketoacidosis (DKA) is also more common. Nausea and vomiting early in gestation or NPO status during labor may also lead to hypoglycemic episodes with ketosis.

Diabetes has far-reaching consequences for the pregnancy. Inadequate glycemic control early in gestation has been associated with diabetic embryopathy. Growth abnormalities are seen quite commonly in the pregnancies of diabetic patients. Maternal hyperglycemia is associated with fetal macrosomia. With increasing vascular disease, growth restriction may be noted due to impaired blood supply leading to decreased fetal nutrition and oxygenation. These women are also at increased risk for hypertensive complications especially toward the end of pregnancy. The perinatal death rate is also increased.

The incidence of spontaneous abortions, pyelonephritis, preterm labor, hydramnios, and postpartum hemorrhage are increased in the diabetic patient as is the rate of cesarean section. The offspring of women with Type II DM and GDM are at increased risk of developing DM in their lifetime.[19]

Antenatal Management of the Woman with Diabetes Mellitus

The antenatal management of the patient with pregestational diabetes is similar to that of the woman class A2 GDM (Table 9-5). Attention must be directed at maintaining euglycemia and detecting and treating maternal and fetal complications that may develop.

At the initial prenatal visit a general health assessment should be made. This includes a general history and physical examination, assessment of blood pressure, retinal examination, glycosylated hemoglobin determinations, 24-hour urine for protein and creatinine clearance,

Table 9-5. Antenatal Management of Pregestational Diabetes

	First Trimester	Second Trimester	Third Trimester
Laboratory evaluation	Glycosylated hemoglobin 24-hour urine for protein and creatinine clearance BUN Creatinine Urine culture	Glycosylated hemoglobin 24-hour urine for protein and creatinine clearance BUN Creatinine Urine culture Triple screen	Glycosylated hemoglobin 24-hour urine for protein and creatinine clearance BUN Creatinine Urine culture
Fetal testing	Ultrasound for dating and viability	Level II ultrasound	Fetal movement counts NST/BPP Ultrasound for growth

BPP, biophysical profile; NST, nonstress test; BUN, blood urea nitrogen.

and serum BUN and creatinine determinations. Oral hypoglycemics are stopped and insulin started. This allows tighter control of glucose levels. There is also a risk of severe neonatal hypoglycemia in the infant of the patient who delivers while on oral hypoglycemic agents. The dietitian is consulted early in gestation and the patient's diet is adjusted for the increased caloric demands of pregnancy (approximately 300 kcal/day). Patients are generally placed on a combination of short- and intermediate-acting insulin after observation of the patient's control on diet or her current insulin regimen.

Glucose is monitored with fasting, preprandial, 2-hour postprandial, and bedtime capillary glucose determinations. Again the goals are preprandial glucose <100 mg/dL and postprandial glucose <120 mg/dL. Insulin is adjusted to maintain these glucose levels. Most of our patients, both gestational and pregestational, are managed on an outpatient basis. Inability to control glucose, inability of the patient to understand home glucose monitoring or insulin administration, and noncompliance may be indications for admission at least temporarily for glucose control. Most patient's are on a schedule of three to four injections of insulin daily.

A retinal examination and laboratory evaluation consisting of BUN and creatinine, 24-hour urine if proteinuria is detected, glycosylated hemoglobin, and a clean voided urine sample for culture are performed each trimester. Also important in the evaluation of these patients is ma-

ternal serum alpha-fetoprotein because these patients are at high risk (19.5/1000 live births) for the development of neural tube defects. The triple screen should be offered to all patients if available.

Ultrasound evaluation is important in the pregnancy of the woman with DM. An initial ultrasound for establishment of the correct obstetrical dating and viability may be necessary. A targeted ultrasound at 18–20 weeks is necessary due to the high incidence of congenital anomalies in these patients. There should be special attention to fetal cardiac anatomy during this ultrasound. Ultrasound is also helpful in evaluation of fetal growth in the third trimester. Patient's with DM are at risk for the development of fetal macrosomia. Patients who have vascular disease in addition to diabetes are also at risk for developing IUGR. Ultrasound can be helpful in identifying these patients as well.

In addition to ultrasound evaluation, at our institution antenatal testing is instituted at 32 weeks in any patient on insulin consisting of twice-weekly nonstress tests. If a patient has hypertension, other vascular disease, other maternal or fetal complications, or inadequate glycemic control, development of a more intensive monitoring protocol or beginning testing earlier in gestation may be necessary. This may include such tests as the biophysical profiles or contraction stress tests. If the patient has a history of an intrauterine fetal demise, antenatal testing is done prior to the time of the previous demise. All patients should also do daily fetal movement counts starting at 28 weeks.

Labor and Delivery in the Woman with Diabetes Mellitus

Important concepts in the management of the labor and delivery of the diabetic pregnant woman are the timing of delivery, glucose control in the puerpeural period and the route of delivery. When to deliver is determined by a number of factors. In the absence of any complications we elect to deliver all women with diabetes at or near term. If, however, glucose control is inadequate, fetal growth disorders are encountered (IUGR or macrosomia), or the development of pregnancy-induced hypertension or mild preeclampsia occurs, amniocentesis (if these conditions occur prior to 39 weeks) is advocated along with delivery with documentation of fetal lung maturity. If abnormal fetal testing occurs it is managed appropriately. Route of delivery becomes an issue with the macrosomic fetus. Consideration must be given to elective cesarean section if the diabetic patient has a fetus that is estimated to be greater than 4000–4500 g due to the greater incidence of shoulder dystocia in these infants as a result of their truncal obesity.[10]

Women with pregestational DM are more likely to require continuous intravenous insulin infusions in labor (Table 9-3). Generally patients require between 0.5 and 1.5 units of regular insulin per hour. The intravenous insulin infusion allows one to prevent DKA and episodes of hypoglycemia in the laboring patient. We aim to maintain blood glucose <100 mg/dL throughout labor. Intravenous regular insulin has a half-life of approximately 30 minutes, allowing for the rapid and accurate adjustment of glucose levels. These patients are maintained on an NPO status with intravenous glucose-containing solutions. Capillary glucose levels are checked hourly. Urine should also be checked for ketones.

If elective cesarean delivery is to be performed the patient withholds her morning insulin and the surgery is performed in the morning. Regional anesthesia is preferred to allow for detection of signs of hypoglycemia.

Concerns for the Neonate

Neonatal complications are encountered more frequently in the infant of the woman with DM. This includes an increased risk of congenital anomalies that may have implications for the neonatal management. For example, certain cardiac lesions may require surgical repair such as ventricular septal defects and atrial septal defects. Prematurity is encountered more frequently due to the early delivery as a result of the development of maternal complications such as preeclampsia, worsening renal function, or fetal complications resulting from uteroplacental insufficiency or acidosis. This prematurity may lead to respiratory distress syndrome in some infants. Metabolic abnormalities are also seen more commonly such as hypoglycemia, hypomagnesemia, hypocalcemia, and hyperbilirubinemia. Polycythemia and its resultant hyperviscosity may also occur. Cardiomyopathy which may be a reflection of poor maternal glycemic control is seen. Disturbances of fetal growth are not uncommon in the infant of the woman with DM such as macrosomia or growth restriction in patients with vascular disease. Stillbirth continues to be seen with a higher frequency in the pregnancies of woman with DM. The hallmark of prevention of all of these complications is the maintenance of maternal euglycemia both antenatally and in the intrapartum period.

Postpartum

In the postpartum period strict glucose control can be relaxed. In the insulin-dependent diabetic, insulin requirements typically decrease dramatically after delivery of the placenta. Usually continuous insulin infusions can be stopped and the patient can be managed with subcutaneous injections of regular insulin as needed. Capillary glucose levels are generally checked every 4–6 hours, however, glucose levels should be maintained at approximately 150–200 mg/dL.

We continue to encourage patients to maintain the antenatal diet; however, the diet can also be liberalized postpartum. Caloric requirements must be adjusted for the postpartum state and lactation.

Contraception remains a concern in women with DM. Barrier methods are the best means of reversible contraception with sterilization being recommended for permanent contraception. Due to the interference of hormonal preparations with glucose metabolism and lipid profiles these agents are not encouraged. However, if a more reliable form of contraception is needed than a barrier method, low-dose oral contraceptives can be used. Monitoring of blood pressure and lipid profiles is important in patients on these medications, especially if vascular disease or other risk factors for cardiovascular disease exists.

Although breast feeding is not contraindicated in diabetic women the clinician must remember that insulin requirements may fall with breast feeding and caloric requirements increase (approximately 500 additional kcal/day). Adjustments should be made for these changes.

The postpartum period also affords the clinician the opportunity to emphasize the importance of preconceptual counseling and maintenance of euglycemia prior to any future pregnancies. The patient also can be counseled about the importance of weight reduction and diet for her long-term health concerns.

Maternal Complications Associated with Diabetes Mellitus

Maternal complications associated with DM include nephropathy, retinopathy, hypertension, hypoglycemia, DKA, and cardiovascular disease, as well as an increased risk of cesarean delivery and birth trauma.

Nephropathy is seen in women with long-standing DM and may be related to long-term glucose control. Management of these patients includes a low-protein diet.[20] There must be vigilant attention to blood pressure in these patients. A 24-hour urine collection for protein and creatinine clearance is obtained in each trimester as well as monitoring BUN, serum creatinine, and fetal growth. Fetal testing is also indicated starting at 28–32 weeks. The natural course of nephropathy does not appear to be accelerated by pregnancy; however, renal function may improve in the first trimester yet worsen in the second or third trimester. Generally renal function returns to baseline in the postpartum period. These patients are at increased risk for hypertensive complications during pregnancies. Poor pregnancy outcome is associated with the co-existence of hypertension, severe proteinuria, renal failure, or increased serum creatinine.

A frequently encountered difficulty in these patients is detecting the presence of preeclampsia and distinguishing it from worsening renal function. We obtain a baseline 24-hour urine specimen for protein and creatinine clearance in all insulin-requiring women to establish a standard upon which one can compare in the event that other signs and symptoms of preeclampsia develop. Twenty-four-hour urinary calcium may also be helpful in making this distinction. Low urinary calcium levels have been associated with preeclampsia.[21]

Retinopathy has also been seen in these patients. Consultation with opthalmology in each trimester to assess the development or progression of proliferative retinopathy is suggested. This complication can impact on the route of delivery as elective cesarean section may be recommended in patients with proliferative retinopathy to prevent rupture due to increased intracranial pressure during the second stage of labor. Proliferative retinopathy may progress in pregnancy despite the rapid institution of tight control of glycemia. For these reasons proliferative retinopathy should be identified and treated during pregnancy. Laser therapy is not contraindicated in pregnancy.[22]

Hypertension and vascular disease is seen more often in these patients and the physician caring for these patients must diligently search for these complications which may first be exhibited as growth restriction of the fetus since uterine and placental vessels may also be affected.

DKA may occur in pregnant women. DKA may occur at much lower glucose levels than in the nonpregnant patient. Glucose levels as low as 200 mg/dL have been associated with DKA in pregnant women. If a pregnant woman presents with nausea, vomiting, abdominal pain, malaise, ketonuria, altered level of consciousness, hypotension, hyperventilation, dehydration, polydipsia, polyuria, or a fruity odor to the breath, one must consider DKA. If DKA is suspected serum ketones should be obtained. Diagnosis is based on blood glucose levels > 300 mg/dL, arterial pH < 7.30, and serum HCO_3 < 15 mEq/L with ketonemia. Measurements of arterial blood gas, serum glucose, and electrolytes should be obtained on these patients. One must be vigilant in searching for infections in patients with DM as these can be the precipitating factors for the development of DKA. Pyelonephritis is particularly common in the pregnant woman with DM. Once the diagnosis of DKA is made these patients should be hospitalized in an intensive care unit. Intravenous hydration with normal saline with the addition of dextrose when blood glucose levels are <200 mg/dL. Regular intravenous insulin is added and glucose levels and electrolytes are monitored on an hourly basis. Electrolyte abnormalities should be corrected. If fetal viability has been reached continuous fetal monitoring is mandatory as there is a 50% risk of fetal death in patients that present with DKA. For a more detailed management scheme for DKA in pregnancy see Golde.[23]

Hypoglycemia may also be encountered if a meal is omitted when insulin has been taken or if too much insulin is taken. We instruct family members or support persons in the recognition and management of hypoglycemia. Patients are given glucagon for home use in the event of hypoglycemia and unresponsiveness. In general, hypoglycemia is much milder than this, only requiring increasing oral intake of glucose through milk or orange juice. Symptoms of hypoglycemia include jitteriness, altered level of consciousness, sweating, tremors, blurry or double vision, hunger, weakness, confusion, paresthesias, palpitations, anxiety, headaches, stupor,

and nausea. Hypoglycemia may be asymptomatic during pregnancy due to the patient acclimating to the tighter control and the pregnancy itself. In patients with longstanding Type I diabetes, a decreased epinephrine response to hypoglycemia may also lead to a lack of symptoms.[19] The goal of treatment is maintain blood sugar above 60 mg/dL.

Obstetrical complications of concern include increased rate of cesarean delivery. Macrosomia leading to cephalopelvic disproportion, unsuccessful induction of labor, and fetal distress probably leads to this increase. Rates range from 20–70% across centers. Patients with diabetes have poor wound healing; therefore, it is imperative that meticulous surgical technique be used using delayed absorbable suture in the closure of fascia with diligent identification and treatment of postoperative infections.

Fetal Complications Associated with Diabetes Mellitus

There is an increased risk of fetal complications in women with DM. These complications include spontaneous abortions, congenital anomalies, macrosomia, polyhydramnios, and IUGR.

There has been debate over whether the rate of spontaneous abortions in women with DM is changed. Although it appears that the rate in well-controlled diabetic women is no different than that of the general population, the rate of spontaneous abortions is increased in women with poorly controlled diabetes and this rate increases with increasing HbAlc.[24]

Congenital anomalies are more frequent in women with DM and the incidence increases with increasing HbAlc levels.[17] Neural tube defects are especially common. Neural tube defects including anencephaly, meningomyelocele, and encephalocele have an incidence of 19.5/1000 live births in diabetic women. Cardiac defects such as ventricular septal defect, atrial septal defects, cardiomyopathy, and septal hypertrophy are seen in the infants of diabetic women.[25] Sacral agenesis or caudal regression syndrome is the lesion thought to be pathognemonic for diabetes although it is also seen in nondiabetic patients. The incidence of sacral agenesis in women with diabetes is 1/200. Rates of malformation increase with impaired glucose control.

Macrosomia is seen in 20–50% of pregnancies complicated by DM compared to 6–7% of controls. These infants exhibit truncal obesity. They have increased glycogen and fat deposition in response to insulin produced by the fetal pancreas. This increases the risk of shoulder dystocia and cesarean delivery for cephalopelvic disproportion.

Polyhydramnios may also be seen in conjunction with macrosomia. This may be related to polyuria from an osmotic diuresis in the fetus related to hyperglycemia.

IUGR may also be seen in diabetic women, particularly in those with vascular disease. These women should be monitored antenatally with serial ultrasounds to detect growth disturbances and fetal testing to detect evidence of fetal compromise.

CONCLUSION

Diabetes is a complex problem in pregnancy which requires the interaction of the obstetrician, perinatologist, or an internist familiar with the changes of diabetes during pregnancy. It is imperative that the physician be diligent in detecting maternal and fetal complications. However, with close follow-up and attention to maintaining euglycemia, successful maternal and fetal outcomes can be achieved.

REFERENCES

1. White P. Pregnancy complicating diabetes. *Am J Med* 1949;7:609–616.
2. Moore TR. Diabetes in pregnancy. In Creasy RK, Resnik R (eds), *Maternal Fetal Medicine: Principles and Practice*, 3rd ed. Philadelphia: Saunders, 1994:934–978.
3. American College of Obstetricians and Gynecologists. Diabetes and Pregnancy. *ACOG Technical Bulletin 200*. Washington, DC: ACOG, 1994.
4. O'Sullivan JB, Mahan CM. Criteria for the oral glucose tolerance test in pregnancy. *Diabetes* 1964;13:278–285.
5. Catalano PM, Tyzbir ED, Wolfe RR, et al. Carbohydrate metabolism during pregnancy in control subjects and women with gestational diabetes. *Am J Physiol* 1993;264:E60–E67.
6. Catalano PM. Carbohydrate metabolism and gestational diabetes. *Clin Obstet Gynecol* 1994; 37:25–38.
7. Abrams RS, Coustan DR. Gestational diabetes update. *Clin Diab* 1990;8:19–24.
8. American Diabetes Association. Principles of nutrition and dietary recommendations for individuals with diabetes mellitus: 1979. *Diabetes* 1979;28:1027–1030.
9. Hollingsworth DR, Moore TR. Postprandial walking exercise in insulin-dependent (type I) diabetic women: Reduction of plasma lipid levels but absence of a significant effect on glycemic control. *Am J Obstet Gyncol* 1987;157:1359–1363.
10. Acker DB, Sachs BP, Friedman EA. Risk factors for shoulder dystocia. *Obstet Gynecol* 1985;66:762–768.
11. Kjos SL, Henry OA, Montoro M, et al. Insulin-requiring diabetes in pregnancy: A randomized trial of active induction of labor and expectant management. *Am J Obstet Gynecol* 1993;169:611–615.
12. Mondanlou HD, Komatsu G, Dorchester W, et al. Large-for-gestational-age neonates: Anthropometric reasons for shoulder dystocia. *Obstet Gynecol* 1982;60:417–423.
13. O'Sullivan MJ, Skyler JS, Raimer KA, et al. Diabetes and pregnancy. In Gleicher N (ed), *Principles and Practice of Medical Therapy in Pregnancy*, 2nd ed. Norwalk CT: Appleton and Lange, 1992;357–378.
14. Langer O. Diabetes in pregnancy. In Cherry S, Merkatz (eds), *Complications of Pregnancy: Medical, Surgical, Gynecologic, Psychosocial, and Perinatal*, 4th ed. Baltimore: Williams & Wilkins, 1991, pp. 979–993.
15. Catalano PM, Vargo KM, Bernstein IM, et al. Incidence and risk factors associated with abnormal postpartum glucose tolerance in women

with gestational diabetes. *Am J Obstet Gynecol* 1991;165:914–919.

16. Goldman JA, Dicker D, Feldberg D, et al. Pregnancy outcome in patients with insulin dependent diabetes mellitus with preconceptual diabetic control: A comparative study. *Am J Obstet Gynecol* 1986;155:293–297.

17. Miller E, Hare JW, Cloherty JP, et al. Elevated maternal HbA1c in early pregnancy and major congenital anomalies in infants of diabetic mothers. *N Engl J Med* 1981;304:1331–1334.

18. Landon MB. Diabetes mellitus and other endocrine diseases. In Gabbe SG, Niebyl JR, Simpson JL (eds), *Obstetrics: Normal and Problem Pregnancies*, 2nd ed. New York: Churchill Livingstone, 1991, pp. 1097–1116.

19. Hagay ZJ, Reece EA. Diabetes mellitus in pregnancy. In Reece EA, Hobbins JC, Mahoney MJ, et al. (eds), *Medicine of the Fetus and Mother.* Philadelphia: Lippincott, 1992, pp. 982–1020.

20. Cohen D, Dodds R, Viberti G. Effect of protein restriction in insulin-dependent diabetics at risk of nephropathy. *Br Med J* 1987;294:795–798.

21. Taufield PA, Ales KL, Resnick LM, et al. Hypocalciuria in preeclampsia. *N Engl J Med* 1987;316:715–718.

22. Dibble CM, Kochenour NK, Worley RJ, et al. Effects of pregnancy on diabetic retinopathy. *Obstet Gynecol* 1982;59:699.

23. Golde SH. Diabetic ketoacidosis in pregnancy. In Clark SL, Cotton DB, Hankins GDV, et al., (eds), *Critical Care Obstetrics*, 2nd ed. Oxford: Blackwell Scientific Publishers, 1991, pp. 329–339.

24. Miodovnik M, Skillmamn C, Holroyde JC, et al. Elevated maternal glycohemoglobin in early pregnancy and spontaneous abortion among insulin-dependent diabetic women. *Am J Obstet Gynecol* 1985;153:439–442.

25. Becerra JE, Khoury MJ, Cordero JF, et al. Diabetes mellitus during pregnancy and the risks for specific birth defects: A population based Case Control Study. *Pediatrics* 1990;85:1–9.

QUESTIONS

1. Which of the following is true:
   a. Benign retinopathy frequently progresses during pregnancy.
   b. Proliferative retinopathy should be treated with laser therapy postpartum if diagnosed during the pregnancy.
   c. Benign retinopathy requires cesarean delivery.
   d. The presence of benign retinopathy changes the patient's White classification to D.

2. Risk factors for the development of gestational diabetes mellitus include all of the following except:
   a. Obesity.
   b. Glycosuria.
   c. Hypertension.
   d. History of an intrauterine fetal demise in a previous pregnancy.
   e. History of a macrosomic infant in a previous pregnancy.

3. All of the following are metabolic abnormalities commonly seen in the infants of diabetic mothers except:
   a. Hypoglycemia.
   b. Hypomagnesemia.
   c. Hypobilirubinemia.
   d. Hypocalcemia.

4. Women with diabetes mellitus are at increased risk of all of the following pregnancy complications except:
   a. Congenital malformations.
   b. Spontaneous abortion.
   c. Premature delivery.
   d. Preeclampsia.
   e. Incompetent cervix.

5. The diagnosis of gestational diabetes mellitus is based on:
   a. Persistent glycosuria.
   b. Two abnormal values on a 75-g oral glucose tolerance test.
   c. Two abnormal values on a 100-g oral glucose tolerance test.
   d. Two abnormal values on a 50-g oral glucose tolerance test.
   e. Fasting blood glucose persistently above 105 mg/dl.

6. Using a cutoff of 130 mg/dl when compared to 140 mg/dl does which of the following?
   a. Increases sensitivity and increases specificity.
   b. Increases sensitivity and decreases specificity.
   c. Decreases sensitivity and increases specificity.
   d. Decreases sensitivity and decreases specificity.

7. Oral hypoglycemic agents are avoided in pregnancy because:

a. An increased risk of fetal anomalies has been seen.

b. It is impossible to control a pregnant woman's glucose levels with oral hypoglycemics.

c. Microcephaly has been seen more frequently in the infants of women taking oral hypoglycemics.

d. There is a risk of neonatal hypoglycemia in the infant of the woman taking oral hypoglycemics.

For questions 8, 9, and 10 use the following:

    a. 1, 2, and 3 are correct.

    b. 1 and 3 are correct.

    c. 2 and 4 are correct.

    d. Only 4 is correct.

    e. All are correct.

8. In the patient with impaired renal function:

    a. Creatinine clearance usually decreases in the second trimester.

    b. Creatinine clearance returns to the prepregnant baseline postpartum.

    c. Creatinine clearance usually decreases in the third trimester.

    d. Creatinine clearance typically increases in the first trimester.

9. Screening laboratory tests obtained in women on insulin therapy include:

    a. Cholesterol.

    b. Glycosylated hemoglobin.

    c. Triglycerides.

    d. Serum creatinine.

10. Shoulder dystocia:

    a. Is more common in the infants of women with diabetes mellitus than in the normal controls even if the birthweights are the same.

    b. May be seen in diabetes more commonly due to increased fetal fat deposition.

    c. May be seen more commonly in the infants of women with diabetes mellitus due to increased glycogen deposition in the liver.

    d. Occurs in 6–7% of diabetic pregnancies.

10

Pulmonary Diseases and Disorders During Pregnancy and the Effects on Mother and Fetus

Yogesh G. Shah

PHYSIOLOGIC CHANGES IN THE RESPIRATORY SYSTEM DURING GESTATION

Changes in pulmonary physiology occurring in pregnancy are well documented, but effects of pulmonary diseases in pregnancy are not well understood. Even though there is significant increase in ventilation in pregnancy, respiratory insufficiency is uncommon.

During pregnancy, oxygen consumption increases by 20–30% due to the needs of the fetoplacental unit and maternal requirements.[1] Despite increased oxygen consumption, arterial oxygen pressure (PaO_2) is maintained at normal levels above 90 mm Hg by virtue of hyperventilation. The hyperventilation of pregnancy is associated with changes in carbon dioxide tension (PCO_2) below 35 mm Hg. This chronic respiratory alkalosis of pregnancy is partially compensated for by increased renal bicarbonate excretion. The arterial pH is, however, not altered from the nonpregnant level of about 7.4.[2] The increase in ventilation and associated fall in PCO_2 that occur in pregnancy are due to respiratory stimulant effect of progesterone. Total oxygen consumption and basal metabolic rate also increase by 20% and 15%, respectively. Oxygenation is significantly reduced in supine position and hence, when arterial blood gas analysis is indicated in pregnancy, the sample should be drawn in an upright position.[3]

The following changes occur in terms of pulmonary function by term[4]:

1. Decrease in residual volume (20%), functional residual capacity (20%), expiratory reserve volume (21%) and total lung capacity (5%).
2. Increase in inspiratory capacity (6%), tidal volume (33%), and respiratory quotient (from 0.76 to 0.83).
3. No changes in vital capacity or forced expiratory volume in 1 second (FEV_1).

During painful labor there is relative hypoventilation between contractions resulting in decreased maternal PO_2. Liberal use of oxygen in laboring patients without regional anesthesia is indicated in any patients with any respiratory impairment. The gravid uterus pushes the diaphragm by 4 cm above its usual resting position and the chest enlarges in its transverse diameter by 2.1 cm. The subcostal angle increases progressively from an average of 68.5° in early pregnancy to 103.5° during the third trimester.[5]

DYSPNEA OF PREGNANCY

Dyspnea is a frequent symptom in normal pregnancy. By 20 weeks, 50% of women are aware of shortness of breath at rest, long before any mechanical effects of the enlarging uterus can be expected. Maximum incidence of breathlessness occurs between 28 and 31 weeks gestation.[6] The two most common explanations offered for dyspnea of pregnancy are that: (1) it is related to hyperventilation of pregnancy and (2) it is due to changes in the thorax.

Dyspnea is a worrisome symptom for the clinician because it can be caused by pulmonary emboli or a diffuse lung condition. In the absence of any other cardiorespiratory symptom, normal findings on examination and a chest x ray should be sufficient to exclude pathology in most cases. Another useful test is to measure transcutaneous oxygen saturation. The normal saturation is greater than 95%, and it should not fall on moderate exercise. Additional test that may be indicated is assessment of arterial blood gases (ABGs).

BRONCHIAL ASTHMA

Asthma is one of the most common illnesses that complicates pregnancy. Approximately 4% of pregnancies are complicated by bronchial asthma. It is estimated that 10% of the population appears to have nonspecific airway hyperreactivity. Uncontrolled asthma can be associated with increases in maternal-fetal morbidity and mortality.

Definition

Asthma is a lung disease with the following characteristics:

1. airway obstruction that is partially or completely reversible either spontaneously or with treatment;
2. airway inflammation; and
3. increases airway responsiveness to a variety of stimuli.[7]

Pathogenesis

Asthma is characterized by airway hyperresponsiveness with bronchoconstriction in response to physical, chemical, and pharmacologic agents. Several mechanisms have been proposed to explain airway hyperresponsiveness in asthma. They include:

1. airway inflammation;
2. bronchial epithelial injury;
3. altered autonomic neural control of airways with abnormal local release of neuropeptides with defective smooth muscle relaxation, mucosal vascular congestion, and edema;
4. hypertrophic smooth muscle with impaired relaxation; and
5. alterations in the volume and composition of airway liquid lining layer, defects in bronchial blood flow, and abnormal airway geometry.[8]

Diagnosis

Asthma may present for the first time during pregnancy and the diagnosis may be confused with physiologic dyspnea of pregnancy. Diagnosis of asthma is based on medical history and physical examination combined with laboratory test results. The symptoms of asthma include cough, wheezing, dyspnea, and tightness in chest. These symptoms may be episodic, waxing and waning, nocturnal, and seasonal. Symptoms may result from specific triggers, for example, infection, allergens, environmental irritants, occupational exposures, drugs, food additives, weather, menses, exercise and gastroesophageal reflux.[7] The history is often positive for rhinitis, sinusitis, eczema, or allergies.

During an acute exacerbation, the physical examination may reveal hyperinflation, prolonged duration of expiration, wheezing, and use of accessory respiratory muscles.

Diagnostic tests include:

• Complete blood count
• Chest x ray
• Sputum examination and stain for eosinophilia

- Nasal secretion stain for eosinophils and neutrophils
- Pulmonary function test
- In selected cases rhinoscopy, sinus x rays, skin testing to determine specific immunoglobulin E (IgE) antibodies to common inhalant allergens

Differential diagnosis should include:

- Upper airway mechanical obstruction
- Laryngeal dysfunction
- Chronic bronchitis
- Chronic emphysema
- Pulmonary edema
- Pulmonary infiltrate with eosinophilia
- Infectious bronchitis and bronchiectasis
- Cystic fibrosis (CF)
- Pulmonary embolism and
- Physiologic dyspnea of pregnancy

Effect of Asthma on Mother and Fetus

Epidemiologic studies have shown a statistically significant increase in preterm births, low-birth-weight infants, growth retardations, and neonatal hypoxia in the pregnancies of women with asthma compared to control pregnancies.[9] Also there is a statistically significant increase in hyperemesis gravidarum, vaginal hemorrhage, toxemia, and a significant increase in induced and complicated labors in the asthmatic gravid patient versus control pregnant patient. Severe asthma during pregnancy may be a cause of maternal mortality. There is no increased incidence of congenital malformations. The most important cause of adverse outcome appears to be poor asthma control.

Effect of Pregnancy on Asthma

The course of asthma may change during pregnancy. In a combined series of 1087 patients from the literature, the course of asthma improved in 36%, worsened in 23%, and remained unchanged in 41%.[10] Women with severe asthma prior to pregnancy are more likely to deteriorate during pregnancy. The peak inci-

dence of exacerbation appears to be between the 24th and 35th weeks of gestation. It is also of interest that severity is often consistent among successive pregnancies in individual women. Asthma generally remains quiescent during labor and delivery.

A number of hypotheses have been offered to explain the variable effect of pregnancy on asthma. Some of the factors that may improve asthma include: increased serum free cortisol, progesterone, prostaglandin E- and prostaglandin I_2-mediated bronchodilation and stabilization, atrial-natriuretic mediated factor, bronchodilation, glucocorticoid mediated increased beta-adrenergic responsiveness. Factors that have been implicated with worsening of asthma are pulmonary refractoriness to cortisol effects, prostaglandin F_2-alpha mediated bronchoconstriction, increased stress, and pulmonary capillary permeability. Leukotrienes may also mediate changes in airway tone during pregnancy.[11]

Management

The goals of asthma therapy in the gravid patient are:

1. To try and maintain normal pulmonary function
2. To control symptoms
3. To maintain normal activity levels
4. To prevent acute exacerbations of asthma
5. To avoid adverse effects from asthma medications with a delivery of a healthy neonate

All asthmatics require close clinical surveillance during pregnancy. The best objective assessment can be provided by peak expiratory flow rate (PEFR). It correlates well with FEV_1 (volume of air expired in 1 second from maximum inspiration). PEFR monitoring is essential for detecting deterioration of asthma, predicting acute exacerbations, and assessing response to therapy. All pregnant women with moderate to severe asthma should monitor their PEFR with a home peak flow meter device. These patients should monitor in the morning and then 12 hours later. Predicted values of PEFR are in the range of 380–550 L/min and do not change dur-

Table 10-1. Drugs and Dosages for Asthma and Associated Conditions Preferred for Use During Pregnancy*

Drug Class	Specific Drug	Dosage
Antiinflammatory	Cromolyn sodium	2 puffs qid (inhalation)
		2 sprays in each nostril bid–qid (intranasal for nasal symptoms)
	Beclomethasone	2–5 puffs bid–qid (inhalation)
		2 sprays in each nostril bid (intranasal for allergic rhinitis)
	Prednisone	Burst for active symptoms: 40 mg/day, single or divided dose for 1 week, then taper for 1 week. If prolonged course is required, single am dose on alternate days may minimize adverse effects.
Bronchodilator	Inhaled beta-agonist	2 puffs every 4 hours as needed
	Theophylline	Oral: dose to reach serum concentration level of 8–12 μg/mL
Antihistamine	Chlorpheniramine	4 mg by mouth up to qid
		8–12 mg sustained-release bid
	Tripelennamine	25–50 mg by mouth up to qid
		100 mg sustained-release bid
Decongestant	Pseudoephedrine	60 mg by mouth up to qid
		120 mg sustained-release bid
	Oxymetazoline	Intranasal spray or drops up to 5 days for rhinosinusitis
Cough	Guaifenesin	2 tsp by mouth qid
	Dextromethorphan	
Antibiotics	Amoxicillin	3 weeks therapy for sinusitis

Source: Report on the Working Group on Asthma and Pregnancy, *Management of Asthma During Pregnancy.* Washington, DC: National Institutes of Health, 1993.

*This table presents drugs and suggested dosages for the home management of asthma and associated conditions.

ing the course of pregnancy. A personal best PEFR should be established when asthma is best controlled.[7]

Most drugs used for treatment of asthma in pregnancy are safe. Most commonly used drugs shown in Table 10-1 are not known to be teratogenic and are not associated with fetotoxic or fetal growth retarding effects. Inhaled beta-agonists are considered drugs of first choice for treatment of asthma in pregnancy. These drugs are more potent bronchodilators than the methylxanthines and are less systemically absorbed.[12] Drugs for asthma that are contraindicated during pregnancy include alpha-adrenergic compounds, epinephrine, iodides, sulphonamides (in third trimester), tetracyclines, and quinolones.[7]

General guidelines for management of:

1. Mild chronic asthma
   a. Assess PEFR—if ≥80% of baseline then most patients are asymptomatic.
   b. Pretreat with a beta-agonist and/or cromolyn for exposure to exercise or allergen.
   c. Symptomatic patient with PEFR varying 20% or more—treat with inhaled beta-agonist with 2 puffs every 3–4 hours prn for the duration of episode until symptoms are controlled.

2. Chronic moderate asthma with following clinical characteristics:
   a. symptoms >1–2 times/week,
   b. exacerbations affecting sleep or activity and/or lasting several days with,
   c. occasional acute care.

   Management of chronic moderate asthma includes:

   d. Assess PEFR which may vary 20–30% when symptomatic;
   e. treatment with antiinflammatory agents—cromolyn 2 puffs 4 times a day or inhaled corticosteroids 2–4 puffs twice a day; and
   f. inhaled beta-agonist prn to 3–4 times per day. Additional therapy may include oral beta agonist and/or sustained-release theophylline and/or increased inhaled corticosteroids.

3. Chronic severe asthma: Includes outline of treatment as for patients with moderate asthma in conjunction with oral steroids. All patients with severe asthma should be evaluated by a pulmonologist.

All patients with asthma should be monitored for abnormal growth and fetal activity with biometric parameters and other tests of fetal well-being which includes ultrasound, electronic fetal monitoring, and daily self-assessment of fetal movements.

During Labor and Delivery

General principles of treatment include continuation of treatment of the patient's scheduled asthma medications, monitor PEFR on admission, hydration, and providing adequate pain relief to limit risk of bronchospasm. Patients who are steroid-dependent should be given 100 mg hydrocortisone every 8 hours until 24 hours postpartum to treat for possible adrenal suppression. For labor induction, oxytocin is the drug of choice. Use of prostaglandin E_2 gel for cervical ripening is not contraindicated.[13] Use of 15-methyl prostaglandin F_2-alpha should be avoided because it has been reported to cause bronchospasm in patients with asthma.[14]

Narcotics should not be used if there is an acute asthma exacerbation. For analgesia, morphine and meperidine should be avoided and the preferred agent may be fentanyl. Lumbar epidural analgesia enhances bronchodilator therapy in patients with asthma exacerbation.[15] Oxytocin remains the drug of choice for postpartum hemorrhage. Ergot derivatives and prostaglandin F_2-alpha are contraindicated because they may cause bronchospasm.[14,16] If prostaglandin treatment is necessary, the safest analog is prostaglandin E_2 which is less likely to cause bronchospasm.

TUBERCULOSIS

The rate of tuberculosis (TB) is increasing in many areas of the world including the United States. In the United States, 25,701 cases of TB were reported in 1990, an increase of 16% since 1985.[17] The three major factors contributing to the increase in reported cases are (1) coexistence with the human immunodeficiency virus (HIV), (2) increase immigration of people to the United States from countries with a high prevalence of TB, thus enlarging the pool of infected individuals, and (3) general decline in public health services and medical access.

From 1986 to 1989, 22% of persons developing TB in United States were foreign-born. In 1989, the estimated tuberculosis rate for foreign-born persons arriving in the United States was 13 times greater than the overall U.S. rate.[18] The majority of these immigrants have had a chest radiograph, but no tuberculin skin test to detect asymptomatic infection.

The epidemiology of TB and pregnancy is unknown. From 1966 to 1972, the incidence of TB during pregnancy at New York Lying-In Hospital ranged from 0.6–1.0%. During this period, 3.2% of the patients with culture-proven pulmonary TB were first diagnosed during pregnancy, a rate equal to that of nonpregnant women of comparable age.[19] However, with increased immigration of foreign-born individuals and an epidemic of HIV infection, it is likely that the number of women in the United States at risk for TB during or after pregnancy is again rising.

The pathogenesis of TB during pregnancy is consistent with transmission in all adults in which the tubercle bacillus is inhaled.[2] Organs most commonly seeded during the lymphohematogenous phase are apices of the lungs, spleen, liver, meninges, bone/joints, genitalia, endometrium, or placenta. Pulmonary TB and asymptomatic Purified Protein Derivative (PPD) skin test conversions are most common manifestations. Tuberculosis in the fetus can be acquired through various routes: (1) hematogenous: from the umbilical vein, (2) aspiration of infected amniotic fluid in utero or infected material at birth, (3) acquisition of infected material from the mother or attendant during neonatal period by inhalation, ingestion or contamination of traumatized skin or mucous membranes.[20] Infection of the newborn through umbilical cord is rare.[21] These infants' mothers frequently suffer from TB meningitis, pleural effusion, or miliary spread during pregnancy or soon after.[22,23]

The liver is a major site of involvement in congenital TB. The next most common site of congenital infection is the lung. A lower incidence of fetal involvement of the lungs compared to the liver may be due to lower oxygen content and hypoaeration of the lungs.[24] The other sites of congenital infection are bone marrow, bone, gastrointestinal (GI) tract, adrenal glands, spleen kidney, abdominal lymph nodes, and skin. The histologic patterns of involvement are similar to those in adults; tubercles and granuloma are common.

Effect of Pregnancy on Tuberculosis

By the early twentieth century, many publications had appeared in the medical literature emphasizing the deleterious effect of pregnancy on TB. Termination of pregnancy was widely recommended for symptomatic pulmonary TB. In 1953, Hedvall[25] reported on 250 pregnant women with abnormal chest radiographs consistent with TB. He noted that there was no significant difference between the patients who improved and whose TB progressed during pregnancy and during a 1-year follow-up period. Most of the patients remained stable (83.9% during pregnancy and 76% during the 1-year follow-up), including those who had advanced pulmonary TB. Hedvall concluded that pregnancy did not alter the course of TB and termination of pregnancy is not recommended. Pregnancy also does not appear to alter the clinical presentation of TB. One half to two thirds of patients were asymptomatic and unaware of the disease in one report.[26]

In summary, the impact of pregnancy on TB appears minimal except for potentially obscuring the diagnosis and possibly increasing the risk of TB activation during the postpartum period.

Effect of Tuberculosis on Pregnancy

Two important issues need to be addressed with respect to the impact of TB on pregnancy. They are (1) impact on pregnancy pertaining to delivery and (2) impact of disease treatment with its effects on the fetus and newborn. There is no evidence that TB affects or complicates either the course of pregnancy or the type of delivery required.[19] With regard to maternal chemotherapy for tuberculosis, none of the drugs used conventionally are teratogenic. Streptomycin and other potential antibiotics should be avoided during pregnancy because of potential ototoxicity in the newborn infant.[27] Isoniazid is known to be associated with hepatitis and women in postpartum period are vulnerable to hepatotoxicity.[28] The effect on the neonate is complex.

Hematogenesis spread can occur via the umbilical vein with the liver being the most common site of infection. When congenital TB occurs, the most common symptoms are fever, hepatosplenomegaly, poor feeding, and irritability. Most newborns will have abnormal chest x rays and about one half will show a miliary pattern. Despite the potential for transmission in utero, a newborn's greatest risk of acquiring TB is in the postpartum period, especially if born to a mother whose sputum contains acid-fast bacilli (AFB) and whose condition is undiagnosed and untreated. Treatment of inactive, symptomless disease with isoniazid is postponed until after delivery. For patients with active disease, chemotherapy at any gestational age is mandatory.

Management

Antepartum Management

Ideally all patients should be screened by Mantoux technique, intradermal injection of 0.1 ml of 5 tuberculin units of PPD. The test is read at 48 to 72 hours. Induration greater than or equal to 5 mm is classified as positive in (1) persons with HIV infection, (2) in those with close, recent contact with persons with infectious TB and (3) in those who have chest x rays consistent with healed TB.

A reaction greater than or equal to 10 mm is positive in immigrants from high-prevalence countries, medically underserved, low-income Americans, and diabetics.[29] A reaction greater than or equal to 15 mm is positive in healthy individuals not at risk for TB. A negative Mantoux test result never rules out tuberculous disease. Negative skin test may be related to age, malnutrition, immunosuppression by disease or drugs, viral infection, and overwhelming TB. Many adults coinfected with HIV and mycobacterium tuberculosis have anergy for tuberculin. A chest film is recommended in (1) recent converters, (2) those with positive skin test and unknown time of conversion, or (3) when symptoms and signs suggest TB.

In women with positive skin test and without clinical evidence of active disease, prophylaxis with INH is withheld until delivery. Prophylaxis with INH 300 mg orally once daily for 12 months although there is evidence that 6 months of therapy is as effective. All women should be monitored for isoniazid (INH)-associated hepatotoxicity. Those over the age of 35 without special risk factors should generally not be given INH prophylaxis. A patient who has received a full course of treatment does not require treatment for a positive skin test. The Advisory Council for the Elimination of Tuberculosis (ACET) recommends prompt treatment for active TB. The initial treatment of untreated disease represents a far greater risk to a gravid patient and her unborn fetus than does appropriate chemotherapy.[30] The initial treatment for drug-susceptible pulmonary TB should consist of isoniazid (INH) 300 mg/day and rifampin 600 mg/day every day for 2 months, followed by INH 900 mg and rifampin 600 mg twice weekly for another 7 months. Pyridoxine 50 mg/day should be prescribed concurrently to reduce neurotoxicity. The total duration of the above treatment regimen is 9 months.

If INH resistance is suspected, ethambutol at 15–25 mg/kg/day is added to the regimen. When drug resistance is excluded, ethambutol can be discontinued.

The other drugs available for treatment of TB include:

- Pyrazinamide 30–40 mg/kg/day PO,
- Streptomycin 20 mg/kg/day IM, with maximum dose of 1 g/day,
- Ethionamide 15–20 mg/kg/day PO,
- Para-aminosalicylic acid (PAS) 4 g, 3 times a day PO,
- drugs like capreomycin, kanamycin, and cycloserine are associated with high incidences of systemic toxicity.

INH, rifampin, and ethambutol are not known to be teratogenic. Infants exposed to streptomycin in utero are at risk for eighth nerve damage. Abnormalities range from mild vestibular damage to bilateral nerve deafness. It is potentially hazardous throughout gestation. Other aminoglycosides with antituberculous activity, could also have similar fetal toxic effects. No data are available regarding use of pyrazinamide in pregnancy.[12]

Breast feeding is not contraindicated with maternal antituberculin therapy. Snider and Powell[31] concluded that a breast feeding infant would receive no more than 20% of the usual therapeutic dose of INH, and less than 11% of other antituberculosis drugs. When the infant is given prophylaxis, concomitant breast feeding should be avoided since the addition of INH in breast milk to the infant prophylactic dose of INH may lead to toxicity.

Neonatal Management

The general principles are preventing or treating early infection contracted in the neonatal period. Congenital infection is most commonly by maternal contact. Congenital tuberculosis is often associated with miliary TB and endometrial involvement in the mother. The risk of active disease during first year of life may be as high as 50% if prophylactic measures are not taken.[32] The two options for newborn protection include INH prophylaxis or Bacille-Calmette Guérin (BCG) vaccination. INH prophylaxis requires daily treatment and should be continued at least until the mother has been shown to be culture negative for 3 months. At that time, a Mantoux skin test is applied; if positive, INH is continued for a total duration of 9–12 months, but if negative, isoniazid is discontinued. If BCG vaccination is opted, the child must be kept out of the household until skin test result becomes reactive marking protection from infection. BCG vaccination is recommended for a neonate where compliance with chemotherapy cannot be assured and who is likely to be lost to follow-up.

CYSTIC FIBROSIS

Cystic fibrosis (CF) is the most common inherited disorder in the while population, affecting 1/2500 births. It has also been diagnosed in blacks, Indians, Native Americans, and Japanese; the incidence in these races is not known precisely. The clinical features of CF are as a result of abnormality of all exocrine glands with pulmonary involvement and pancreatic insufficiency. Of those infants reaching adult life, 20% will have evidence of portal hypertension and cardiovascular complications are encountered with larger survival of patients. The pathophysiologic abnormalities result from obstruction of glands or their ducts by abnormally viscous secretions.

The most severe manifestation of CF is bronchiectasis. The disease is characterized by frequent exacerbation with infection by *Pseudomonas aeruginosa*, *Staphylococcus aureus*, and *Hemophilus influenzae*. In most cases the pseudomonas is present in its usual ''rough'' form, but in time the dominant organism becomes the mutant mucoid pseudomonas which is found as a pathogen except in the CF lung. The respiratory dysfunction is the result of airway obstruction. Vital capacity is reduced, while residual volume and functional residual capacity are increased.[33] Other clinical manifestations include malabsorption, diabetes mellitus, hepatic and biliary disease, and interference with fertility.

Effect of Cystic Fibrosis on Pregnancy

Maternal disease affects the fetus and neonates. Kent et al.[34] reviewed 20 reports citing cases of pregnancy in women with CF. The rate of spontaneous abortion in 217 pregnancies in 162 women was 4.6%. The rate of preterm deliveries in the review was reported to be 24.3% and 82% of pregnancies progressed beyond 20 weeks. Perinatal death rate was 7.9%. Maternal death rate did not exceed that among age-related women with CF who were not pregnant. Edenborough et al.[35] reviewed outcomes of 22 pregnancies in 20 women with CF. In their retrospective study, they observed that weight gain during pregnancy, duration of gestation, birth weight, and maternal survival were positively correlated with prepregnancy %FEV_1 (forced expiratory volume in 1 second). Pancreatic insufficiency may be associated with poor perinatal outcome depending upon duration and severity of disease.[36,37]

Another area of concern would be with effects of antimicrobial therapy during pregnancy. Tetracyclines and ciprofloxacin should be avoided throughout pregnancy. Aminoglycosides are safe as long as serum levels are monitored. They can be used by both intravenous and inhaled routes. Cohen et al.[36] reported no congenital anomalies in 129 pregnancies, in 26 of which the mothers received aminoglycosides during pregnancy.

All children born to women with CF will be carriers of the CF gene. Also, 2.5% of births to women with CF will have CF.

Effect of Pregnancy on Cystic Fibrosis

There is no unamity of clinical opinion regarding the advisability of pregnancy in women with CF. Success of pregnancy depends on presence or absence of pulmonary emphysema, cor pulmonale, and measures of lung function. Maternal pulmonary hypertension is associated with a maternal mortality of 53%[38] and for Eisemenger's syndrome it is 31%.[39] In a study by Edenborough et al.,[35] mothers with prepregnancy %FEV_1 of >60% did well, while two-thirds of those with pre-pregnancy %FEV_1 of <60% died within 3.2 years of delivery. Pregnancy itself caused a significant decline in pulmonary function along with natural progression of lung disease. Mothers with mild prepregnancy pulmonary disease tolerated pregnancy well.

Management

Management of CF begins with preconceptual counseling and should include assessment of pulmonary function, presence or absence of pulmonary hypertension, pancreatic insufficiency, diabetes, and hepatobiliary disease. Patients with cor pulmonale, Eisemenger's syndrome, and FEV_1 of less than 60% should be counseled regarding increased perinatal morbidity and mortality along with increased maternal mortality. Cardiorespiratory management should be continued as in the nonpregnant patient. Caloric intake and maternal weight should be monitored closely. Enzyme replacement with oral pancreatic enzymes is safe and effective. Preterm labor and delivery presents a significant obstetrical risk. Patients should be counseled and educated regarding symptoms and signs of preterm labor. During labor, attention should be directed to fluid and electrolyte balance. Patients with CF lose large quantities of sodium in sweat and may easily become hypovolemic. Oxygen may be administered freely. Regional anesthesia is recommended for labor and delivery.

SARCOIDOSIS

Sarcoidosis is a chronic granulomatous disease of unknown etiology presenting with bilateral hilar lymphadenopathy, pulmonary infiltrates, and occasionally with skin and eye lesions. It is an uncommon complication of pregnancy affecting at most 1/2000 of all pregnancies. Blacks are affected at a rate tenfold that of whites. Most cases have an insidious onset of disease followed by progressive pulmonary fibrosis. Respiratory complaints are the presenting symptoms in 50% of all patients with sarcoidosis. Other clinical features include weight loss, fever, anorexia, skin lesion, eye disease, or neurologic abnormalities.

If sarcoidosis changes during pregnancy it usually improves, due to increase in free cortisol as well as total cortisol level. The condition may relapse in the puerperium.[2] The relapse is usually not serious and should not be a contraindication to pregnancy.

There is no known effect of sarcoidosis on the fetus or the pregnancy. There is no contraindication for pregnancy unless maternal pulmonary function is compromised secondary to pulmonary fibrosis. No special management is necessary for sarcoidosis. Determination of angiotensin-converting enzyme levels is not indicated in monitoring patients with sarcoid who become pregnant since the enzyme levels vary markedly independent of the disease activity.[40] Sarcoid granulomas can synthesize vitamin D, which occasionally causes hypercalcemia, and postpartum hypercalcemia sarcoidosis has been reported.[41] Hence, sarcoidosis patient should be cautioned not to take extra vitamin D supplements. Steroids for severe systemic or ocular, myocardial, or central nervous system (CNS) disease are not contraindicated. Steroid therapy for pulmonary disease is based on pulmonary function impairment and respiratory symptoms. When therapy is begun, the starting dose is 40–60 mg prednisone per day.

PNEUMONIAS

The prevalence of antepartum pneumonias has fallen from a rate in the preantibiotic era (before 1956) of 1/118[42] deliveries to 1/2288 deliveries.[43] The most recent review reported a rate of 1 per 1287 deliveries.[44] This increase attributed to a greater number of women with chronic respiratory disease, drug addiction, and altered immune state are achieving pregnancy. The lower lobes are most commonly involved with multilobar disease in 42% of patients.[45]

Bacterial

The most common of these are *Streptococcus pneumoniae*, *Hemophilus influenzae*, and *My-*

coplasma pneumoniae. Diagnosis requires high index of suspicion in women with respiratory complaints, including fever, chills, pleuritic chest pain, and productive cough. Bacteremia is present in 30% of cases. Effusions occur in 5% of cases. Diagnostic studies should include a complete blood count (CBC) with differential, chest x ray, Gram stain, and culture of sputum, diagnostic thoracentesis, if effusion is present, and with blood cultures and oxygen saturation in hospitalized patients.

Treatment includes appropriate antibiotics, hydration, oxygenation to prevent maternal and fetal hypoxemia and symptomatic treatment. The drug of choice is penicillin, given orally, Penicillin-VK 500 mg four times a day, or in the ill patient, parenterally 1.2–2.4 million units/day in divided doses. The duration of therapy should be 7–14 days. Patients allergic to penicillin should be treated with erythromycin. Erythromycin is also useful in the patient for whom pneumonias and mycoplasma both remain diagnostic possibilities. If gram-negative pneumonia is suspected, ceftriaxone is a good choice. Pneumococcal vaccine is indicated for the pregnant patient with CF, sickle cell anemia, asthma, or asplenia. Preterm labor and delivery in hospitalized patient is uncommon.[45]

Mycoplasma Pneumonias

Mycoplasma pneumonia is the most common type of pneumonia in the ambulatory patient. Onset of symptoms are usually gradual and includes sore throat, nonproductive cough, headache, and fever. Usual clinical findings are rales, patchy, unilateral or bilateral infiltrates, or frank consolidation. Complications that can occur include bullous myringitis, hemolytic anemia, skin eruptions, and either cardiac or neurologic involvement.[46] Diagnosis is dependent upon the presence of cold agglutinins and/or presence of complement-fixing antibodies to mycoplasma. These serologic tests often do not reveal significant titres until the second week of illness. The drug of choice for treatment during pregnancy is erythromycin. Tetracyclines are contraindicated.

Fungal Pneumonias

Of the fungal infections that may be encountered during pregnancy, coccidiodomycosis has generated the most interest in North America. *Coccidioides immitis* is endemic in the southwestern United States and northern Mexico. It is a widely prevalent disease in the San Joaquin Valley of California ("valley fever"). Dissemination is 40–100 times more common during pregnancy than in the general population and occurs in approximately one third of cases of disease in pregnancy. The increased risk of dissemination has been proposed on the basis of a study investigating the effects of progesterone and estradiol on *C. immitis*. This study showed an increase rate of the fungus and rate of release of endospores in the presence of 17B-estradiol and progesterone.[47] Untreated disseminated disease is associated with a maternal mortality of 100% compared to 50% mortality among untreated nonpregnant patients.[48] In Smale and Waechter's[49] series of 15 cases of disseminated coccidiodomycosis during gestation, fetal loss was 50%.This was due to prematurity or fetal death in utero secondary to maternal death. Congenital disease is rare, but it does occur.

Diagnosis requires a high index of suspicion in endemic areas and demonstration of delayed hypersensitivity to coccidioidin or the presence in the serum of complement-fixing or precipitating antibodies. Other studies include direct examination of sputum and sputum cultures. When scalene node lymphadenopathy is present, biopsy is diagnostic.

The drug of choice for treatment is amphotericin. The dosage is 1.0–1.5 mg/kg/day tapering to 1.0–1.5 mg/kg/day, three times a week to a total of 0.5 to 1.5 g IV. Amphotericin's nephrotoxic effect is dose-dependent and reversible. Amphotericin does not appear to have any detrimental effects on fetal or neonatal course.

The other fungal diseases reported during pregnancy include histoplasmosis, caused by histoplasma capsulatum, and blastomycosis, caused by *Blastomyces dermatitidis*. In most cases, infection is mild and self-limited and recovery occurs without therapy.

Viral Pneumonias

Influenza

There are two types of influenza virus, Type A and Type B. Influenza virus is an RNA virus and infections may be asymptomatic or they may vary from mild upper respiratory infection to pneumonia and death. Outbreaks typically occur in late autumn or early spring. There are two broad patterns of respiratory involvement, pure influenza-virus pneumonia and influenza-associated bacterial pneumonias.

Clinical manifestations usually are malaise, myalgia, fever, chills, headaches, pain on ocular movement, and sore throat. Development of cough, dyspnea, hemoptysis and chest pain herald onset of clinical deterioration. Purulent sputum indicates superimposed bacterial infections. Bacterial infection is usually due to staphylococci, streptococcus, and *Escherichia coli*. Marked cyanosis secondary to pulmonary decompensation and shock due to cardiovascular collapse precede death. Fetal death usually precedes maternal death.

Diagnosis of influenza pneumonia is presumptive and is based on characteristic pattern of disease occurring at a time when influenza infection is prevalent in the community. Treatment of maternal influenza is directed at symptomatic relief. The patient with pneumonia should be hospitalized and antibiotics are indicated when bacterial superinfection is suspected.

The Centers for Disease Control considers influenza vaccine safe for use in pregnancy and recommends its use when indicated for underlying chronic disease such as diabetes, renal failure, or asthma.[50] The vaccine should not be given routinely to all pregnant women. There is no relationship between influenza and abortions, prematurity, stillbirths, congenital anomalies, or an increase in malignant disease in offspring.[51] Amantadine hydrochloride prophylaxis has limited applicability in a gravid population. It protects only against influenza A infection. It is reported to be embryotoxic and teratogenic in animal model.[12]

Varicella-Zoster Pneumonia

Varicella pneumonia in women of childbearing age is uncommon since 90% are immune.[52] In a review of 17 cases, Harris et al.[52] reported a maternal mortality of 41%. In a series of 43 patients with varicella complicating pregnancy, Paryani et al.[53] reported a mortality of 25% in those with varicella pneumonia. Most cases of varicella pneumonia occur in the third trimester at a time when maternal cell-mediated immunity is depressed. Acyclovir has been used in the gravid patient with varicella pneumonia in late second or third trimester. Most reports involve use of intravenous acyclovir 5–18 mg/kg every 8 hours for 5–10 days.[54]

However, adequate data demonstrating efficacy in modifying the natural history of the disease, safety for the fetus, optimum dosage, and duration of therapy are lacking.

PULMONARY EDEMA

Pregnancy complicated with pulmonary edema can be associated with increased morbidity and, rarely, mortality. The characteristic clinical features are shortness of breath, cough, tachypnea, tachycardia and pulmonary rales and rhonchi on auscultation with decreased breath sounds. High index of suspicion is the key to diagnosis. Diagnosis is confirmed by arterial blood gas evaluation and chest x-ray. Pulse oximetry can help in the early diagnosis of hypoxemia.

Factors that predispose to pulmonary edema in pregnant women include (1) preeclampsia,[55] (2) tocolytic therapy with or without steroid therapy,[56] (3) underlying maternal cardiac disease, (4) multiple gestation, (5) pyelonephritis-related pulmonary injury,[57] (6) aspiration pneumonitis, (7) amniotic fluid embolism, (8) sepsis, and (9) drug abuse.

Management includes placing the patient in upright position with basic laboratory evaluation consisting of a CBC, serum electrolytes, chest x rays, arterial blood gas(es), and electrocardiogram.[58] Hourly recordings of fluid administered and urine output should be implemented. One hundred percent oxygen should be administered via a face mask with a rebreather apparatus to help increase the inspired concentration of oxygen. Aggressive diuresis is indicated with furosemide starting at 20–40 mg IV push. The dose can be doubled every 30 minutes until urine output improves. Administration of IV morphine 10 mg will allay maternal anxiety but also increases capacitance of large vessels in the venous system. All patients should be monitored with pulse oximetry[59] since oxygen percent saturation (arterial) (SaO_2) levels of 90% may reflect a significant hypoxemia. Electronic fetal monitoring should be implemented if the fetus is at a viable gestational age. Inadequate response to aggressive diuresis and oxygen therapy warrants invasive management which includes transfer of patient to an intensive care unit and placement of pulmonary artery catheter.

Endotracheal intubation must be considered in a patient with respiratory rate of >35/min, carbon dioxide partial pressure (PCO_2) > 55 mm Hg, and partial pressure of oxygen (PO_2) < 70 mm Hg with face mask at 40% oxygen.[60] Patients intubated should be placed in 100% oxygen and should be ventilated with small tidal volumes (7–8 mL/kg) and high respiratory rates of 30/minute. The patient should be kept in a lateral decubitus position to prevent a decrease in venous return.

In conclusion, it is important to aggressively treat the underlying disease leading to pulmonary edema.

PULMONARY EMBOLISM

The clinical features of pulmonary embolism include (1) shortness of breath with or without pleuritic chest pain, (2) hemoptysis, pleural effusion, and pulmonary infiltrate on chest x-ray, (3) right-sided failure with dyspnea and tachypnea, and (4) severe chest pain with hypotension and syncope associated with massive embolism occluding at least 50% of pulmonary arterial circulation. The cardiac manifestations and chest signs of pulmonary embolism include pleural effusion, rales, elevated jugular venous pressure with a prominent A-wave, right ventricular heave, accentuated pulmonary second sound, and gallop rhythm.[61]

Diagnostic tests include (1) chest x-ray—it is frequently normal or it may show nonspecific abnormalities such as pleural effusion, infiltrate, or atelectasis. (2) Electrocardiogram—tachycardia is the most common abnormality. The electrocardiogram may show signs of right heart strain such as right axis deviation or an $S_1Q_3T_3$ pattern. Nonspecific T-wave inversion is also seen. (3) Arterial blood gas analysis may reveal hypoxemia and hypocapnia. A PaO_2 of 90 mm Hg makes the diagnosis of pulmonary embolism unlikely, if signs and symptoms persist. (4) Lung scanning with labeled technetium is a safe procedure during pregnancy. The specificity of lung scan is significantly improved with a ventilation study.[62] Pulmonary angiography is the definitive method for diagnosing pulmonary embolism.

When a family history of repeated thromboembolism is encountered, levels of protein C and protein S should be evaluated.[63]

Management includes (1) oxygen therapy, (2) morphine or other narcotics may be used for pain management and allaying anxiety; (3) bedrest for 5–7 days to allow organization of clot, (4) prevention of constipation, and (5) anticoagulation therapy with intravenous heparin. A baseline CBC, platelet count, prothrombin time (PT), and activated partial thromboplastin time (aPTT) should be obtained. A loading dose of heparin is 5000–10,000 units IV by rapid administration.[64] This is followed by a continuous infusion at 1000–1500 units/hr to achieve aPTT 1.5–2.0 times control. An aPTT should be obtained every 6 hours until stable. Continuous intravenous heparin should be given for at least 5 days and then patient should be instructed to self-administer heparin every 12 hours. The dose must be sufficient to prolong the aPTT to 1.5 times control at the midpoint of dosing interval.

At the time of delivery, the patient can remain fully anticoagulated during vaginal delivery.[65] Regional analgesia is contraindicated. The dose of heparin can be reduced to 5000 units every 12 hours. After delivery, full anticoagulation should be reinstituted within 12 hours. Then heparin and warfarin should be given until a therapeutic warfarin effect is achieved. Heparin is then discontinued while warfarin therapy is maintained for 6 months.[66] Warfarin is compatible with breast feeding.

ADULT RESPIRATORY DISTRESS SYNDROME (ARDS)

ARDS is a syndrome of noncardiogenic pulmonary edema with diffuse injury to pulmonary alveolar epithelial and capillary endothelial cells. It occurs as a result of obstetric complications like inhalation of gastric contents during anaesthesia, disseminated intravascular coagulopathy in preeclampsia/eclampsia, sepsis, abruptio placentae, amniotic fluid embolism, pyelonephritis, and shock from hemorrhage.[67] It is associated with a maternal mortality rate of 50–60%.[68]

The clinical features of ARDS include severe hypoxemia with a high inspired oxygen concentration with ''stiff lungs'' and diffuse infiltrates resembling pulmonary edema on chest x rays. Patients often develop refractory hypoxemia and respiratory insufficiency and require mechanical ventilation. Peripheral edema, elevated jugular pressure, and cardiomegaly are unusual findings in ARDS. A normal wedge pressure by Swan-Ganz catheterization rules out primary cardiac abnormality. The Swan-Ganz catheter also permits monitoring of cardiac output and pulmonary arterial pressures.

Management includes correction of underlying maternal disorder, mechanical ventilation, administration of vasoactive drugs, inotropes, and steroids. Implementation of positive end-expiratory pressure (PEEP) is believed to force extravasated water back into the circulation and reverse atelectasis. Monitoring fluid balance is crucial in management of patient with ARDS. The role of steroids is controversial since the study of Bernard et al. suggests that it does not affect outcome.[68]

CIGARETTE SMOKING

Cigarette smoking is the most common drug addiction among pregnant women. Maternal smoking is detrimental to mother and fetus, but only 20% of women smokers quit during pregnancy.[69] For the mother, smoking increases airway irritability and mucous production, and impairs respiratory tract mucociliary function. Inhalation of carbon monoxide from smoke produces carboxyhemoglobin, shifting maternal and fetal oxyhemoglobin dissociation curves to the left. This shift limits oxygen exchange between maternal and fetal compartment. In addition, smoking is the leading risk factor for development of chronic obstructive pulmonary disease (COPD). Increased maternal smoking is associated with increased risk of placental abruption, placenta previa, bleeding during pregnancy, and premature rupture of membranes. Placentas of smoking mothers are larger than those of nonsmoking mothers and are reported to have abnormal histology.[70]

The effect of smoking on fetus and newborn and future development of infant and child is proportional to the intensity of smoking. Light smoking increases risk of fetal death by 20% and heavy smoking increases the risk by 35%.[71] Fetal hazards include growth retardation, directly proportional to the number of cigarettes smoked, prematurity, and spontaneous abortion.[71] The fetal effects are related chiefly to chronic fetal hypoxemia and uteroplacental insufficiency (from increased fetal carboxyhemoglobin and nicotine-induced vasospasm). Several studies have reported a positive association between maternal smoking and SIDS.[72,73] Cessation of smoking is vital for optimal maternal and fetal outcome.

REFERENCES

1. Pernoll ML, Metcalfe J, Schlenker T, et al. Oxygen consumption at rest and during exercise in pregnancy. *Respir Physiol* 1975;25:285–293.
2. Weinberger SE, Weiss ST, Cohen WR, et al:

State of the art: Pregnancy and the lung. *Am Rev Respir Dis* 1980;121:559–581.

3. Awe RJ, Nicotra MB, Newsom TD, et al. Arterial oxygenation and alveolar-arterial gradients in term pregnancy. *Obstet Gynecol* 1979; 53:182–186.

4. Bonica J, McDonald JS. *Principles and practice of Obstetric Analgesia and Anesthesia.* Malvern, Pa: Williams & Wilkins, 1992, pp. 1063–1075.

5. Thomson KH, Cohen ME. Studies on the circulation in pregnancy. II. Vital capacity observations in normal pregnant women. *Surg Gynecol Obstet* 1938;66:591–603.

6. Milne JA, Howie AD, Pack AI. Dyspnoea during normal pregnancy. *Br J Obstet Gynaecol* 1978;84:448–451.

7. *Report of the Working Group on Asthma and Pregnancy Management of Asthma During Pregnancy.* Washington, DC: National Institutes of Health (NIH) Publication No. 93-3279. National Asthma Educational Program. National Heart, Lung and Blood Institute, 1993.

8. Widdicombe JG (ed). Supplement: Airway hyperreactivity. National Asthma Education Program. *Am Rev Respir Dis* 1991;143:S1–S82.

9. Bahna SL, Bjerkedal T. The course and outcome of pregnancy in women with bronchial asthma. *Acta Allergol* 1972;27:397–406.

10. Gluck JC, Gluck P. The effects of pregnancy on asthma: A prospective study. *Ann Allergy* 1976; 37:164–168.

11. Schatz M, Zeiger RS. Management of asthma, rhinitis, and anaphylaxis during pregnancy. *Curr Obstet Gynecol* 1991;1:65–73.

12. Briggs GG, Freeman RK, Yaffe SJ. Drugs in pregnancy and lactation, 4th ed. Baltimore, MD: Williams & Wilkins, 1994.

13. Rayburn WF. Prostaglandin E_2 gel for cervical ripening and induction of labor: A critical analysis. *Am J Obstet Gynecol* 1989;160:529–534.

14. Fishburne JI Jr, Brenner WE, Braaksma JT, et al. Bronchospasm complicating intravenous prostaglandin F_2'a for therapeutic abortion. *Obstet Gynecol* 1972;39:892–896.

15. Younker D, Clark R, Tessem J, et al. Bupivacaine-fentanyl epidural analgesia for parturient in status asthmaticus. *Can J Anaesth* 1987;34: 609–612.

16. Crawford JS. Bronchospasm following ergometrine (letter). *Anesthesiology* 1980;35:397–398.

17. Centers for Disease Control. Tuberculosis morbidity in the United States: Final data, 1990. *MMWR* 1992;40:1–19.

18. Centers for Disease Control. Tuberculosis among foreign-born persons entering the United States. *MMWR* 1990;39:1–21.

19. Schaefer G, Zervoudakis IA, Fuchs FF, et al. Pregnancy and pulmonary tuberculosis. *Obstet Gynecol* 1975;46:706–715.

20. Jacobs RF, Abernathy RS. Management of tuberculosis in pregnancy and the newborn. *Clin Perinatol* 1988;15:305–319.

21. Smith MHD, Teele DW. Tuberculosis. In Remington JS, Klein JO (eds), *Infectious Diseases of the Fetus and Newborn*, 4th ed. Philadelphia: Saunders, 1995, pp. 1074–1086.

22. Nemir RL, O'Hare D. Congenital tuberculosis. *Am J Dis Child* 1985;139:284–287.

23. Petrini B, Gentz J, Winbladh B, et al. Perinatal transmission of tuberculosis: Meningitis in mother, disseminated disease in child. *Scand J Infect Dis* 1983;15:403–405.

24. Hageman J, Shulman S, Schreiber M., et al. Congenital tuberculosis: Critical reappraisal of clinical findings and diagnostic procedures. *Pediatric* 1980;66:980–984.

25. Hedvall E. Pregnancy and tuberculosis. *Acta Med Scand* 1953;147:1–101.

26. Wilson EA, Thelin TJ, Dilts PV. Tuberculosis complicated by pregnancy. *Am J Obstet Gynecol* 1972;115:526–529.

27. Robinson GC, Cambon KG: Hearing loss in infants of tuberculous mothers treated with streptomycin during pregnancy. *N Engl J Med* 1964; 271:949–951.

28. Snider DE Jr, Garas GJ: Isoniazid-associated hepatitis deaths: A review of available information. *Am Rev Respir Dis* 1992;145:494–497.

29. American Thoracic Society: Diagnostic standards and classification of tuberculosis. *Am Rev Respir Dis* 1990;142:725–735.

30. American Thoracic Society: Treatment of tuberculosis and tuberculous infection in adults and children. *Am Rev Respir Dis* 1994;149: 1359–1374.

31. Snider DE Jr, Powell KE. Should mothers taking antituberculosis drugs breast-feed? *Arch Intern Med* 1984;144:589–590.

32. Kendig EL. The place of BCG vaccine in the management of infants born to tuberculous mothers. *N Engl J Med* 1969;281:520–523.

33. Wood RE, Boat TF, Doeshuk CF. Cystic fibrosis. State of the art. *Am Rev Respir Dis* 1976; 113:833–875.

34. Kent NE, Farquharson DF. Cystic fibrosis in pregnancy. *Can Med Assoc J* 1993;149:808–813.

35. Edenborough FP, Stubleforth DE, Webb AK, et al. Outcome of pregnancy in women with cystic fibrosis. *Thorax* 1995;50:170–174.

36. Cohen LF, diSant'Agnese PA, Friedlander J. Cystic fibrosis and pregnancy: A national survey. *Lancet* 1980;2:842–844.

37. Corkey CWB, Newth CJL, Corey M, et al. Pregnancy in cystic fibrosis: A better prognosis in patients with pancreatic function? *Am J Obstet Gynecol* 1981;140:737–742.

38. McCaffrey RM, Dunn LJ. Primary pulmonary hypertension and pregnancy. *Obstet Gynecol Surv* 1964;19:567–591.

39. Morgan Jones A. Eisenmenger syndrome in pregnancy. *Br Med J* 1965;1:1627–1631.

40. Erskine KJ, Taylor KJ, Agnew RAL. Serial estimation of serum angiotensin converting enzyme activity during and after pregnancy in a woman with sarcoidosis. *British Medical Journal* 1985;290:269–270.

41. Wilson-Holt N. Postpartum presentation of hypercalcaemic sarcoidosis. *Postgrad Med J* 1985;61:627–628

42. Oxorn H. The changing aspects of pneumonia complicating pregnancy. *Am J Obstet Gynecol* 1955;70:1057–1063.

43. Benedetti TJ, Valle R, Ledger W. Antepartum pneumonia in pregnancy. *Am J Obstet Gynecol* 1982;144:413–417.

44. Madinger NE, Greenspoon JS, Gray-Ellrodt A. Pneumonia during pregnancy: Has modern technology improved maternal and fetal outcome? *Am J Obstet Gynecol* 1989;161:657–662.

45. Berkowitz K, LaSala A. Risk factors associated with the increasing prevalence of pneumonia during pregnancy. *Am J Obstet Gynecol* 1990; 163:981–985.

46. Weinberger, SE, Weiss ST. Pulmonary diseases. In Burrow GN, Ferris TF (eds), *Medical Com-* *plications During Pregnancy*, 3rd ed. Philadelphia: Saunders, 1988, pp. 448–484.

47. Powell BL, Drutz DJ, Huppert M, et al. Relationship of progesterone and estradiol binding proteins in coccidiodes immitis to coccidiodal dissemination in pregnancy. *Infect Immun* 1983; 40:478–485.

48. Harris RE. Coccidioidomycosis complicating pregnancy. *Obstet Gynecol* 1966;28:401–405.

49. Smale LE, Waechter KH. Dissemination of coccidioidomycosis in pregnancy. *Am J Obstet Gynecol* 1970;107:356–361.

50. Advisory Committee on Immunication Practices. Prevention and Control of influenza: Part 1, Vaccines. *MMWR* 1989;38;297–309.

51. MacKenzie JS, Houghton M. Influenza infections during pregnancy: Association with congenital malformations and with subsequent neoplasms in children, and potential hazards of live virus vaccines. *Bacteriol Rev* 1974;38: 356–370.

52. Harris R, Rhoades E. Varicella pneumonia complicating pregnancy: Report of a case and review of the literature. *Obstet Gynecol* 1965;25: 734–740.

53. Paryani S, Arvin A. Intrauterine infection with varicella zoster virus after maternal varicella. *N Engl J Med* 1986;314:1542–1546.

54. Boyd K, Walker E. Use of acyclovir to treat chickenpox in pregnancy. *Br Med J* 1988;296: 393–394.

55. Sibai BM, Mabie BC, Harvey CJ, et al. Pulmonary edema in severe preeclampsia-eclampsia: Analysis of thirty-seven consecutive cases. *Am J Obstet Gynecol* 1987;156:1174–1179.

56. Hankins GDV. Complications of b-sympathomimetic tocolytic agents. In Clark SL, Cotton DB, Hankins GDV, et al. (eds), *Critical Care Obstetrics*, 2nd ed. Boston: Blackwell, 1991, pp. 233–250.

57. Cunningham FG, Lucas MJ, Hankins GD. Pulmonary injury complicating antepartum pyelonephritis. *Am J Obstet Gynecol* 1987;156:797–807.

58. Mabie WC, Hackman BB, Sibai BM. Pulmonary edema associated with pregnancy: Echocardiographic insights and implications for treatment. *Obstet Gynecol* 1993;81:227–234.

59. Stoneham MD, Saville GM, Wilson IH. Knowl-

edge about pulse oximetry among medical and nursing staff. *Lancet* 1994;344:1339–1342.

60. Hankins GDV. Acute pulmonary injury and respiratory failure during pregnancy. In Clark SL, Cotton DB, Hankins GDV, et al. (eds), *Critical Care Obstetrics*, 2nd ed. Boston: Blackwell, 1991, pp. 340–370.

61. Sasahara AA, Sharma GVRK, Barsamian EM, et al. Pulmonary thromboembolism. *JAMA* 1983;249:2945–2950.

62. Hull RD, Hirsh J, Carter CJ, et al. Pulmonary angiography, ventilation lung scanning, and venography for clinically suspected pulmonary embolism with abnormal perfusion lung scan. *Ann Intern Med* 1983;98:891–899.

63. Comp PC, Esmon CT. Recurrent venous thromboembolism in patients with partial deficiency of protein S. *N Engl J Med* 1984;311:1525–1528.

64. Pridmore BR, Murray KH, McAllen PM. The management of anticoagulant therapy during and after pregnancy. *Br J Obstet Gynaecol* 1975;82:740–744.

65. Rutherford SE, Phelan JP. Thromboembolic disease in pregnancy. *Clin Perinatol* 1986;13:719–739.

66. Schulmen S, Rhedin A, Lindmaker P, et al. A comparison of six weeks with six months of oral anticoagulation therapy after a first episode of venous thromboembolism. *N Engl J Med* 1995;332:1661–1665.

67. Divertie MD. The adult respiratory distress syndrome. *Mayo Clin Proc* 1982;57:371–378.

68. Bernard GR, Luce JM, Spring CL, et al. High dose corticosteroids in patients with adult respiratory distress syndrome. *N Engl J Med* 1987;317:1565–1570.

69. Prager K, Malin H, Spiegler D, et al. Smoking and drinking behavior before and during pregnancy of married mothers of liveborn infants and stillborn infants. *Public Health Rep* 1984;99:117–127.

70. Asmussen J. Ultrastructure of the human placenta at term. Observations on placentas from newborn children of smoking and non-smoking mothers. *Acta Obstet Gynecol Scand* 1977;56:119–125.

71. Meyer MB, Tonascia JA. Maternal smoking, pregnancy complications, and perinatal mortality. *Am J Obstet Gynecol* 1977;128:494–502.

72. Naeye RL, Ladis B, Drage JS. Sudden infant death syndrome: A prospective study. *Am J Dis Child* 1976;130:1207–1210.

73. Lewak N, van den Berg BJ, Beckwith B. Sudden infant death syndrome risk factors: Prospective data review. *Clin Pediatr* 1979;18:404–411.

QUESTIONS
(choose the single best answer)

1. All parameters of pulmonary function change during pregnancy except:
   a. Respiratory quotient.
   b. Total lung capacity.
   c. Vital capacity.
   d. Residual volume.
   e. Functional residual capacity.
2. The best objective assessment of asthma during pregnancy can be provided by:
   a. Serial pulmonary function test.
   b. Peak expiratory flow rate.
   c. Continuous transcutaneous oxygen saturation.
   d. Serial chest x rays.
3. Drugs listed below are safe for treatment of asthma in pregnancy include all except:
   a. Alpha-adrenergic compounds.
   b. Cromolyn sodium.
   c. Betamimetics.
   d. Prednisone.
   e. Antihistamines.
4. The most common site of congenital tuberculosis is the:
   a. Lung.
   b. Kidneys.
   c. Spleen and lymph nodes.
   d. Liver.
   e. Skin.
5. Perinatal outcome in pregnant patients with cystic fibrosis is positively correlated with maternal:
   a. Malabsorption.
   b. Prepregnancy percentage of FEV_1.
   c. Diabetes mellitus.
   d. Hepatic and biliary disease.
   e. All of the above.
6. The most common type of pneumonia in the ambulatory pregnant patient is:
   a. Streptococcus pneumonia.
   b. Viral agent.
   c. Hemophillus influenza.
   d. Mycoplasma.

e. Fungal.

7. The proper initial therapy of proven pulmonary edema includes all except:
   a. Upright position, complete blood count, electrolytes, EKG.
   b. Oxygen therapy with intravenous Lasix.
   c. Intravenous narcotics.
   d. Endotracheal intubation.
   e. Pulse oximetry.

8. The most accurate diagnostic test for pulmonary embolism during pregnancy is:
   a. Chest x ray.
   b. Electrocardiogram.
   c. Lung scanning.
   d. Pulmonary angiography.

9. Adult respiratory distress syndrome can occur as a result of maternal:
   a. Inhalation of gastric contents during anaesthesia.
   d. Sepsis.
   c. Placental abruption.
   d. Preeclampsia/eclampsia.
   e. All of the above.

10. Maternal cigarette smoking is associated with increased predisposition to all except:
    a. Preeclampsia.
    b. Placenta previa.
    c. Placental abruption.
    d. Low birth weight.
    e. Fetal death.

11

Pregnancy Complicated by Maternal Cardiac Disease

Elliot H. Philipson

INTRODUCTION

Advances in cardiology and maternal fetal medicine have changed many facets in the approach to cardiac disease in pregnancy. Particularly important is the concept of patient individualization using new technologies for accurate prenatal assessment of cardiac and respiratory function. With improvement in our understanding of maternal cardiovascular physiology, antenatal and intrapartum monitoring, and neonatal resuscitation and evaluation, pregnancies complicated by cardiac disease often result in successful outcomes. The constant challenge for obstetrics is to care for two patients. Maternal health and safety need to be maintained and, similarly, a fetal environment suitable for normal growth and development needs to be provided. Before discussing specific disorders of cardiac diseases in pregnancy, a concise review of basic cardiovascular physiology is presented.

CARDIOVASCULAR PHYSIOLOGY

Hemodynamic changes during pregnancy labor and delivery, and the postpartum period have been well described.[1-4] Maternal blood volume, both plasma and the number of erythrocytes, increase during pregnancy. Because the plasma volume increases to a greater extent than the erythrocyte mass, the hematocrit may decrease causing a relative *anemia* of pregnancy. The increase in blood volume is secondary to a rise in progesterone and estrogen. These changes lead to an increase in the renin-aldosterone system, which causes an increase in sodium and water retention. The resultant edema is often a normal finding in pregnant women. Stroke volume, maternal heart rate, and pulse also increase. Beginning in the first trimester, cardiac output increases until the midsecond trimester when the cardiac output peaks to 30–40% above resting, nonpregnant levels.[3] Cardiac output has been reported to be relatively constant at approximately 8.0 L/min throughout the third trimester,[5] although a recent review indicates that cardiac output is widely divergent.[6] Individual factors including a change in maternal position, compression of the vena cava by an enlarging pregnant uterus, and, possibly, variation in collateral channels, may lead to a reduction, an increase, or no change in cardiac output in the third trimester. Early in pregnancy, systemic vascular resistance falls. With a fall in vascular resistance and an increase in cardiac output, maternal blood pressure generally remains unchanged or falls slightly during normal pregnancy. Diastolic blood pressure tends to decrease more than the systolic pressure so that pulse pressure widens.

During labor and after delivery, contractions of the uterine muscle result in significant blood volume changes. This is often referred to as *autotransfusion*, in which a uterine contraction results in a bolus of 300–500 ccs of blood into the circulation from the uterus. This can increase the stroke volume, blood pressure, cardiac output, and risk of heart failure. In one study, a 31% increase in cardiac output has been reported.[7] Following delivery of the fetus and placenta, cardiac output is lower than at any time during pregnancy.[5,6] Maternal hemodynamic changes can be influenced by blood loss, hypovolemia, position, infection, and anesthesia. Depending on the specific cardiac abnormality, not necessarily identified antenatally, postpartum monitoring can be critical. The patient's cardiovascular status may gradually return to the nonpregnant state in several weeks. However, echocardiographic changes may not regress until 12 weeks postpartum.[8]

One important recent contribution to the understanding of the hemodynamic changes that occur during pregnancy has been the use of invasive monitoring with the pulmonary artery catheter (Swan-Ganz catheter).[9] A landmark report of central monitoring in obstetrics reported various hemodynamic parameters in normal pregnancy.[10] These normal parameters are compared to nonpregnant values in the same patients (Table 11-1) indicating that normal pregnancy late in the third trimester is not associated with hyperdynamic left ventricular function. Pulmonary capillary wedge pressure is unchanged reflecting the decrease in systemic vascular resistance in spite of the marked increase in intravascular volume. This data is important when evaluating critically ill pregnant patients.

RISK ASSESSMENT

Patients with preexisting cardiac disease are often referred for counseling prior to pregnancy. A comprehensive review of the records and

Table 11-1. Central Hemodynamic Changes

	Nonpregnant	Pregnant
Cardiac output (L/min)	4.3 + 0.9	6.2 + 1.0
Heart rate (beats/min)	71 + 10.0	83 + 10.0
Systemic vascular resistance (dyne · cm · sec^{-5})	1530 + 520	1210 + 266
Pulmonary vascular resistance (dyne · cm · sec^{-5})	119 + 47.0	78 + 22
Colloid oncotic pressure (mm Hg)	20.8 + 1.0	18.0 + 1.5
Colloid oncotic pressure — pulmonary capillary wedge pressure (mm Hg)	14.5 + 2.5	10.5 + 2.7
Mean arterial pressure (mm Hg)	86.4 + 7.5	90.3 + 5.8
Pulmonary capillary wedge pressure (mm Hg)	6.3 + 2.1	7.5 + 1.8
Central venous pressure (mm Hg)	3.7 + 2.6	3.6 + 2.5
Left ventricular stroke work index (g · m · m^{-2})	41 + 8	48 + 6

Source: From ref. 10, reprinted with permission.

a detailed history and physical examination should be performed. Additional diagnostic testing or evaluation can be performed as needed, including an electrocardiogram, M-mode or two-dimensional echocardiography, Doppler echocardiography, radionucleotide techniques, X-ray studies, or cardiac catheterization. If patients with cardiac disease are pregnant or if cardiac disease is diagnosed during pregnancy, appropriate consultation may include a cardiologist, anesthesiologist, nutritionist, geneticist, or maternal-fetal medicine specialist. Depending on the abnormality and symptomatology, further cardiac evaluation may be necessary and intrapartum monitoring and delivery at a facility with expertise in maternal fetal medicine may be appropriate.

Risk assessment has traditionally been based on maternal age, history of congestive heart failure, or the presence of cyanotic congenital heart disease. In 1929, the New York Heart Association (NYHA) functional classification during pregnancy (Table 11-2) was proposed and revised in 1979 in which patients with functional classes I and II can have successful pregnancies, class III require special expertise and care, and class IV should not conceive.[1,11] In general, these functional classes provided reasonable guidelines for clinicians. However, this system may not be particularly accurate as it is based on the initial symptoms described by the patient or family, does not allow for progressive changes in symptomatology, and is independent of the specific cardiac disease. In one report, 40% of patients in whom congestive heart failure develops were in NYHA class I.[12] More recently, the American College of Obstetricians and Gynecologists[1,12] proposed three groups of maternal mortality risk based on the specific cardiac abnormality. Mortality rates from less than 1% for NYHA class 1 and 2 and other cardiac defects to rates as high as 50% for some other cardiac conditions are reported. This type of risk assessment appears to be more accurate and useful for patient counseling and prognostic risk assessment. Undoubtedly, this type of specific cardiac risk assessment will become more detailed and refined with more clinical experience and development of new technology.

In addition to maternal risk assessment, patients with congenital heart disease should receive counseling for fetal risks. Epidemiologic data indicate that most congenital heart disease is not part of any recognizable genetic syndrome. However, recurrence rates of congenital heart disease range from 1% to 17.9% depending on the specific cardiac abnormality, the number of siblings affected, the time period, and the investigator.[13,14] Multifactorial or polygenic inheritance has been suggested. It is important to note that the specific cardiac anomaly of the mother is not necessarily similar to the abnormality of the fetus/neonate. Also, the risk is greater if the mother rather than the father has the heart defect, suggesting that mitochondrial genetics may be involved.[15,16] Fetal risk should also be considered as some genetic disorders are associated with congenital heart disease and inheritance patterns may follow traditional Mendelian genetics. An example of this would be

Table 11-2. Maternal Mortality Associated with Pregnancy

Group 1—Mortality < 1%
  Atrial septal defect
  Ventricular septal defect
  Patent ductus arteriosus
  Pulmonic/tricuspid disease
  Tetralogy of Fallot, corrected
  Bioprosthetic valve
  Mitral stenosis, NYHA class I and II
Group 2—Mortality 5–15%
  2A
    Mitral stenosis, NYHA class III and IV
    Aortic stenosis
    Coarctation of aorta, without valvular involvement
    Uncorrected tetralogy of Fallot
    Previous myocardial infarction
    Marfan syndrome with normal aorta
  2B
    Mitral stenosis with atrial fibrillation
    Artificial valve
Group 3—Mortality 25–50%
  Pulmonary hypertension
  Coarctation of aorta, with valvular involvement
  Marfan syndrome with aortic involvement

Source: From ref. 1, reprinted with permission.

the autosomal dominant pattern in Marfan's syndrome (see below). Some drug therapy and use has been associated with fetal cardiac risk. One of the best known associations was first described after careful history taking: the association between lithium use and Ebstein's anomaly (although recently disputed).[17] In summary, the important clinical message is that a detailed and thorough history be obtained, genetic counseling offered, and a level 2 ultrasonographic exam with fetal echocardiography be performed.

VALVULAR DISEASE

The majority of congenital heart disease has historically been secondary to complications from rheumatic heart disease. With the use of antibiotics, this type of congenital heart disease has decreased. This section will highlight important practical considerations of valvular disease and pregnancy.

Mitral Stenosis

Mitral stenosis is the most common rheumatic valvular disease and the most important hemodynamic valvular lesion in pregnancy.[4] With a stenotic mitral valve, the left atrium will become dilated and over time, left atrial pressure will increase. This can lead not only to pulmonary edema, hypertension, and ventricular failure, but also intramural thrombus formation. In patients with mitral stenosis, the cardiac output is fixed and, therefore, fluid management and balance is critical. Hypovolemia can significantly reduce cardiac output and volume overload can lead to pulmonary edema. Pulmonary capillary wedge pressure can be elevated or falsely elevated due to the stenotic valve (i.e., the pulmonary capillary wedge pressure may not reflect left ventricular filling pressure) so that following the trend through labor and delivery is important. Maintaining the pulmonary capillary wedge pressure less than 14 mm Hg (high normal range) is desirable.[18] Because an increased maternal heart rate may decrease cardiac filling time, maternal tachycardia (greater than 90–100 beats per minute) should be avoided with the use of beta-blockade.[3] Intrapartum management should also include subacute bacterial endocarditis prophylaxis and adequate pain relief. Epidural anesthesia is very useful, but hypotension needs to be avoided by appropriate volume expansion and the use of ephedrine. Vaginal birth is the mode of choice with Cesarean birth when obstetrically indicated. Historically, shortening the second stage of labor with the use of forceps or vacuum extraction has been suggested but probably is not necessary if patients are hemodynamically stable. If atrial fibrillation occurs, digoxin can be used and anticoagulation with heparin should be initiated. For hemodynamically unstable patients or patients with persistent incapacitating symptoms despite medical treatment, percutaneous balloon commissurotomy has become an alternative to open-heart or closed mitral commissurotomy. Maternal percutaneous mitral commissurotomy, performed in 13 pregnant patients at a mean gestational age of 26 weeks, has been shown to be efficacious and well-tolerated by the fetus.[19]

Mitral Insufficiency

Mitral insufficiency is usually rheumatic and often associated with other valvular lesions. During pregnancy, mitral insufficiency is generally well tolerated because the decreased systemic vascular resistance in pregnancy favors forward flow.[3] These patients can be managed in labor as uncomplicated pregnancies. However, with long-standing disease, left atrial dilation and left ventricular hypertrophy may limit myocardial function. Close hemodynamic monitoring may be necessary if pulmonary hypertension or atrial fibrillation develops. Invasive monitoring may be indicated to optimize preload and reduce afterload. Bacterial endocarditis prophylaxis is recommended.

Mitral Valve Prolapse

Mitral valve prolapse is estimated to occur in 17% of healthy, asymptomatic young women.[20] Some patients may develop palpitations, chest pain, or premature ventricular contractions. The diagnosis is often made by auscultating a characteristic midsystolic click and murmur. Beta blockades or other antiarrhythmic agents are effective for symptoms. If the murmur is present indicating regurgitant flow, bacterial endocarditis prophylaxis is recommended during labor and delivery.[1] Without a murmur, prophylaxis is generally not recommended.

Aortic Stenosis

Aortic stenosis is usually a congenital lesion if isolated and rheumatic if associated with other lesions.[3] As left ventricular hypertrophy develops and myocardial work increases, maintenance of cardiac output becomes more difficult. With severe lesions, i.e., gradients greater than

100 mm Hg, there is an increased risk of myocardial infarction. Historically, congenital aortic stenosis has been considered a contraindication to pregnancy with high maternal and perinatal mortality.[21] More recent reappraisals of aortic stenosis and pregnancy generally indicate good pregnancy outcomes.[22,23] Antenatal management includes limitation of physical activity and rest. For patients with severe aortic stenosis, meticulous fluid balance during labor and delivery is essential to maintain adequate preload and avoid volume overload. Pulmonary artery catheterization may be necessary. Vaginal birth and shortening the second stage of labor with the use of forceps or vacuum extraction to avoid the Valsalva maneuver is recommended. Postpartum monitoring is important as these patients may experience pulmonary edema from the autotransfusion or redistribution of volume. Critical aortic stenosis can be improved by percutaneous balloon commissurotomy.

Aortic Insufficiency

Aortic insufficiency is most often rheumatic and often coexists with mitral valve disease. As blood refluxes into the left ventricle from the aorta, left ventricular hypertrophy may develop. However, pregnancy often improves aortic insufficiency as the normal pregnancy decrease in systemic vascular resistance decreases afterload, hence limiting regurgitant flow. Improvement also occurs as the more rapid maternal heart rate decreases the time for regurgitant flow during diastole. Intrapartum management is similar to normal parturients. With left ventricular hypertrophy, good analgesia and vaginal delivery are appropriate. If pulmonary edema occurs, afterload reduction should be administered. Bacterial endocarditis prophylaxis is indicated.

Pulmonary/Tricuspid Lesions

Pulmonary and tricuspid lesions are relatively uncommon, although they have been associated with intravenous drug use. Pregnant patients with right-sided valvular lesions generally tolerate pregnancy and delivery well because pregnancy is associated with an increased preload. The increased preload maintains pulmonary perfusion and oxygenation. Intrapartum management involves careful fluid balance.

Prosthetic Valves

Prosthetic heart valves are often used in young patients with severe valvular disease. When these patients become pregnant, the type of prosthetic valve is important. Tissue valves offer an advantage in that anticoagulation is not necessary. The disadvantage lies in the fact that these valves are more likely to need replacement requiring reoperation. The mechanical valves, while less likely to require reoperation, require lifelong anticoagulation. The use of anticoagulants in pregnancy remains controversial due to increased risk of warfarin embryopathy with Coumadin and bleeding with heparin.

SPECIFIC CARDIAC DEFECTS AND MEDICAL CONDITIONS

Advances in surgery have permitted many women with other types of congenital heart disease to pursue pregnancy. Several of the more common congenital heart diseases and their significance in pregnancy are as follows.

Atrial Septal Defect (ASD)

Atrial septal defects are the most common cardiac defects unrecognized until adult life.[24] The secundum type is the most common, usually occurring in the region of the fossa ovalis and separated from the atrioventricular valves by a rim of septal tissue.[25] Fortunately, ASD is well tolerated in pregnancy due to the normal decrease in systemic vascular resistance, which can improve cardiac performance by decreasing left-sided pressure and decreasing the left to right shunt. Labor and delivery are generally uncomplicated, although supplemental oxygen, lateral recumbent position, and avoiding fluid overload have been suggested. Subacute bacterial endocarditis (SBE) prophylaxis appears to be controversial, although recommended by some authors.[4] Acute blood loss can increase the shunt and, therefore, hypovolemia needs to be monitored carefully. With large and uncorrected defects, patients can develop pulmonary hypertension. Atrial fibrillation, congestive heart failure, and death are rare but reported.[1]

Ventricular Septal Defects (VSD)

Ventricular septal defects are the commonest of all congenital heart lesions, alone or in combination with other malformations.[1,24] The majority of VSDs are the membranous type, inferior to the crista near the base of the interventricular septum. Hemodynamic changes are determined by the size of the defect and associated malformations. Small defects are often asymptomatic and well tolerated in pregnancy. Larger defects alone or those associated with tetralogy of Fallot, transposition of the great vessels, or coarctation of the aorta are most frequently complicated by arrhythmias, congestive heart failure, or pulmonary hypertension.[1] Management during labor and delivery is similar to patients with ASD. SBE prophylaxis is recommended.

Patent Ductus Arteriosus (PDA)

Patent ductus arteriosus is a persistent fetal communication between the pulmonary artery and the aorta, usually from the proximal portion of the left pulmonary artery to the descending aorta just distal to the origin of the left subclavian artery.[25] Significant hemodynamic PDA is rare today as most defects are corrected in childhood. Large uncorrected PDA can lead to pulmonary hypertension with maternal risk. Small PDAs, generally asymptomatic, are well tolerated during pregnancy, labor, and delivery.

Ebstein's Anomaly

Ebstein's anomaly is a rare congenital cardiac defect in which the tricuspid valve is atypically displaced downward.[25] This malformation leads to tricuspid regurgitation and right atrial enlargement. The clinical significance of this lesion has been the association with maternal lithium use during pregnancy.[26] Recently there has been some question regarding the association of lithium use and this specific cardiac defect.[17] As a result, women who are exposed to lithium during pregnancy should have a level 2 ultrasound and fetal echocardiographic evaluation.

The outcome of pregnancy in women with Ebstein's anomaly was studied in 44 women who had 111 pregnancies.[27] In general, pregnancy is well tolerated although the risk of prematurity, fetal loss, and congenital heart disease are increased, particularly in cyanotic patients. Male patients with Ebstein's anomaly also have a higher risk of children with congenital heart disease.

Eisenmenger's Syndrome

Eisenmenger's syndrome is the right-to-left intracardiac shunting of blood through an atrial septal defect (ASD), foramen ovale, or large ventral septal defect (VSD) in the presence of pulmonary hypertension, right ventricular hypertrophy, or ventricular failure.[25] Pulmonary hypertension is regarded as a contraindication to pregnancy with maternal mortality rates of 30–50% and sudden death at any time.[28,29] In a 1979 review, maternal mortality was 34% and 75% with vaginal delivery and Caesarean births respectively.[28] Mortality risk was also higher when the defect involved a large VSD compared to an ASD or PDA. Any decrease in systemic vascular resistance, by blood loss, hypotension, or even that in normal pregnancy, can lead to decreased right ventricular filling pressure, decreased cardiac output and further right-to-left shunting and compromise of the pulmonary arterial bed.[1] For these reasons, pregnancy termination is recommended for patients with Eisenmenger's syndrome. For patients with this syndrome who continue pregnancy, bed rest, oxygen therapy, and hospitalization are appropriate. Serial ultrasonographic assessments are important as intrauterine growth restriction is common.[29,30] Intrapartum management should include pulmonary artery catheterization if possible. Decreases in preload or cardiac output should be avoided.[1] A slightly elevated capillary wedge pressure; i.e., 16–18 mm Hg is recommended to maintain cardiac output.[24] Vaginal birth is preferred with second stage assistance by vacuum extraction or forceps to avoid the Valsalva maneuver. Cesarean birth should be based on obstetrical indications. Because thromboembolism has been associated with 43% of maternal deaths, anticoagulation has been suggested although data is very limited Pitts et al.[31] Sudden cardiovascular collapse within one week of delivery or even four to six weeks postpartum is well known.[1]

Marfan's Syndrome

Marfan's syndrome is a connective tissue disorder with an autosomal dominant mode of inheritance.[32] Characteristics of this type of inheritance include variable expressivity and penetrance so that a wide diversity of system involvement is often observed. The most common systems involved are the skeletal, ocular, and cardiovascular.[33,34] Skeletal changes may involve the anterior chest wall (pectus excavatum or carinatum), spine (kyphoscoliosis), long extremities, or abnormally long, slender fingers (arachnodactyly). Ocular changes may include displacement of the lens (ectopia), severe nearsightedness, or spontaneous retinal detachment. Cardiovascular alterations involve the aortic media with dilation, aneurysm formation, and dissection. Aortic regurgitation as well as bacterial endocarditis, mitral valve prolapse and insufficiency are also problematic for these patients. With cardiovascular disease, life expectancy is shortened.[35] Echocardiography is used to evaluate the cardiovascular manifestations. More recently, digital subtraction angiography has been shown to be effective in diagnosing and monitoring the aorta.[36] Surgical correction of the ascending aorta with composite graft repair has been associated with low operative morbidity and long-term mortality. Prophylactic surgical repair even in asymptomatic

patients is now recommended when an aortic aneurysm reaches a diameter of 6 cm.[37] Medical therapy with the use of long-term B-adrenegic blockade has recently been shown to slow the rate of aortic dilation and reduce aortic complications in some patients.[38] These medical and surgical accomplishments have improved the quality of life and allowed some patients to enter the reproductive age group.

There are two important obstetrical implications of Marfan's syndrome. First, as an autosomal dominant disorder, 50% of the offspring may be affected. It is estimated that 15% of the cases may be due to new mutations; therefore, this should be part of the prenatal counseling for the parents. Second, the maternal cardiovascular system needs to be evaluated initially and serially throughout pregnancy with particular attention to the diameter of the ascending aorta. In one report, pregnant women with minimal cardiac involvement and an aortic diameter of less than 4 cm had a small but potential risk of aortic dissection.[39] An ascending aorta greater than 4 or 4.5 cm is more likely to rupture; therefore, pregnancy should be avoided or surgical correction should be encouraged prior to pregnancy. Frequent reports of pregnancies with good outcomes are well described.[40] In a recent report of 45 pregnancies in 21 women with Marfan's syndrome, the maternal and fetal outcomes were favorable when the cardiovascular involvement was minor (no evidence of aortic regurgitation or dissection) and the aortic root diameter was less than 4 cm.[39] Long-term follow-up of these patients showed no significant worsening or accelerated dilatation of the ascending aorta when compared to age-matched nonpregnant women with Marfan's syndrome.

Tetralogy of Fallot

Tetralogy of Fallot is a cyanotic congenital heart lesion characterized by the combination of usually a large ventral septal defect, severe obstruction to right ventricular outflow (often pulmonary stenosis), right ventricular hypertrophy, and overriding of the aorta.[25] If uncorrected, the ventricular septal defect can augment a right-to-left shunt. As systemic vascular resistance decreases in normal pregnancy, the shunt can increase and cyanosis can become more severe. Poor prognosis has been associated with congestive heart failure, an elevated hematocrit, syncope, cardiomegaly, low oxygen saturation, and elevated right ventricular pressure.[1] Older studies have reported a maternal mortality range from 4% to 15%, with a 30% fetal mortality due to hypoxia.[1] Cardiac arrhythmias may be present and require monitoring. Intrapartum care involves maintaining preload and systemic vascular resistance, avoiding hypotension, and minimizing blood loss. If cases of Tetralogy of Fallot that have been corrected, good outcome has generally been reported.[29,41]

Myocardial Infarction

Myocardial infarction is uncommon during pregnancy and reported to occur in 1 of 10,000 pregnancies in a frequently cited 1970 reference.[42] In spite of the significant cardiovascular changes of pregnancy that increase cardiac work, relatively few cases of myocardial infarction have actually been reported during pregnancy.[43–45] This most likely reflects the young age and general good health of reproductive age women. However, in a 1985 review of 70 cases of myocardial infarction in pregnancy, only 13% of the patients had coronary artery disease prior to pregnancy.[45] In addition, the maternal mortality rate was 35% with the majority of deaths occurring at the initial infarction. Mortality was the greatest in the third trimester of pregnancy and when delivery occurred within two weeks of the infarction. Therefore, pregnancy associated with ischemic heart disease or myocardial infarction has substantial risk. Precipitating events can include severe pregnancy-induced hypertension, embolism, cardiac arrhythmias, and cocaine use. Myocardial infarction has been described after prostaglandin to induce labor, ergonovine for postpartum hemorrhage, and bromocriptine to suppress lactation.[4]

Antenatal care of women with a history of ischemic heart disease or myocardial infarction is best managed by a multidisciplinary team including a cardiologist, anesthesiologist, obstetrician, and dietitian. Initial therapy consists of strict limitation of activity and rest. Maternal echocardiography can be performed to determine ventricular function. Diagnostic radionucleotide cardiac imaging and cardiac catheterization can be performed if further diagnostic testing becomes necessary.[1] Pharmacologic therapy may include sublingual nitrates for angina and morphine sulfate for chest pain and anxiety. Beta blockade may be used to reduce myocardial oxygen demand. Heparin therapy may be added to reduce mural thrombi and embolization with the development of ventricular dyskinesis or aneurysms. Intravenous lidocaine to reduce the risk of post myocardial infarction arrhythmias is controversial. For patients with continued symptoms despite therapy, percutaneous transluminal coronary angioplasty, aortocoronary bypass grafting, and balloon angioplasty have been successfully performed.[46,47]

Intrapartum care consists of supplemental oxygen, lateral recumbent position, and pain relief with epidural anesthesia.[1,49] Vaginal birth is the preferred mode of delivery with instrumental assistance to avoid the Valsalva maneuver. Maternal hypotension and afterload reduction need to be avoided. Pulmonary artery catheterization may be required to optimize preload, afterload, and cardiac output for some patients. However, invasive central monitoring appears to be unnecessary for patients with good cardiac function and reserve.[43] Transfer to an intensive cardiac care unit may also be necessary.

Peripartum Cardiomyopathy

Peripartum cardiomyopathy is defined as the development of cardiomyopathy in the last month of pregnancy or first six months postpartum in a patient with no prior history of cardiac disease.[1] The heart is enlarged with ventricular dilatation, ventricular failure, and arrhythmias with histological findings of lipid deposition, hydropic degeneration, and swelling of the myofibrils.[25] This condition occurs in 1 of 15,000 deliveries.[50] A higher incidence between 1 in

1500–4000 deliveries has been reported, probably indicating population differences or the difficulty in making an accurate diagnosis.[51] The diagnosis is made by excluding other causes of cardiac disease such as hypertension or any valvular, metabolic, or infectious diseases. Mortality ranges from 25–50% (52). Typical symptoms include progressive dyspnea, orthopnea, fatigue, and edema.

Management consists of aggressive treatment for heart failure including supplemental oxygen, digoxin to improve cardiac performance and prevent ventricular arrhythmias, diuretics, limitation of sodium intake, and heparin to prevent pulmonary embolism. Since these patients are prone to congestive heart failure, pulmonary artery catheterization should be considered to avoid both volume overload and hypovolemia. Intrapartum management includes vaginal delivery with assistance to avoid the Valsalva maneuver. Epidural anesthesia is appropriate. In one study, a high recurrence risk for survivors was reported.[53] With persistent cardiomegaly, the mortality was between 40% and 80%. Pregnancy would appear to be contraindicated in this group of patients.

Antibiotic Prophylaxis

There are no clinical trials supporting prophylactic antibiotic use in pregnancy.[1,54,55] However, the American Heart Association provided updated antibiotic guidelines to prevent bacterial endocartiditis for patients with congenital heart disease.[55] Antibiotic prophylaxis should be administered for patients with most congenital cardiac malformations, prosthetic heart valves, and most acquired valvular lesions. The standard antibiotic regimen in these patients at risk is Ampicillin 2 g IV (or IM) plus Gentamycin 1.5 mg/kg IV (or IM) 30 minutes before the procedure, followed by Amoxicillin 1.5 g orally six hours after the initial dose. Alternatively, the parenteral regimen may be repeated once eight hours after the initial dose. For penicillin allergic patients, Vancomycin 1 g IV administered over one hour plus Gentamycin 1.5 mg/kg IV (or IM) (not to exceed 80 mg) one hour before

the procedure. This may be repeated once eight hours after the initial dose.

An alternative oral regimen for low-risk patients would consist of Amoxicillin 3 g orally one hour before the procedure, then 1.5 g six hours after the initial dose.

REFERENCES

1. American College of Obstetricians and Gynecologists. Cardiac disease in pregnancy. *ACOG Technical Bulletin 168*. Washington, DC: ACOG, 1994.
2. Sullivan JM, Ramanathan KB. Management of medical problems in pregnancy—Severe cardiac disease. *NEJM*. 1985;313:304–309.
3. Elkayam U, Gleicher N, eds. Cardiovascular physiology of pregnancy. *Cardiac Problems in Pregnancy*. New York: Alan R Liss, 1982, 5–26.
4. Cunningham FG, MacDonald PC, Gant NF, et al, eds. Cardiovascular diseases. *Williams Obstetrics*, 19th Ed. Norwalk, CT: Appleton & Lange, 1993, 1083–1104.
5. Mabie WC, DiSessa Tg, Crocker LG, et al. A longitudinal study of cardiac output in normal human pregnancy. *Am J Obstet Gynecol*. 1994; 170:849–856.
6. van Oppen ACA, Stigter RH, Bruinse HW. Cardiac output in normal pregnancy: a critical review. *Obstet Gynecol*. 1996;87:310–318.
7. Henricks CH, Quilligan EJ. Cardiac output during labor. *Am J Obstet Gynecol*. 1956;71:953–972.
8. Capeless EL, Clapp JF. When do cardiovascular parameters return to their preconception values? *Am J Obstet Gynecol*. 1991; 165:883–886.
9. American College of Obstetricians and Gynecologists. Invasive hemodynamic monitoring in obstetrics and gynecology. *ACOG Technical Bulletin 121*. Washington, DC: ACOG, 1988.
10. Clark SL, Cotton DB, Lee W, et al. Central hemodynamic assessment of normal term pregnancy. *Am J Obstet Gynecol*. 1989;161:1439–1442.
11. Criteria Committee of the New York Heart Association. *Nomenclature and Criteria for Di-*

agnosis of Diseases of the Heart and Great Vessels, 8th Ed. Boston: Little Brown, 1979.

12. Clark SL. Structural cardiac disease in pregnancy. In: Clark SL, Cotton DB, Phelan JP, eds. *Critical Care Obstetrics*, Oradell, NJ: Medical Economics Books, 1987, 97–113.

13. Whittemore R, Hobbins JC, Engle MA. Pregnancy and its outcome in women with and without surgical treatment of congenital heart disease. *Am J Cardiol.* 1982;50:641–651.

14. Nora JJ, Nora AH. Update on counseling the family with a first-degree relative with a congenital heart defect. *Am J Med Genet.* 1988;29: 137–142.

15. Nora JJ, Nora AH. Maternal transmission of congenital heart disease: new recurrence risk figures and the questions of cytoplasmic inheritance and vulnerability to teratogens. *Am J Cardiol.* 1987;59:459–463.

16. Pyeritz RE, Murphy EA. Genetics and congenital heart disease: perspectives and prospects. *J Am Coll Cardiol.* 1989;13:1458–1468.

17. Jacobson SJ, Jones K, Johnson K et al. Prospective multicentre study of pregnancy outcome after lithium exposure during first trimester. *Lancet.* 1992;339:530–533.

18. Clark SL, Phelan JP, Greenspoon J, et al. Labor and delivery in the presence of mitral stenosis: central hemodynamic observations. *Am J Obstet Gynecol.* 1985;157:984–988.

19. Lung B, Cormier B, Elias J, et al. Usefulness of percutaneous balloon commissurotomy for mitral stenosis during pregnancy. *Am J Cardiol.* 1994;73:398–400.

20. Markiewicz W, Stoner J, London E, et al. Mitral valve prolapse in one hundred previously healthy young females. *Circulation.* 1976;53: 464–473.

21. Arias F, Pineda J. Aortic stenosis and pregnancy. *J Reprod Med.* 1978;20:229–232.

22. Lao TT, Sermer M. MaGee L, et al. Congenital aortic stenosis and pregnancy—a reappraisal. *Am J Obstet Gynecol.* 1993;169:540–545.

23. Easterling TR, Chadwick HS, Otto CM, Benedetti TJ. Aortic stenosis in pregnancy. *Obstet Gynecol.* 1988;72:113–118.

24. Clark SL. Cardiac disease in pregnancy. In: Medicine of the Mother and Fetus, Reece EA, et al, eds. 1st ed., Philadelphia: Lippincott, 1992, 943–954.

25. *Nomenclature and Criteria for Diagnosis of Diseases of the Heart and Great Vessels*, 9th Ed. Boston: Little, Brown and Co., 1994.

26. Weinstein MR, Goldfield MD. Cardiovascular malformations with lithium use during pregnancy. *Am J Psychiatry.* 1975;132:529–531.

27. Connolly HM, Warnes CA. Ebstein's anomaly: outcome of pregnancy. *JACC.* 1994;23:1194–1198.

28. Gleicher N. Midwall J, Hochberger D, Jaffin H. Eisenmenger's syndrome and pregnancy. Obstet Gynecol Surv. 1979;34:721–741.

29. Patton DE, Lee W, Cotton DB, et al. Cyanotic maternal heart disease in pregnancy. *Obstet Gynecol Surv.* 1990;45:594–600.

30. Shime J, Mocarski EJM, Hastings D, et al. Congenital heart disease in pregnancy: short- and long-term implications. *Am J Obstet Gynecol.* 1987;156:313–322.

31. Pitts JA, Crosby WM, Basta LL. Eisenmenger's syndrome in pregnancy. Does heparin prophylaxis improve the maternal mortality rate? *Am Heart J.* 1977;93:321–326.

32. Pyeritz RE, McKusick VA. The Marfan syndrome: diagnosis and management. *N Engl J Med.* 1979;300:772–776.

33. Marsalese DL, Moodie DS, Vacante M, et al. Marfan's syndrome: natural history and long-term follow-up of cardiovascular involvement. *JACC.* 1989;14:422–428.

34. Geva T, Hegesh J, Frand M. The clinical course and echocardiographic features of Marfan's syndrome in childhood. *AJDC.* 1987;141: 1179–1182.

35. Murdoch JL, Walker BA, Helpern BL, et al. Life expectancy and causes of death in the Marfan syndrome. *N Engl J Med.* 1972;286:804–808.

36. Detrano, R, Moodie DS, Gill CC, et al. Intravenous digital subtraction aortography in the preoperative and postoperative evaluation of Marfan's aortic disease. *Chest.* 1985;88:249–253.

37. Gott, VL, Pyeritz RE, Magovern GJ, et al. Surgical treatment of aneurysms of the ascending aorta in the Marfan syndrome. *N Engl J Med.* 1986;314:1070–1074.

38. Shores J, Berger KR, Murphy EA, Pyeritz RE. Progression of aortic dilatation and the benefit of long-term B-adrenergic blockade in Marfan's

syndrome. *N Engl J Med*. 1994;330:1335–1341.

39. Rossiter JP, Repke JT, Morales AJ, et al. A prospective longitudinal evaluation of pregnancy in the Marfan syndrome. *Am J Obstet Gynecol*. 1995;173:1599–1606.

40. Mor-Yosef S, Younis J, Granat M, et al. Marfan's syndrome in pregnancy. *Obstet Gynecol Sur*. 1988;43:382–385.

41. Hseih TT, Chen KC, Soong JH. Outcome of pregnancy in patients with organic heart disease in Taiwan. *Asia-Oceanic J Obstet Gynaec*. 1993;19:21–27.

42. Ginz B. Myocardial infarction in pregnancy. *J Obstet Gynaecol Br Commonw*. 1970;77:610–615.

43. Sheikh AU, Harper MA. Myocardial infarction during pregnancy: management and outcome of two pregnancies. *Am J Obstet Gynecol*. 1993;169:279–284.

44. Samra D, Samra Y, Hertz M, Maier M. Acute myocardial infarction in pregnancy and puerperium. *Cardiol*. 1989;76:455–460.

45. Hankins GDV, Wendel GD, Leveno KJ, Stoneham J. Myocardial infarction during pregnancy. a review. *Obstet Gynecol*. 1985;65:139–146.

46. Hands ME, Johnson MD, Saltzman DH, Rutherford JD. The cardiac, obstetric, and anesthetic management of pregnancy complicated by acute myocardial infarction. *J Clin Anesth*. 1990;2:258–268.

47. Sanchez-Ramos L. Chami YG, Bass TA, et al. Myocardial infarction during pregnancy: management with transluminal coronary angioplasty and metallic intracoronary stents. *Am J Obstet Gynecol*. 1994;171:1392–1393.

48. Frenkel Y, Barkai G, Reisin L, et al. Pregnancy after myocardial infarction: are we playing safe? *Obstet Gynecol*. 1991;77:822–825.

49. Nolan TE, Hankins GDV. Myocardial infarction in pregnancy. *Clin Obstet Gynecol*. 1989;32:68–75.

50. Cunningham FG, Pritchard JA, Hankins GDV, et al. Peripartum heart failure: idiopathic cardiomyopathy or compounding cardiovascular events? *Obstet Gynecol*. 1986;67:157–168.

51. Homans DC. Peripartum cardiomyopathy. *N Engl J Med*. 1985;312:1432–1437.

52. Veille JC. Peripartum cardiomyopathies: a review. *Am J Obstet Gynecol*. 1984;148:805–818.

53. Demakis JG, Rahimtoola SH, Sutton GC, et al. Natural course of peripartum cardiomyopathy. *Circulation*. 1971;44:1053–1061.

54. Uyemura MC. Antibiotic prophylaxis for medical and dental procedures. *Postgraduate Medicine*. 1995;2:137–147.

55. Dajani AS, Bisno A, Chung KJ. Prevention of bacterial endocarditis: recommendations by the American Heart Association by the Committee on Rheumatic Fever, Endocarditis, and Kawasaki Disease. *JAMA*. 1990;264:2919–2922.

QUESTIONS
(choose the single best answer)

1. Physiologic changes in pregnancy include all of the following except
   a. Increased cardiac output peaking at 30–40% of prepregnant levels
   b. Increased plasma volume
   c. Increased blood flow
   d. Increased systemic vascular resistance
   e. Widened pulse pressure
2. Compared to normal nonpregnant subjects, pulmonary artery catheterization in the third trimester of normal pregnancy indicates that all of the following are true except
   a. Pulmonary artery pressure remains unchanged
   b. Pulmonary capillary wedge pressure remains unchanged
   c. Pulmonary capillary wedge pressure is normally 6–12 mm/Hg
   d. Pregnancy is associated with hyperdynamic left ventricular function
   e. Pulmonary vascular resistance is decreased
3. The highest risk of maternal mortality is associated with
   a. Aortic stenosis
   b. Mitral stenosis
   c. Pulmonary hypertension
   d. Ventricular septal defects
   e. Atrial septal defects
4. Intrapartum management of patients with severe mitral stenosis include all of the following except
   a. Lateral uterine displacement
   b. Large volumes of fluid to maintain preload

c. Supplemental oxygen
d. Pulmonary artery catheterization
e. Bacterial endocarditis prophylaxis
5. Marfan's syndrome is
   a. An autosomal recessive disorder
   b. Inherited as an X-linked disorder
   c. Associated with overriding of the aorta
   d. Often involved in dilation of the ascending aorta
   e. A right to left shunting of blood

12

Endocrine Disorders During Pregnancy

Ming-xu Lu and Marsha D. Cooper

INTRODUCTION TO THYROID DISEASE DURING PREGNANCY

Thyroid disease is common in women during their reproductive years. Abnormal thyroid function can significantly affect the course of the pregnancy and the health of the fetus. Pregnancy also significantly alters the course of autoimmune disease in general and thyroid disease in particular. There is evidence that changes induced by pregnancy may actually stimulate remission and exacerbation of preexisting thyroid disease.[1]

Diseases of the thyroid affect the pregnant woman (Table 12-1). The fetal thyroid is autonomous and maternal thyroid hormones have minor effect on it, however, treatment of thyroid disease during pregnancy can be very complicated since the fetal thyroid responds to the same pharmacological agents as does the maternal thyroid.

Thyroid gland influences pregnancy through various mechanisms. Pregnancy with its associated hormonal and metabolic changes, makes the evaluation of thyroid function very complex. Therefore, knowledge of normal thyroid hormone physiology and how pregnancy affects thyroid function is essential for the accurate diagnosis and management of thyroid disease during pregnancy.

Normal Thyroid Physiology

Thyroid hormones are largely responsible for controlling the general level of cellular metabolism. Thyroid hormone diffuses across the cell membrane and cytoplasm to enter the nucleus, where it binds to the nuclear receptor and controls metabolism largely by regulating gene expression and synthesis.[2]

Thyroid hormones are critically important in fetal development, particularly of the neural and skeletal systems.[3] They also have marked chronotropic and inotropic effects on the heart, which are similar to those induced by catecholamines. Thyroid hormones may amplify catecholamine action. Thyroid hormones are necessary for normal hypoxic and hypercapnic drive to the respiratory centers. They have a potent stimulatory effect on bone turnover, increasing bone formation and resorption.

The thyroid gland is responsible for synthesizing and secreting thyroid hormones, L-thyroxine (T4) and L-triiodothyronine (T3). The concentration of circulating free thyroid hormone is regulated by the hypothalamic-pituitary-thyroid axis. Thyrotropin-releasing hor-

Table 12-1.   Common Thyroid Diseases in Relation
to Pregnancy

Graves' hyperthyroidism
Autoimmune hypothyroidism
Postablative hypothyroidism
Postpartum thyroid disease
Thyrotoxicosis
Hypothyroidism

mone (TRH) from hypothalamus brings about
the secretion of thyrotropin or thyroid-stimulating hormone (TSH), from the anterior lobe of
the gland. TSH in turn controls the iodine uptake, the synthesis and the release of the two
major thyroid hormones, T4 and T3. On the
other hand, TSH is regulated by circulating levels of free T4 and T3 as negative feed-back
mechanism. Thyroid hormones mostly bind to
plasma proteins, mainly thyroxine binding globulin (TBG). Thyroid hormones also combine
with thyroglobulin for their storage as colloid
contained in the thyroid follicles and are released from the colloid under the control of
TSH.

Maternal Thyroid Physiology

The basal metabolic rate increases progressively during normal pregnancy by as much as
25%, which accompanies moderate enlargement
of the thyroid gland as a result of hyperplasia
of the glandular tissue and increased vascularity.
Most of this increase is due to metabolic activity
during pregnancy. In healthy pregnant women,
the regulation of thyroid function depends upon
various factors. An important factor is the direct
stimulation of the thyroid by human chorionic
gonadotropin (hCG), which shares some structural similarities with human TSH and acts as a
thyrotropic hormone especially in the first trimester of pregnancy. Moreover, one of the most
notable changes in maternal thyroid physiology
during pregnancy is an increase in serum TBG
level in response to hyperestrogenemia by its
sialylation and decreasing hepatic clearance.[1]
The net result is that T3 uptake by the thyroid
follicles is decreased and the total serum T4 and

T3 are increased. However, serum levels of free
T4 and T3 and thyrotropin (TSH) are within a
normal range, and thus there is no overt functional hyperthyroidism (see Table 12-2 for summary).

Placental Fetal Thyroid Physiology

Many questions still remains about how maternal thyroid hormones affect fetal development. Although it has been thought that T4 and
T3 did not cross the placental barrier, the exis-
tence of thyroid hormone receptors and the measurement of thyroid hormone in fetal tissues before fetal serum T4 levels increase imply that
placental transfer of hormones occurs. Indeed,
T4 crosses the placenta in the third trimester at
least in fetuses which cannot synthesize the hormone in the fetal thyroid.[4] There is no doubt that
low maternal T4 concentration during early
pregnancy results in impairment of fetal brain
development.[5]

Placenta can further influence the fetal hypothalamic-pituitary-thyroid axis development
by readily transferring several agents affecting
thyroid function. These include iodide, thionamides (propylthiouracil and carbimazole), β-
adrenergic receptor blockers (propanolol), somatostatin, exogenous TRH, and dopamine
agonist and antagonists (bromocriptine). However there is no transfer of TSH across placenta.
The placenta also contains deiodinase which
presumably regulate the quantity of thyroid hormones that can cross to the fetus.[6]

Fetal thyroid starts hormone production at 12
weeks gestation.[7] At this time fetal TSH is detectable but remains low until about 20 weeks,
hence, a functional fetal pituitary-thyroid axis
exists at 12 weeks gestation. The studies of maturation timing of thyroid function during human
fetal development has shown that total T4, free
T4, TBG and TBG and TSH levels increase
with gestational age, free T4 reached adult values by 28 weeks and TGB at 30 weeks. These
are important for the intrauterine diagnosis and
treatment of fetal thyroid disorders.

Table 12-2.   Useful Thyroid Function Tests in Normal Pregnancy, Hypothyroidism, and Hyperthyroidism

Test	Normal Pregnancy	Hypothyroidism	Hyperthyrodism
Basal metabolic rate	increased	decreased	increased
T3 resin uptake (T3 RU)	decreased	decreased	increased
Total T4	increased	decreased	increased
T4 binding globulin	increased	decreased	no change
Free T4	no change	decreased	increased
Total T3	increased	decreased	increased
Free T3	no change	decreased	increased
T7 (free thyroxine index)	no change	decreased	increased
Absolute iodine uptake	no change	decreased	increased
Serum cholesterol level	increased	?	decreased
TSH	no change	increased	decreased

LABORATORY EVALUATION OF THYROID FUNCTION IN PREGNANCY

Testing of thyroid function consists of laboratory studies performed on peripheral blood and testing of thyroid status in vivo. Laboratory studies routinely used to determine thyroid functions include (a) tests related to the binding of thyroid hormones in the blood; (b) measurement of the concentration of circulating thyroid hormones or biologically inactive products secreted by the thyroid gland; (c) evaluation of the hypothalamic-pituitary-thyroid axis, such as measurement of serum TSH; and (d) determination of antithyroid antibodies for diagnosis of autoimmune diseases. The easiest and least costly screening tests of thyroid function in pregnancy are TSH, total T4 and T3 resin uptake. The product of T3 and T4 is termed the free thyroxine index (T7), which is approximately equal to free T4 and is unchanged during pregnancy. Values of useful thyroid function tests are summarized in Table 12-2.

Measurement of TSH with the highly sensitive ELISA would form a useful first line test for thyroid dysfunction in pregnancy. A normal TSH value virtually excludes the possibility of thyroid dysfunction. Performing radioactive thyroid uptake studies and scans is contraindicated during pregnancy.

OTHER DIAGNOSTIC APPROACHES OF THYROID DISEASE

The radioactive diagnostic methods should be avoided for pregnant women, these are radionuclide scanning, fluorescent scanning, and radioactive thyroid uptake studies. Ultrasonography is used to differentiate between cystic and solid thyroid lesions. Cordocentesis is a direct access to the fetal circulation for evaluating fetal well-being and thyroid function.[8]

HYPERTHYROIDISM AND PREGNANCY

Next to the diabetes, untreated or previously treated hyperthyroidism is the most common endocrine disorder encountered during pregnancy. The prevalence of hyperthyroidism in pregnancy is 0.05–0.2%, and the disease is associated with a significant increase in neonatal mortality.[9] The commonest cause of hyperthyroidism in pregnancy is Graves' disease, accounting for over 85% of cases.[10] Graves' disease is an organ-specific autoimmune process usually associated with thyroid-stimulating antibody (TSAb) activity. These auto-antibodies mimic TSH in its ability to stimulate thyroid function. This condition may spontaneously remit during pregnancy because of the maternal

Table 12-3.   Major Etiology of Hyperthyroidism in Pregnancy

1. Graves' disease
2. Subacute thyroiditis
3. Toxic multinodular goiter
4. Toxic adenoma
5. Gestational trophoblastic neoplasia(s)
6. Exogenous T4 and T3

immunosuppression in response to fetal cytokines (7, 34). Other causes (Table 12-3) of hyperthyroidism include toxic multinodular goiter, toxic uninodular goiter and gestational trophoblastic tumor in which the hyperthyroidism is presumed due to the high level of hCG produced by the trophoblastic tumors, acting as a thyroid stimulator as hCG and TSH share some structural as well as functional similarities.

Clinical Presentation and Diagnosis

As expected, mild thyrotoxicosis may be difficult to diagnosis during pregnancy. The clinical presentation of thyrotoxicosis is nonspecific and independent of the cause of the hyperthyroidism. It is difficult to distinguish thyrotoxicosis from the apparent ''hypermetabolic'' state of pregnancy, particularly in the second and third trimesters. Many of the classic signs of hyperthyroidism—including heat intolerance, diaphoresis, warm skin, fatigue, anxiety, emotional liability, tremulousness, tachycardia, and a wide pulse pressure—are also seen during a normal pregnancy. Helpful differentiating signs seen in thyrotoxicosis, but rarely in a normal pregnancy, are eye signs and pretibial myxedema, weight loss, and a heart rate faster than 100 beats/min that does not decrease with the Valsalva maneuver.[11]

Maternal thyroid function should be assessed by measuring free T4, free T3, and TSH (see Table 12-2 for detail). A total serum thyroxine level of greater than 15 μg/dL or a greatly elevated free thyroxin index are diagnostic. (Careful attention should be paid to the normal ranges of these hormones in pregnancy when interpreting the results).

It is well recognized that TSH-receptor antibodies are heterogeneous and can have stimulating or blocking activity resulting in fetal hyper- or hypothyroidism.[12] Thyroid stimulating immunoglobulins (auto-antibodies) which can cross the placenta are present in Graves' disease and their detection at 36 weeks' gestation is a good guide to the likelihood of transient neonatal hyperthyroidism.[13]

Fetal and Neonatal Thyrotoxicosis

The fetal thyroid may be affected by maternal thyroid disease due to substances, including drugs, which cross the placenta (Table 12-4). Careful fetal monitoring is recommended during a thyrotoxic pregnancy, so the hypo- or hyperthyroidism in the fetus might be avoided. The level of thyroid-stimulating immunoglobulins (TSH) should be measured in the third trimester in all pregnant women with either active or quiescent Graves' disease. TSH levels of five times normal are seen more commonly in the mother of babies with neonatal hyperthyroidism.[12] The fetal thyroid becomes susceptible to maternal stimulating immunoglobulins between 20 to 24 weeks gestation. Fetal thyrotoxicosis is suggested by a heart rate greater than 160 beats per min (bpm), growth retardation and craniosynostosis in utero, all of which can be detected by ultrasonography.

Treatment of Hyperthyroidism

Hyperthyroidism is best treated prior to conception because the outcome for early treatment before pregnancy is better than that for treatment administered during pregnancy. There is an increased risk of abortion and minor fetal anomalies in untreated pregnant thyrotoxics. Treatment of hyperthyroidism during pregnancy is best done using antithyroid drugs. Medical treatment may cause fetal complications because both propylthiouracil and methimazole readily cross the placenta and can induce fetal hypothyroidism and goiter. The goal of treatment is to gain control of the thyrotoxicosis

Table 12-4. Fetal Transplacental Diseases

Fetal diseases	Maternal Diseases	Causes
Hyperthyroidism	Graves	TSH receptor stimulating Ab*
Hypothyroidism	Hashimoto's thyroiditis	TSH receptor blocking Ab*
		Anti-thyroid drugs, or iodides
Goiter	Goiter or Hashimoto's	Iodides, antithyroid drugs

Abbreviation: *Ab, antibody.

while avoiding any fetal or neonatal transient hypothyroidism. The aim should be to maintain the dose of carbimazole or propylthiouracil at the lowest level compatible with euthyroidism, or a dose that maintains maternal free thyroxine levels in a mildly thyrotoxic range in order to protect the fetus.

Thionamide Therapy

The thionamide drugs (Category D) are used most commonly for treatment of thyrotoxicosis during pregnancy. Propylthiouracil (PTU) theoretically cross the placenta and into breast milk to a lesser degree, so it is prescribed most frequently in the United States. The thionamides inhibit the iodination of thyroglobulin and thyroglobulin synthesis by competing with iodine of the enzyme peroxidase. PTU also inhibits the conversion from T4 to T3. As emphasized by Burrow,[14] the dose of PTU is empirical, and depending upon symptoms, the starting dose is 300 to 450 mg daily. If necessary, this dose should be increased until the woman, by clinical assessment, appears to be only minimally thyrotoxic, and the total serum thyroxine level is reduced to the upper normal range for pregnancy. Some patients may require doses of 600–900 mg per day. The risk of uncontrolled maternal thyrotoxicosis is greater than that of high-dose thionamide therapy. Once the patient is rendered euthyroid, free T4 and T3, and TSH levels should be measured monthly and the dose of thionamides should be adjusted accordingly. As pregnancy is associated with remission of the disease it is possible that no further therapy will be required although the patient should be monitored regularly. The most serious side effect of thionamide therapy is blood dyscrasias

—leukopenia and agranulocytosis, which occur in 0.3% of the patients. The development of agranulocytosis, is a contraindication to further thionamide therapy.[15] Routine CBC is advisable with PTU treatment. Surveillance cultures should be obtained and antibiotic treatment should be administered if signs of infection exist.

Iodides

Iodide therapy is an important adjunctive therapy in severe cases of hyperthyroidism, however, iodide crosses the placenta, and fetus is very sensitive to the inhibitory effect of excessive iodine. Goiter will occur after long-term use. Therefore it should only be used for a short-term course lasting no longer than two weeks.[16]

β-adrenergic Blocker (e.g., Propranolol)

β-adrenergic blockers are particularly useful for rapid control of the symptoms of thyrotoxicosis. Propranolol, 20 to 40 mg two to three times per day, or atenolol, 50 to 100 mg per day, will keep the maternal heart rate at 80 to 90 bpm.[16] Administration of propranolol for prolonged periods may be associated with small placenta and neonatal hypoglycemia, bradycardia, and depressed respiration, therefore it is not recommended as sole therapy.[10,17]

β-agonists often used to treat premature labor must never be given to women who are or have been thyrotoxic because of maternal fetal risks.

Surgery

Treatment of the hyperthyroidism by bilateral subtotal thyroidectomy may be undertaken most conveniently in the second trimesters, however, surgery should be performed only as a last resort after a trial of drug therapy or in the case of side effects to all antithyroid drugs. Patients should be preoperatively prepared for two weeks with iodine to decrease the vascularity of the gland, and thionamides and β-adrenergic blockers for symptomatic control (see above medical treatment).

HYPOTHYROIDISM AND PREGNANCY

Maternal hypothyroidism is relatively uncommon in pregnancy because hypothyroid females are relatively infertile. The prevalence rate of hypothyroidism in the United States is 0.6%. Women with hypothyroidism have higher incidence of gestational hypertension, preeclampsia, and placental abruption, which are the risk factors of premature labor. It has also been shown there is higher rate of low-birth-weight infants, stillbirths, abortions and congenital anomalies in babies born to mothers with untreated disease.[18] The commonest cause is Hashimoto's autoimmune thyroiditis (Table 12-5), which is characterized by the presence of antimicrosomal and antithyroglobulin antibodies. Hashimoto's thyroiditis occurs in patients with other autoimmune diseases including Addison's disease, diabetes mellitus, and pernicious anemia.

Clinical Presentation and Diagnosis

Prompt diagnosis and treatment of hypothyroidism can prevent the neonatal morbidity associated with the complications of premature labor due to gestational hypertension, preeclampsia and placental abruption (Leung et al.[19]).

Table 12-5.   Major Etiology of Hypothyroidism in Pregnancy

1. Hashimoto's thyroiditis
2. Post-therapy hypothyroidism
3. Suppurative and subacute thyroiditis
4. Drugs
5. Iodine deficiency

The symptoms of hypothyroidism in the adult are insidious without definable onset, and they are often masked by the hypermetabolism of the pregnant state. In most of these women, a history of surgical or radioiodine treatment, usually for Graves' thyrotoxicosis, and family history of thyroid disease will be evaluated. Hypothyroid women may complain of cool, dry skin, coarse hair, constipation, cold intolerance, fatigue, irritability, or altered mentation. In addition, gestational hypertension and preeclampsia are more common in women with hypothyroidism as mentioned above (Leung et al.[19]).

Laboratory parameters offer the most sensitive and specific means for diagnosing hypothyroidism. If the expected rise during pregnancy in the level of circulating thyroxine (T4) does not occur, and the level of TSH is elevated, primary hypothyroidism is diagnosed. In secondary or pituitary hypothyroidism, the TSH will be normal or low in the setting of a low free T4. The thyroid autoantibodies may lend confirmation to the diagnosis of autoimmune hypothyroidism.

Fetal and Neonatal Hypothyroidism and Neonatal Screening

Deficiency of thyroid hormones during fetal development or the first two years of life can cause irreversible brain damage, with the severity of disease related to the severity, duration, and age at which the hypothyroidism occurs. The most common cause of congenital primary sporadic hypothyroidism is thyroid dysgenesis, occurring approximately once in every 4000 births (Table 12-6).[20] Iodine deficiency is a com-

Table 12-6.   Etiology of Congenital Hypothyroidism

Primary hypothyroidism
   Thyroid dysgenesis
   Inborn errors of thyroid function
   Drug-induced
   Endemic hypothyroidism (iodine deficiency)
Secondary hypothyroidism (TSH deficiency)
Tertiary hypothyroidism (TRH deficiency)

mon cause of hypothyroidism in many parts of the world, although it is extremely rare in the United States. Cretinism is a syndrome of severe mental retardation, abnormal growth, deaf-mutism, spasticity, strabismus, and abnormal asexual maturation secondary to iodine deficiency occurring in utero.

No matter what the cause of neonatal hypothyroidism, it is important that the infant should be treated as early as possible.

The clinical diagnosis of congenital hypothyroidism during the neonatal periods is difficult to make and often is missed. However, the neonatal screening programs of all infants diagnose most cases of congenital hypothyroidism, and prompt treatment usually prevents mental retardation.[21]

The screening techniques rely on a sample of cord or heel prick blood. A T4 measurement is followed by a measurement of TSH in specimens. Ideal timing for screening is between day 2 and day 6 of life. A low T4 level (less than 7 ug/mL) and TSH concentrations greater than 40 uU/mL is indicative of congenital hypothyroidism. Borderline TSH levels (20–40 uU/mL) should be repeated.[22]

Clinical Management

As soon as the diagnosis of hypothyroidism during pregnancy has been established, an adequate replacement dosage of L-thyroxine should be started immediately, the aim of the therapy is to normalize the serum TSH level. Most patients require usually 0.125 to 0.15 mg per day with readjustment of dosage based on clinical and laboratory reevaluation at two to three weeks. Pregnant women with adequate replacement of L-thyroxine should have normal TSH levels (<6 uU/mL) as well as normal T4 levels for pregnancy. Subnormal level can be readjusted by increasing L-thyroxine dosage of 0.05 mg per day every two to three weeks until optimal levels of TSH and T4 are reached. Because of the increased amount of TBG binding during normal pregnancy, it may be necessary to modestly increase the amount of L-thyroxine replacement during pregnancy. However, L-thy-roxine replacement dosage should not normally exceed 0.30 mg per day.[16]

THYROID NODULES, MALIGNANT TUMORS, AND NONTOXIC GOITER AND PREGNANCY

Thyroid nodules are more common in women than in men, and most nodules are discovered in the course of routine examinations. The finding of a solitary nodule during pregnancy requires fine-needle aspiration to investigate the possibility of malignancy, especially in those patients who present before 20 weeks of gestation with rapidly enlarging thyroid nodules, nodules associated with palpable cervical adenopathy, solid nodules larger than 2 cm, or cystic nodules larger than 4 cm.[23] Although ultrasonography can define whether the nodule is solid or cystic, it has low specificity for thyroid pathology. Free T4 and TSH levels should be obtained to rule out the possibility of a toxic nodule or an unusual presentation of Hashimoto's thyroiditis. Thyroid carcinoma rarely presents during pregnancy. Growth of a nodule while a patient is receiving thyroid hormone suppression therapy is highly suspicious for malignancy, biopsy should performed later in gestation (stage II and III).[23] On the other hand, pregnancy may have a small impact on the progression of thyroid cancer. In the rare case of thyroid carcinoma diagnosed during pregnancy, surgery is recommended. Radiation therapy should be postponed until after delivery. Nontoxic goiter may enlarge during pregnancy. Some authors recommend treatment with L-thyroxine to prevent further enlargement.[24]

POSTPARTUM THYROIDITIS

Postpartum thyroiditis is usually caused by painless lymphocytic thyroiditis that may be identified in 5% to 9% of women about 12 months following delivery.[25,26] The hallmark of postpartum thyroiditis, or silent thyroiditis is its transient nature.[27] Postpartum thyroid dysfunction is diagnosed infrequently, largely because it typically developed after the traditional postpartum examination and because it results in vague and nonspecific symptoms which are commonly attributed to the postpartum state.[28] The postpartum thyroiditis is thought to relate to the immunologic rebound that occurs following the natural immunosuppression during pregnancy.[29] In addition, transient postpartum hypothyroidism associated with autoimmune thyroiditis was described by Amino et al.[30] and Ginsberg and Walfish.[31]

Clinical Presentation

There is a typical clinical course for this disease (Table 12-7). Initially, 75% of women will experience a thyrotoxic phase beginning about two to four months postpartum. Symptoms of fatigue, weight loss, palpitations, and dizziness experienced in the thyrotoxic phase are accepted by many new mothers as a natural part of a normal postpartum course. The following hypothyroid phase, seen about four to eight months postpartum, is usually more clinically evident with complaints primarily of fatigue and weight loss. Dry skin, constipation, and cold intolerance are not common. Goiter, which appears in 50% of the patients, may be noted at

Table 12-7. Clinical Presentation of Postpartum Thyroiditis

Thyrotoxic phase
  2–4 months postpartum
  Usually mild symptoms or asymptomatic
    (dry skin, weight loss, dizziness & constipation)
  Transient elevation of free T4 or free T3
  Low radioiodine uptake
  Negative thyroid stimulating antibody
Hypothyroid phase
  4–8 months postpartum
  Symptomatic—psychiatric symptoms such as depression
  Clinically hypothyroid—goiter with lymphocytic infiltration by tissue biopsy
  High titers of antimicrosomal antibodies
  Treatment with T4 often required
  Recurrence of disease in subsequent pregnancy
  Long-term hypothyroidism may occur in 25%

---

this time, and some women experience depression. Most patients return to the euthyroid states after three to five months, although 10 to 30% is marked variability in presentations between patients, recurrence in a single patient with a similar course and intensity usually occurs after subsequent pregnancies.[30,32] There is marked variability in presentations between patients, those who develop marked symptoms early in the postpartum period without goiter are more likely to have permanent hypothyroidism.[27]

Pathogenesis and Diagnosis

The etiology of postpartum thyroid dysfunction is almost certainly immunological, reflecting the phenomenon of immunologic rebound from the relative immune tolerance during pregnancy. The disease has been well characterized histologically as a destructive, lymphocytic thyroiditis. The diagnosis of postpartum thyroiditis is made by abnormal free T4 and TSH values in the postpartum period coupled with a positive titer of antimicrosomal antibodies and/or antithyroglobulin antibodies (76%).[26] When microsomal autoantibody titers are followed sequentially in seropositive women during pregnancy and postpartum, a characteristic pattern emerges.[33] These titers decrease somewhat during pregnancy, rise to a peak 4 to 6 months after delivery, and then decline to early pregnancy levels by 10 to 12 months postpartum. The level of antimicrosomal antibody in first trimester of pregnancy may be used to predict the development of postpartum thyroiditis in those with a personal or family history of thyroid disease. Hemagglutination titers of 1:6400 or higher routinely predict postpartum thyroiditis, while those less than 1:100 virtually exclude it.[33] If the titer is positive, the patient should be followed throughout pregnancy and the postpartum period, carefully monitoring the TSH and free T4 concentrations.[28] The thyrotoxic phase should be distinguished from postpartum relapse of Graves' disease by obtaining a radioactive iodine uptake. Uptake is extremely low in patients with postpartum thyroiditis and normal to high in patients with Graves' disease.

Treatment

Treatment of postpartum thyroiditis is based on symptoms and usually is not necessary. If symptoms of hypothyroidism become prominent, replacement therapy with L-thyroxine should be initiated.

DISEASES OF THE PITUITARY

The normal pituitary gland enlarges and has numerous physiologic changes in function during pregnancy, which make the diagnosis of pituitary disease difficult. Gonadotropin (FSH & LH) levels are decreased as a result of elevated estrogen and progesterone. Growth hormone release in response to standardized stimulation is decreased. Circulating adrenocorticotropic hormone (ACTH) concentrations increase during pregnancy despite the concomitant rise of free cortisol. Thyroid-stimulating hormone (TSH) concentrations are slightly decreased during the first trimester and return to normal during the second and third trimesters. Serum prolactin concentrations increase dramatically during pregnancy (presumably the result of lactotrope hyperplasia secondary to the increasing serum estrogen and progesterone concentration). Levels increase from approximately 20 ng/mL at 5 to 8 weeks gestation to up to 200 to 400 ng/mL at term. Menses resume after normalization of prolactin levels, expected by the latest 4 to 6 months postpartum in a nonlactating mother. A failure of menstrual periods to return by this time may indicate underlying pathology such as pituitary prolactinemia.

Disorder resulting in either hyperfunction or hypofunction of the pituitary gland may occur during pregnancy. Most commonly hyperprolactinemia secondary to a pituitary microadenoma, or panhypopituitarism due to postpartum ischemic necrosis (Sheehan's syndrome).[34]

Pituitary Microadenomas

Of those functional pituitary tumors, growth hormone-producing tumors resulting in acromegaly, ACTH-producing tumors give rise to Cushing's disease. Prolactin-secreting microadenomas are by far the most common pituitary tumors (40%) encountered in pregnancy.[35] Moreover, prolactin-secreting microadenomas and hyperprolactinemia are among the abnormalities reported for women exposed prenatally to diethylstilbestrol (DES).[36]

Prolactin-secreting microadenomas are often associated with the syndrome of amenorrhea and galactorrhea. Diagnosis of the lesion is made by history, elevated levels of prolactin, and radiological identification of a sellar or suprasellar mass. The most accurate radiographic technique is magnetic resonance imaging (MRI), which can identify a lesion smaller than 3 mm in diameter. Arteriography may occasionally be useful. Neurologic findings such as changes in the visual fields can occur with larger lesions, but they are uncommon because most tumors are small.

Possible methods of management of pituitary microadenomas include observation alone and medical management with dopamine agonists (bromocriptine). A relatively large number of pregnancies have not been observed in women treated with bromocriptine.[34] Bromocriptine does not affect the fetus adversely. Surgery is reserved for women with no response to this drug.

Sheehan's Syndrome

Sheehan's syndrome is the most common cause of anterior pituitary insufficiency in the adult woman associated with pregnancy. This syndrome of postpartum pituitary necrosis is associated with postpartum hemorrhage. Presumably the hyperplastic gland in pregnancy is more vulnerable to an inadequate blood supply. The diagnosis and the extent of pituitary damage can be determined by tests of target organ function, such as thyroid function tests, cortisol concentration, as well as tests of pituitary reserve (e.g., GnRH, TRH, GHRH, and CRF).[37] Treatment of pituitary insufficiency during pregnancy with replacement doses of L-thyroxine (0.1 to 0.2 mg/day) and cortisol (20 mg AM, 10 mg PM) or prednisone (5 mg AM, 2.5 mg PM) are administrated to maintain well-being.[16,20]

Anencephaly and Congenital Pituitary Hypofunction

Low levels of amniotic fluid estriol, cortisol, 17-hydroxysteroids, and other steroid products are associated with anencephaly. It reflects the absence of the hypothalamus and its releasing hormones, resulting in lack of pituitary ACTH secretion and absence of adrenal stimulation, thus small adrenal glands.

However, the adrenals of the anencephalic fetus are normal until 20th week of pregnancy,[38] amniotic fluid studies would not be useful for the early diagnosis of anencephaly at midpregnancy, reliance should be placed on measuring α-fetoprotein concentrations and ultrasonographic studies.

DISEASES OF ADRENAL GLANDS

Plasma cortisol levels rise progressively at the second and third trimester during pregnancy, as well as plasma corticotropin-releasing factor (CRF) and ACTH concentrations (Table 12-8). The diurnal variation of both cortisol and ACTH is maintained. Corticosteroid-binding globulin (CBG) concentrations increase threefold during pregnancy, resulting in an increase in the total plasma cortisol and a fall in its metabolic clearance. The unbound fraction also increases, and thus a rise in urinary free cortisol. Although free cortisol is increased during pregnancy, the elevated progesterone concentrations in pregnancy compete for the same cellular binding sites.

Thus, the elevated plasma cortisol fraction may represent a relative diminution in intracellular cortisol binding. Renin activity also increases during pregnancy and is positively correlated with rising of aldosterone concentrations which is five to eight times that of nonpregnant women.

Adrenocortical Insufficiency (Addison's Disease)

The disease may first present in pregnancy, although most cases are diagnosed outside of pregnancy. The signs and symptoms are nonspecific and include persistent fatigue, nausea, vomiting, weight loss, postural hypotension and personality changes. Laboratory findings of Addison's disease include decreased serum sodium; increased serum potassium, BUN, creatinine, hypoglycemia, and other specific tests as summarized in Table 12-8.

In patients with already recognized adrenal disorders, replacement hormone therapy is continued throughout gestation, using cortisol (20 mg AM, 10 mg PM) along with fludrocortisone (0.05 to 0.1 mg per day) for hyperkalemia and postural hypotension, and the patient should be monitored regularly.

Cushing's Syndrome in Pregnancy

Cushing's syndrome describes the combination of symptoms and signs caused by excessive exposure to glucocorticoids.[39,40] Features of mineralocorticoid excess may also be present, depending on the cause of the syndrome. The coincidence of untreated Cushing's syndrome

Table 12-8. Laboratory Diagnosis of Adrenocortical Insufficiency (Addison's Disease) During Pregnancy

Test	Normal Response	Addison's
Corticotropin stimulation	>doubling of cortisol at one hour	<doubling of cortisol at one hour
Plasma ACTH	Increases during pregnancy	+/− (+ with primary disease, − with secondary disease)
A.M. plasma cortisol	Increase during pregnancy	Decrease
Plasma CBG	Increase during pregnancy	
Urine-free cortisol (24-hour excretion)	Increase during pregnancy	Decrease

Table 12-9. Causes of Cushing's Syndrome

Administration of glucocorticoid or ACTH
ACTH overproduction
   Pituitary: Adenoma
               Hyperplasia
   Ectopic: Small cell carcinoma of lung
               Bronchial carcinoid
               Pancreatic islet cell tumor
               Thymoma
Adrenal adenoma and carcinoma

and pregnancy is rare. Causes of Cushing's syndrome are listed in Table 12-9.

Cushing's syndrome during pregnancy is associated with an increased incidence of miscarriage, premature labor, and stillbirth.

Clinical features of Cushing's syndrome include classically truncal and facial obesity, plethoric cheeks, striae, "buffalo hump," osteoporosis, and hypertension. Hirsutism and acne tend to be particularly prominent. There are some common complaints of weakness, easy bruising, an increased tendency to peptic ulcers and gastrointestinal bleeding, and sometimes mental changes including depression and euphoria. Glucose intolerance is frequent.

Lab tests include screening tests, confirmatory tests, and definitive diagnosis (Table 12-10).

Treatment of Cushing's syndrome depends on the cause. Not one of the many modalities of treatment seems suitable. Surgical resection

Table 12-10. Investigation of a Suspected Case of Cushing's Syndrome

Screening test:	Overnight dexamethasone suppression test
Confirmatory test:	24-hour urinary free cortisol level
	Diurnal plasma cortisol values
Definitive diagnosis:	Plasma ACTH measurement
	Four-day dexamethasone suppression test
	Abdominal and cerebral CT scan if carcinoma suspected
	Chest x-ray looking for tumor
	Surgical exploration during pregnancy if suspect adrenal carcinoma

of the adrenal hormone source in cases of urgent treatment needed still remains the method of choice as it is in the nonpregnant state. Some people suggest Metyrapone treatment in doses up to 2 g per day from the 29th week to delivery.

Congenital Adrenal Hyperplasia (CAH)

The congenital adrenal hyperplasia (CAH) results from inherited defects in enzymes required in the biosynthetic pathways of steroid hormones of all three groups. Cortisol synthesis is diminished, and there is accumulation of intermediate metabolites due to the absence or reduced activity of an enzyme required for their further processing.

Over 90% of patients with CAH have defective 21-hydroxylase, which may present as severe salt-wasting, simple virilizing, attenuated or cryptic disease, which is manifested at birth with ambiguous genitalia in the female and normal genitalia in the male.

11-β-hydroxylase deficiency accounts for approximately 5% of cases of CAH. This defect results in diminished cortisol but elevated levels of deoxycorticosterone and adrenal androgens. Hypertension may be a feature of this disorder, along with masculinization of the female fetus.

The only satisfactory treatment of all forms is life-long administration of cortisol or other glucocorticoids. Cortisone acetate of 25 mg in the morning and 12.5 mg in the afternoon is adequate for maintenance. Malformation of the external genitalia in girls is the only symptom which cannot be influenced by postnatal cortisol. Surgical correction of the external female genitalia is indicated for ambiguous genitalia.[20]

DISORDER OF PARATHYROID GLANDS

Physiology of the Parathyroid Glands During Pregnancy

The majority of the calcium requirement for the fetus occurs in the third trimester of pregnancy, when fetal skeletal growth reaches an accelerated phase. The full-term fetus contains between 25 and 30 g of calcium which are obtained from the mother via the placenta. To prepare for this large demand and also for the loss of calcium during lactation, maternal calcium accretion begins early in gestation by increasing calcium absorption. Another source of calcium from the mother is from mobilization of her own stores in the skeleton. Maternal concentration of serum calcium during pregnancy is dependent on a complex interaction of parathyroid hormone (PTH), calcitonin, and vitamin D and its metabolites. It is believed that the rise in 1,25 dihydroxycholecalciferol together with increased calcium absorption from the gut is responsible for the transfer of the necessary calcium to the developing fetus.[35] Total serum calcium and phosphorus actually decrease in pregnancy. The decrease in serum calcium is accompanied by a similar decrease in serum proteins such as albumin during pregnancy. The release of PTH is stimulated by decrease in plasma calcium or magnesium. Conversely, increases in plasma calcium and magnesium levels suppress PTH.

Disorder of Hypersecretion of Parathyroid Hormone

Hyperparathyroidism is a rare condition during pregnancy caused by excessive PTH production. The majority of hyperparathyroidism involves a single parathyroid adenoma, but adenomatous hyperplasia may also occur, especially in familial syndromes. Pregnancy may exacerbate preexisting hyperparathyroidism, and spontaneous abortion and late fetal deaths occur much more commonly than normal.[41] The symptoms may include fatigue, prolonged and intractable nausea and vomiting, constipation, polyuria and bone pain. The diagnosis is confirmed by finding elevated serum free calcium levels, low serum phosphorous levels, and high PTH. Localized radiological studies should be kept to minimum. Treatment choice is surgical removal of the tissue. If surgery is contraindi-

cated, the serum calcium may be controlled by thiazide diuretics and oral phosphate therapy.

Neonates born to women with hyperthyroidism experience subnormal calcium levels after birth. This is due to the excessive calcium suppressed by the fetal PTH. More than 50% of such infants will develop tetany. However, in this case, tetany is usually short-lived as the parathyroid glands recover their normal function spontaneously. Intravenous calcium gluconate and oral 1-α-OH-vitamin D3 should be considered in the severe case of tetany.

Disorder of Hyposecretion

Hypoparathyroidism usually results from inadvertent removal at the time of thyroid surgery, but rarely autoimmune destruction may occur. Symptoms are related to subnormal serum calcium, such as paresthesias, numbness and tingling, muscle cramps, and even tetany. Diagnosis is made by subnormal serum calcium level with a low PTH serum determination. Treatment includes calcium supplementation and vitamin D. The dosage of both need to be increased with advancing gestation.

If maternal hypoparathyroidism is poorly controlled during pregnancy, then the fetus suffers from hypocalcemia and osteopenia (skeletal undermineralization). At birth, such neonates may exhibit elevated PTH levels with widespread osteitis fibrosa cystica, hypotonia, poor feeding, constipation, and failure to thrive, and the mother who is treated with vitamin D should avoid breastfeeding.

REFERENCES

1. Lowe TW, Cunningham FG. Pregnancy and thyroid disease. *Clin Obstet Gynecol.* 1991; 34(1):72–81.

2. Oppenheimer JH. Thyroid hormone action at the nuclear level. *Ann Intern Med.* 1985;102: 374–377.

3. Scott, JR, DiSaia PJ, et al. *Danforth's Obstetrics and Gynecology*, 7th Ed. Philadelphia: Lippincott 1994, 427–435.

4. Vulsma T, Gons MH. Maternal-fetal transfer of thyroxine in congenital hypothyroidism due to a total organification defect or thyroid agenesis. *N Engl J Med.* 1989;321:13–21.

5. Pharoah POD, Connolly KJ. Maternal thyroid hormones and fetal brain development. In: *Iodine and the Brain.* New York: Plenum Press, 1989, 333–352.

6. Roti E, Gnudi A. The placental transport, synthesis and metabolism of hormones and drugs which affect thyroid function. *Endocr Rev.* 1983;4:131–149.

7. Fisher DA, Klein AH. Thyroid development and disorders of thyroid function in the newborn. *N Engl J Med* 1981;16:1361–1364.

8. Hare JY. Cordocentesis: direct access to the fetal circulation for evaluating fetal well-being and thyroid function. *Current Opinion in Obstet & Gynecol.* 1994;6(5):440–444.

9. Hollingsworth D. Hyperthyroidism in pregnancy. In: The Thyroid, Hollingsworth, D, ed. Philadelphia: J. B. Lippincott, 1986, 1043–1063.

10. Mestman JH, Goodwin TM, et al. Thyroid disorders of pregnancy. *Endocrinol Metab Clin North Am.* 1995;24:41–71.

11. Burrow GN. Thyroid diseases in pregnancy. *Thyroid Function and Disease.* Philadelphia: WB Saunders, 1989, 292–323.

12. Clavel S, Madec AM. Anti TSH-receptor antibodies in pregnant patients with autoimmune thyroid disorder. *Br J Obstet Gynecol* 1990;97:1003–1008.

13. Munro DS, Dirmikis SM. The role of thyroid stimulating immunoglobulins of Graves' disease in neonatal thyrotoxicosis. *Br J Obstet Gynecol.* 1978;85:837–843.

14. Burrow GN. The management of thyrotoxicosis in pregnancy. *Endocrinologist.* 1991;1:409–417.

15. Bishnoi A, et al. Thyroid disease during pregnancy. *Am Family Physician.* 1996;53:215–220.

16. Creasy R, Resnik R. *Maternal Fetal Medicine, Principles and Practice,* 3rd Ed. Philadelphia: WB Saunders, 1994, 979–1025.

17. Burrow GN. Thyroid function and hyperfunction during gestation. *Endocr Rev.* 1993;14:194–202.

18. Montoro M, et al. Successful outcome of preg-

19. Leung AS, Miller LK, Koonings PP, et al. Perinatal outcome in hypothyroid patients. *Obstet Gynecol.* 1993;81:349–353.

20. Reece EA, Hobbins JC, et al. *Medicine of the Fetus and Mother, Endocrine Disease in Pregnancy.* Philadelphia: Lippincott, 1992, 1025–1044.

21. Fisher DA. Effectiveness of newborn screening for congenital hypothyroidism: recommended guidelines. *Pediatrics.* 1987;80:745–749.

22. Gomella TL. *Neonatology—A Large Clinical Manual,* 1st Ed. Norwalk, CT: Appleton & Lange, 1994, 463–465.

23. Snitzer JL. Maternal and fetal thyroid function. *N Engl J Med.* 1995;332(9):613–614.

24. Koutras DA. Prevention and treatment of nontoxic goiter during pregnancy. In: Beckers C, Reinwein D, eds. *The Thyroid and Pregnancy.* New York: Wiley, 1992.

25. Walfish PG, Chan JYC. Postpartum hyperthyroidism. *J Clin Endocrinol Metab.* 1985;14:417–425.

26. Learoyd DL, et al. Postpartum thyroid dysfunction. *Thyroid.* 1992;2(1):73–80.

27. Jansson R, Dahlberg PA, et al. Postpartum thyroiditis. *Ballieres Clin Endocrinol Metab.* 1988;2:619–626.

28. Ramsey I. Postpartum thyroiditis: an underdiagnosed disease. *Br J Obstet Gynecol.* 1986;93:1121–1126.

29. Stagnaro-Green A. Postpartum thyroiditis: prevalence, etiology and clinical implications. *Thyroid Today.* 1993;16:1–11.

30. Amino N, Mori H, Iwatani Y, et al. High prevalence of transient postpartum thyrotoxicosis and hypothyroidism. *N Engl J Med.* 1982;306:849–853.

31. Ginsberg J, Walfish PG. Postpartum transient thyrotoxicosis with painless thyroiditis. *Lancet.* 1977;1:1125–1127.

32. Tachi J, Amino N, et al. Long-term follow-up and HLA associations in patients with postpartum hypothyroidism. *J Clin Endocrinol Metab.* 1988;66:480–488.

33. Jansson R, Bernander S, et al. Autoimmune thyroid dysfunction in the postpartum period. *J Clin Endocrinol Metab.* 1984;58:681–688.

34. Molitch ME. Pregnancy and the hyperprolacti-

nemic women. *N Engl J Med.* 1985;312:1364–1369.

35. Steichen JJ, et al. Vitamin D homeostasis in the perinatal period. *New Engl J Med.* 1980;302:315–318.

36. Potter EL. A historical review: DES use during pregnancy. *Ped Pathology.* 1991;11(5):781–789.

37. Lufkin EG, Kao PC, et al. Combined testing of anterior pituitary gland with insulin, thyrotropin-releasing hormone and luteinizing hormone-releasing hormone. *Am J Med.* 1983;75:471–479.

38. Tulchinsky D and Ryan KJ. Maternal-Fetal Endocrinology, W. B. Saunders, part III—the fetal endocrine system, Philadelphia: W. B. Saunders Company, 1980.

39. Koerten JM, et al. Cushing's syndrome in pregnancy: a case report and literature review. *Am J Obstet Gynecol.* 1986;154:626–629.

40. Gold EM. The Cushing syndromes: changing views of diagnosis and treatment. *Ann Intern Med.* 1979;90:829–836.

41. Pellegrino SV. Primary hyperparathyroidism exacerbated by pregnancy. *J Oral Maxillofac Surg.* 1977;35:915–921.

QUESTIONS

1. Prolactin-secreting pituitary adenomas (prolactinomas) usually
   a. Diminish in size during pregnancy
   b. Increase in size over time
   c. Are symptomatic during lactation
   d. Impinge upon the olfactory nerve
   e. Respond to medical therapy
2. Which of the following is most likely to be born to a woman with Graves' disease currently under control?
   a. Hypothyroid infants
   b. Infertile infants
   c. Hyperthyroid infants
   d. Infants with ambiguous genitalia
3. A 35-year-old woman has recently experienced fatigue, sleepiness, dry skin, constipation, and a 10-pound weight gain. Her thyroid is form and twice the normal size. Which one of the following laboratory tests is most likely to confirm the suspected diagnosis of hypothyroidism?
   a. Serum thyroxine (T4)
   b. Serum triiodothyroxine (T3)
   c. T3 resin uptake
   d. Serum thyroid-stimulating hormone (TSH) measurement
   e. Antithyroid antibodies
4. Hypothyroidism should be treated with daily administration of which one of the following thyroid hormone preparations
   a. Thyroid extract
   b. Thyroglobulin
   c. Thyroxine (T4)
   d. Triidothyronine (T3)
   e. T3 and T4
5. Congenital hypothyroidism is most commonly due to:
   a. Inborn errors of metabolism
   b. Aplasia of the thyroid gland
   c. Hypoplasia of a thyroid gland in the normal position
   d. Inadequate function in an ectopic thyroid gland
   e. Medication given to the mother during pregnancy

For each of the findings (a–d) on a neonatal thyroid screening test carried out on the third day of life, select the one that is most suggestive of each of the following conditions:

	T4	TSH
a.	Low	High
b.	Normal	High
c.	Low	Low
d.	Low	Normal

6. Secondary hypothyroidism
7. Primary hypothyroidism

For each result of thyroid function tests, select the clinical condition with which it is most likely to be associated:

8. Elevated serum T4, low T3 resin uptake
9. Elevated serum T4, elevated radioactive iodine uptake
   a. Graves' disease
   b. Hypothyroidism
   c. Pregnancy

13

Drug Abuse in Pregnancy

Diana Smigaj

ILLICIT DRUGS IN GENERAL

The use of recreational drugs, legal and illegal, is widespread in our society. Use during pregnancy can have detrimental effects for the mother, the fetus, and the child after birth. Such effects vary with the substance, with the magnitude and timing of use, and with associated phenomena such as malnourishment and infection. Some general characteristics of drug use are worth noting before considering specific drugs in detail.

Users of illegal drugs and alcoholics often attempt to hide this by misrepresentation and by minimizing prenatal care; it is fairly common to have heavy users present in labor with no prior prenatal care.

Users often take other drugs in addition to their primary drug of choice; this can be random, with the user taking whatever is available, and also includes some common pairings:

- Alcoholics frequently smoke cigarettes.
- Cocaine or amphetamine users take tranquilizers and barbiturates to minimize the "crash."
- Heroin users turn to alcohol when their heroin supply is limited.

Users are often malnourished. Cigarette smokers can have deficiencies in vitamins C, E, and zinc. Alcohol abusers often undereat because they obtain so many calories from alcohol. Cocaine and other stimulants depress the appetite. Heavy drug users are often preoccupied with maintaining their habit rather than with eating properly.

Promiscuity is common in heavy drug users.

Risk of infections in general is increased because of malnourishment, promiscuity, unsanitary needle use, and unstable living environment.

An increased risk of physical abuse is a feature of the drug scene.

Patients who are intoxicated or "stoned" during labor and delivery present special problems.

While withdrawal from some drugs can be risky for any patient, there are additional risks during pregnancy.

The serious consequences of substance abuse make it imperative that practitioners pay attention to indicators of abuse (see Table 13-1). Drug screens can be useful in diagnosis and management but should be done consistent with patient consent and the policies of the hospital and laws of the state involved. Management should be multidimensional and should address all aspects of the drug abuse problem (see Table 13-2).

Table 13-1.   Signs and Symptoms of Substance Abuse

Physical Findings
  Track marks and other evidence of intravenous drug use
  Alcohol on the breath
  Scars, injuries
  Hypertension
  Tachycardia or bradycardia
  Tremors
  Slurred speech
  Self-neglect or poor hygiene
  Liver or renal disease
  Runny nose
  Chronic cough
  Cheilosis
  Nervous mannerisms (e.g., frequently licking lips, jitters, foot tapping)
  Pinpoint or dilated pupils
  Reproductive dysfunction (hypogonadism, irregular menses, miscarriage, infertility, fetal alcohol syndrome)
Psychologic Problems
  Memory loss
  Depression
  Anxiety
  Panic
  Paranoia
  Unexplained mood swings
  Personality changes
  Intellectual changes
  Sexual promiscuity
  Dishonesty
  Unreliability

Source: From ref. 92. Reprinted with permission.

Table 13-2.   General Principles of Management for the Pregnant Drug Abuser

Drug Management
  Watch for multiple drug use
  Sheltered, controlled withdrawal:
    Cocaine
    Alcohol
    Amphetamines
    Barbiturates
  Outpatient withdrawal:
    Minor tranquilizers and sedatives
    Tobacco
    Marijuana
  Maintenance therapy for narcotics:
    Methadone
Psychosocial
  Establish contact with support services
  Watch for suicidal depression
  Low threshold for hospitalization or protective study
Nutrition
  Prevent deficiency states (calories, vitamins, protein)
  Prevent maternal ketosis
Infection
  Examine for and treat sexually transmitted disease
  Examine for hepatitis B, AIDS
  Watch for and treat intercurrent illness
Fetus
  Watch for intrauterine growth retardation
  Watch for toxemia

Source: From ref. 12.

ALCOHOL

Sixty percent of American women drink alcoholic beverages. During pregnancy 2% of women drink at least two drinks a day.[1] There are regional differences in heavy drinking (usually defined as 3 or more drinks a day) varying from 1/2% to 16%.[2,3] The amount of ethanol in beverages varies. A drink can be defined as the volume of a beverage that contains 12–15 ml of absolute alcohol, which is equivalent to one 12 oz. beer, 4 oz. wine, or one shot of 100 proof hard liquor.

Alcohol crosses the placenta freely. Amniotic fluid may function as a reservoir for both ethanol and its toxic metabolite, acetaldehyde, exposing the fetus long after alcohol has been cleared from the maternal system. Alcohol and its metabolites are cleared by a number of different enzyme systems and genetic differences between individuals may account for variability in fetal effects with the same level of intake. An example of variability is with fraternal twins where only one fetus develops serious effects.

Alcohol causes an increase in cellular peroxidase activity, decrease in DNA synthesis, disruption of protein synthesis and impairment of cell growth, differentiation, and neuronal cell migration in the fetus. Alcohol interferes with fetal growth by impairing placental transfer of amino acids and glucose, and by inhibiting protein synthesis in the fetus. It can cause hypoglycemia, hypoinsulinemia and decrease in fetal thyroid hormones and liver glycogen stores. It also causes alterations in prostacyclin-thromboxane ratio which may lead to vasoconstriction and chronic hypoxia.

The negative effects of alcohol are dose related and extensive (Tables 13-3, 13-4). Fetal alcohol syndrome (FAS), a constellation of mental and physical abnormalities (Jones et al.[4]) occurs in cases where 6 or more drinks a day are consumed over time.[5] Other alcohol-related effects can occur when consumption is 3–6 drinks/day (Harlap and Shiono,[2] Emhart et al.[6]). Some studies find effects at doses of 1–2 drinks/day, including lowered birth weight,[7] abnormal neural development and spontaneous abortion.[2] These effects have been questioned, however, because of the data analysis methods used in the studies and because drinkers tend to under report usage. These studies do not demonstrate effects for less than one drink a day. The issue of a safety threshold is unresolved, and thus it is best to advise pregnant women to abstain from drinking, or if this is not acceptable to the patient, to limit consumption to less than one drink a day. The focus should be to identify and treat

Table 13-3. Reported Effects of Alcohol on Pregnancy

Anatomic birth defects
   Craniofacial anomalies (see Table 13-4)
   Cardiac septal defects
   Hemangiomas
   Undescended testes
   Hernias
   Unusual finger print patterns
   Palmer creases
Neurological abnormalities
   Microcephaly (frequently in FAS) from decreased brain growth
   Hydrocephalus
   Absence of corpus callosum
   Abnormal migration of nerve & supportive glial cells
Neurobehavioral abnormalities
   Neonates restless during sleep and sleep less
   Abnormal EEG during sleep up to 6 weeks after birth
   Slower mental development
   Mental retardation in fetal alcohol syndrome & heavy drinkers
   Cerebral palsy
   Hyperactivity
Fetal death — 8 times more frequent in alcoholic mothers
Intrauterine growth retardation — dose dependent, more severe effects in third trimester, from direct effects of acetaldehyde and chronic fetal hypoxia
Spontaneous abortion
Preterm delivery — controversial

Table 13-4. Fetal Alcohol Syndrome (FAS)

At least one characteristic from each of the following categories:
   1. Growth retardation before and/or after birth, failure to thrive (weight, length, and/or head circumference <10th percentile)
   2. Facial anomalies, epicanthic folds; flattened nasal bridges; short length of nose; thin upper lip, low-set unparallel ears; retarded midfacial development, microphthalmia and/or short palpebral fissures, poorly developed philtrum, thin upper lip and flattening or absence of the maxilla
   3. Central nervous system dysfunction, including microcephaly (head circumference <3rd percentile), varying degrees of mental retardation or other evidence of abnormal neurobehavioral development, such as attention deficit disorder with hyperactivity

Source: from ref. 41.

those patients who are clearly at risk, those consuming 2 or more drinks/day, and to counsel all patients about the risks of heavy drinking.

Alcohol accounts for 5% of all congenital anomalies[8] and has been cited as the most common cause of mental retardation in the Western world.[9] Different effects are related to various times of gestation; there is no time where risk is absent. Craniofacial anomalies may occur during embryogenesis,[6] disorders of central nervous system function later in gestation, growth disturbances may be related to alcohol exposure over a broad range of gestation.

Diagnosis and Treatment

Prevention is the only course since there is no cure for alcohol-related birth defects. There are several questionnaires used to identify problem drinkers. T-ACE is a four question screen which is reported to identify 69% of pregnant problem drinkers (Table 13-5).[10] Identification and counseling initiated during pregnancy is beneficial and should include family members. In one study two-thirds of pregnant problem drinkers reduced their alcohol intake when enrolled in a counseling program.[11]

Each patient should be screened for HIV, other STDs, alcoholic hepatitis, and pancreatitis. Thiamine and vitamins should be administered. Identification and treatment for other drug use

Table 13-5.   T-ACE Questions Found to Identify Women Drinking Sufficiently to Potentially Damage the Fetus

T	How many drinks does it take to make you feel high? (tolerance)
A	Have people annoyed you by criticizing your drinking?
C	Have you felt you ought to cut down on your drinking?
E	Have you ever had to drink first thing in the morning to steady your nerves or to get rid of a hangover (eye opener)?

For the tolerance question, an answer of more than two drinks is considered a positive response. A score of 2 is assigned for a positive response to the tolerance question, and a score of 1 is assigned to all others for a positive response. A T-ACE score of 2 or greater is considered positive for problem drinking, which is considered to be 2 or more drinks a day.

Source: From ref. 96. Reprinted with permission.

(tobacco and alcohol are frequent pairs) should be attempted. An early ultrasound to establish dating, one at 20 weeks to screen for anomalies, and additional evaluations, as needed during the course of pregnancy, to detect intrauterine growth retardation (IUGR) are useful. Nonstress tests (NSTs) are also useful to assure fetal well-being in the latter part of pregnancy.

There are three manifestations of alcohol withdrawal[12]:

- Tremulousness and irritability occur within 48 hours of the last drink and last for several days.
- Delirium tremens (DTs), a life-threatening symptom of withdrawal marked by sympathetic overactivity, fever, encephalopathy, and hallucinations, is a serious and sometimes fatal manifestation.
- Alcohol withdrawal seizures can occur after 12–48 hours and usually manifest as one or two grand mal seizures. No anticonvulsants are needed. If seizures are multiple, another etiology should be sought.

Heavy drinkers should undergo inpatient withdrawal over a 3–4 day period. If medication is required, 2–6 days of treatment with a short-acting barbiturate, such as pentobarbital, is acceptable in pregnancy.[12] Preterm labor can occur with severe withdrawal and the fetus should

be carefully monitored. Neonates of alcoholics who were heavy users in late pregnancy may also undergo withdrawal after delivery, requiring treatment if severe.

Alcoholics develop a high tolerance for pain medications. Large doses may be used during labor, resulting in neonatal respiratory depression.

Disulfiram (Antebuse), a medication used to treat the nonpregnant chronic alcoholic, inhibits many enzyme systems, is a suspected teratogen, and is contraindicated in pregnancy.

Acute intoxication causes vomiting, atonia, nystagmus, acute psychosis, shock, cardiac dysfunction, hypothermia, and hypoglycemia. Alcoholic ketoacidosis (ketosis and dehydration) occurs more frequently in pregnant patients in response to an abrupt alteration of food or alcohol intake. The treatment of acute intoxication is the same in pregnant women and includes gastric lavage, charcoal, and cathartic administration. Thiamine 100 mg IM should be given prior to administration of dextrose for hypoglycemia.

Breast-Feeding

Alcohol crosses into breast milk easily and levels approximate those of the mother (Briggs et al.[13]). Questions of delayed motor development measured at one year in breast-fed infants of alcoholic mothers have been raised. For this reason breast-feeding may be contraindicated, depending on the level of maternal alcohol ingestion.

TOBACCO

One-fourth of women of reproductive age smoke and 19% to 30% of smokers continue to some extent during pregnancy.[14] Most pregnant smokers are chronic, regular users who maintain their habit with high enough levels to produce adverse effects. These effects are dose related, and occur at relatively low levels of chronic consumption.

Physiological Effects

Tobacco smoke contains 2500 different substances, including nicotine, carbon monoxide, and various carcinogenic agents.[14] Many of these biologically active compounds cross the placenta freely and some accumulate in the fetus. Nicotine and carbon monoxide build up in the fetal circulation and HbCO levels in umbilical cord blood are 2.5 times higher than in maternal blood.[15]

Nicotine is a vasoconstrictor, effecting both the maternal placental flow and that of the fetus.[15] When carbon monoxide binds to hemoglobin to form carboxyhemolobin, the oxygen-carrying capacity of the blood is reduced. CO also increases the affinity of hemoglobin for oxygen, which inhibits oxygen release to the tissue.[16]

One effect of tobacco smoking is inhibition of steroidogenesis, thereby decreasing maternal levels of estradiol, sex hormone binding globulin, and human chorionic gonadotropins (hCG). Maternal and fetal hemoglobin are increased secondary to carbon monoxide related impairment of oxygen transport.[15] The normal compensation in pregnancy of 2,3 DPG does not occur in smokers, resulting in a mild decrease of oxygen delivery to maternal and fetal tissues. Diabetics already have this impairment in 2,3 DPG compensation, which may be compounded by smoking.

There is an increase in platelet reactivity and a decrease in prostacyclin which may cause vasoconstriction and decreased uteroplacental perfusion.[17] Characteristic placental changes include large and small infarcts, fibrinoid changes in arteries, avascular stem villa, thickened basement membranes of trophoblast, smaller vessels in terminal villa, and necrosis at placental margins.[18]

Smokers tend to have lower intakes of most nutrients, and nutritionally poor diets. Chronic smokers are often deficient in the antioxidants (vitamins A, C, E) and certain minerals. Zinc deficiency is known to cause growth retardation in humans, and cadmium (from cigarette smoke) interferes with zinc absorption. This has been proposed as a mechanism of IUGR in infants of smokers.[19]

Tobacco use causes a decreased baseline fetal heart rate variability and increased fetal heart rate.[20] The incidence of a nonreactive NST may be increased[21] or unchanged.[22] Fetal breathing movements may also be increased.[23]

Maternal and Fetal Effects

There is an increase in fetal and infant death which appears to be dose related.[24] One study found a 25% increase in fetal and infant mortality in primaparous women smoking less than one pack per day. This increased to 56% in those smoking greater than one PPD.[25] Kleinman in a study of 360,000 births, 2500 fetal deaths, and 3800 infant deaths in Missouri from 1979–1983, estimated that fetal and infant deaths would decrease by 10% if all women quit smoking.[25]

Decreased birth weight is dose related and occurs with smoking at any gestational age. On the average, smoking decreases birth weight 150–200 gms and smokers have twice the rate of infants less than 2500 grams.[26] The decrease appears to be in lean, not fat tissue.[15,27] This may be because of decreased placental perfusion, vasoconstriction, relative hypoxia, direct toxicity of nicotine and thiocyanate, or nutritional deficiencies. Passive smoke is linked to IUGR[28] and one study has suggested a tobacco-caffeine interaction which results in decreased birth weight.[29]

The risk of spontaneous abortion is twice that of nonsmokers, has a higher proportion of normal karotypes, and tends to occur later.[30]

Prematurity was 2.3 times higher with 20 cigarettes/day in one study,[31] in part due to an increased incidence of premature rupture of the membranes (PROM). There is a lower incidence of respiratory distress syndrome (RDS) in smoking mothers, and the enhanced lung maturity may be secondary to the stress of chronic fetal hypoxia.[32,33]

Abruptio placenta is well documented[26,34] with the risk in light smokers increased 24%, and the risk in heavy smokers (>20 cigarettes/

day) increased 68%. This may be from degenerative changes in arteriole lining of decidual vessels.

Placenta previa is increased 25% in light smokers and 92% in heavy smokers.[26,34] The etiology of this finding is not clear.

SIDS (Sudden Infant Death Syndrome) occurs twice as often in those infants whose mothers are smokers.[35] It is not clear whether prenatal or postnatal smoking is the risk factor. Animal research shows histologic brain stem damage in rat fetuses exposed to maternal smoke. This is consistent with brain stem gliosis reported in human SIDS cases and may suggest a prenatal etiology.

It is unclear whether tobacco smoke is a teratogen. Some congenital malformations including neural tube defects, orofacial clefts, congenital heart disease, and limb reduction defects have been reported, but studies don't control for important confounders and results are contradictory.

Maternal smoking is associated with a wide variety of serious childhood diseases. Delayed neurologic and intellectual development at age 14 years, including shorter stature and poorer mean school performance, was found in 1800 children of smokers in Finland.[36] Animal research supports the idea that antenatal exposure contributes more than postnatal.[37] There is an increased incidence of lower respiratory track infection, even when mothers stopped smoking postpartum. A study of 12,000 children in England suggested that prenatal smoke may be more correlated than passive postnatal smoke.[38] Also, increased incidence of asthma has been correlated to maternal smoking.[39] Some investigators found an increase in childhood cancers including lymphoblastic leukemia, non-Hodgkin's lymphoma and Wilm's tumor[40] but other researchers did not detect higher cancer rates. Childhood asthma, pneumonia, and bronchitis are more common in infants exposed to in utero and environmental tobacco smoke.[39]

Treatment

Encouragement by physicians and other medical staff to decrease or quit smoking has been shown to decrease maternal smoking.[41] Early identification and treatment of smokers is desirable since quitting before 20 weeks eliminates many complications of smoking. Damage is done throughout gestation and after delivery through decreased lactation and passive smoke exposure, so quitting or decreasing consumption is to be stressed at all times. Avoidance of passive smoke should be encouraged, for the mother during pregnancy and for the infant after delivery. Nutritional counseling and augmentation should be emphasized, especially if the habit is continued. Other drug use should be identified (alcohol and heavy coffee consumption are common) and treated to decrease this use.

Breast-Feeding

Tobacco smoking causes a decrease in milk volume. This is dose related and may impact on the adequacy of milk supply in women smoking heavily.[42]

CAFFEINE

Caffeine is an alkaloid found in coffee, tea, chocolate, various soft drinks, and many over-the-counter analgesics and cold remedies. There may be a dose related decrease in birth weight, with heavy users (>450 mg/day, approximately 4 cups coffee) showing a decrease in birth weight of 121 gm in one study.[43] Cigarette smoking also causes decreased birth weight, and the effects of smoking plus caffeine consumption may be additive. A smoking-caffeine interaction causing a decreased birth weight in women who are heavy smokers and heavy coffee drinkers has been proposed.[29] Pregnant patients should be advised to limit their intake to the equivalent of 2 cups of coffee/day, especially if they also smoke cigarettes.

COCAINE

Cocaine, a naturally occurring alkaloid, is extracted from the leaves of Erythroxylen Coca. It is strongly addictive psychologically but has relatively few abstinence symptoms. A relative tolerance develops with increased usage, requiring larger doses to achieve the euphoria, with more associated depression, exhaustion, and anxiety. Users tend to compulsively binge to avoid the "crash."

The powder form of cocaine can be injected intravenously or "snorted" (intranasal). Alkaloidal cocaine (free base), also known as crack, is heat stable, and can be smoked. Up until the early 1970s cocaine was an expensive drug used by an affluent population. The cheapness and availability of crack resulted in its present epidemic use.

Cocaine is a sympathomimetic that blocks the presynaptic reuptake of norepinephrine and dopamine, thereby increasing these transmitters at receptor sites. Immediate effects include euphoria (probably from the CNS effect of dopamine), increased blood pressure, tachycardia, and vasoconstriction.[44] It crosses the placenta and metabolites are found in fetal urine. It is metabolized by cholinesterases whose activity is diminished in pregnancy and in the fetus. This may lead to accumulation of cocaine and increased toxicity. Metabolites are excreted in urine and can be detected for 48–72 hours after ingestion.

Cocaine, a potent stimulant and vasoconstrictor interferes with the low-pressure, high-flow hemodynamics of pregnancy. Chronic use, and the accompanying interference in flow, can lead to such expected effects as reduced birth weight and placental dysfunctions. Any use of cocaine can produce immediate, sometimes fatal, maternal and fetal effects. Cocaine users may participate in a "drug scene" that includes promiscuity, violence, multiple drug use, and malnourishment, which can exaggerate the effects of cocaine and increases the risk of infections.

Maternal Complications

Among serious maternal complications of cocaine use are cerebral vascular accident, seizures, acute myocardial infarction, arrhythmias, and sudden death. The increased incidence of placental abruption is well established[45–50,52] as is a high risk for PROM.[52]

Chronic use can cause a cardiomyopathy which can be confused with peripartum cardiopathy. Bronchitis, broncospasm, and "crack lung" (which includes hemoptysis, chest pain, and diffuse alveolar infiltrates) occur. This may be secondary to a hypersensitivity reaction to cocaine or contaminants. Cocaine use can also induce a pseudo preeclampsia with acute elevation of blood pressure, proteinuria and hematologic abnormalities resembling HELLP (hemolysis, elevated liver enzymes, and low platelets). This should be considered in a suspected cocaine user who presents as a severe preeclamptic, with symptoms rapidly disappearing after admission without delivery.

Fetal Complications

Cocaine is associated with an increased incidence of spontaneous abortion and fetal death in utero.[47] A substantial increase in preterm labor and delivery is well documented.[48–51,53–57]

Decrease in fetal weight and intrauterine growth restriction (IUGR) occurs,[48,49,51–54,56,57] independent of maternal weight. In one study a mean birth weight reduction of 376 gms was seen in 366 cocaine using women compared to controls. This is probably a direct effect from vasoconstriction of uteroplacental circulation. Decreased fetal head circumference was seen by numerous investigators[51,53,55,57,58] in infants of cocaine using women.

Fetal CNS effects include periventricular/intraventricular hemorrhage, cerebral infarction,[59,60] EEG changes and seizure activity[61,62] possibly from in utero cerebral hemorrhage. Fetal tachycardia and hypoxia are also reported.[48,51]

The presence of increased fetal anomalies is controversial. Congenital anomalies appear to be higher in this population but these are hard to attribute to cocaine alone. Some investigators have reported anomalies involving the CNS and cardiovascular system.[63] Other investigators failed to find increased rates of these fetal anomalies.[49,56,64]

Infant Complications

Neonatal withdrawal can occur but is less common than with opiate withdrawal. Sudden infant death syndrome (SIDS) was not increased in one investigation[65] but this study lacked the power to detect any difference less than a 12-fold increase. A second study has linked use to SIDS,[66] but has been criticized as having significant confounders. Thus the issue of SIDS is unresolved.

Long-term consequences are controversial. Increased neurobehavioral abnormalities (sleeping patterns, feeding problems, hypertonia, tremors, and poor interactive behaviors) occur,[57] but infants seem to perform in the expected range on Bayley Scales and Standard Binet Test at age 2–3 years.[67]

Treatment

One-half of users who do not receive prenatal care deliver prematurely.[68,69] The principal objectives of treatment are early identification, good prenatal care, and sheltered withdrawal from the drugs and the drug scene. Cocaine users frequently use other drugs, especially tranquilizers and barbiturates. Detection of cocaine and associated drug use, screening for infections, counseling, social services, and attention to nutritional needs are important.

Treatment of acute crisis is generally supportive. Diazepam can be used to treat seizures and agitation. Propranolol has been used for treatment of the adrenergic phenomena.[70]

Breast-Feeding

Cocaine crosses into breast milk. While the milk/plasma ratios have not been established, there are reports of breast-feeding infants with measurable levels of cocaine and symptoms of intoxication. Because of this reason, and the risk of HIV in this population, breast-feeding is generally discouraged.

AMPHETAMINES

Amphetamines ("uppers") are sympathomimetic drugs that stimulate the central nervous system, producing depressed appetite, wakefulness, and euphoria. These drugs, including amphetamine, dextroamphetamine, and methamphetamine can be taken orally or intravenously. Crystal methamphetamine ("ice") can also be smoked and is similar to "crack" cocaine in potency and intended effects. Use can result in increased alertness, anorexia, and euphoria without intellectual compromise but higher doses or prolonged use results in agitation, paranoia, hallucinations, and violent behavior. Methamphetamine users often binge, taking repeated doses and staying "up" for days before finally "crashing," with depression and discomfort which they may attempt to alleviate with use of narcotics, sedatives, and alcohol.

Amphetamine use can cause serious, occasionally fatal, arrhythmias. There is an increased risk of ventricular tachycardia and asystole during obstetric anesthesia.[12] Users who inject the drug are at high risk for HIV, hepatitis, and other infections. Chronic users can be severely malnourished, which, combined with the vasoconstrictive effects, can produce intrauterine growth retardation (IUGR). Amphetamine use has been related to fetal death in utero, placental abruption, IUGR, and decreased fetal head circumference.[57,71] Maternal and fetal complications of usage are similar to those of cocaine and likewise their teratogenic potential is not clear. Discontinuation results in depression and prostration, and withdrawal can occur in the neonate.

Treatment is supportive and similar to that of cocaine, with the primary goals being detoxification, removal from drug milieu, good nutrition, identification and treatment of associated infections, and identification and treatment for other drug use.

OPIATES

Codeine and morphine are naturally occurring opiates from the poppy, Papaversomni Ferum.

Heroin, the most commonly thought of opiate, is semisynthetic. Opiate use, while more prevalent in lower socioeconomic classes, involves all levels of society. It has been reported that 5% of the middle class used opiates at some point during pregnancy.[72] Fentanyl, commonly used in anesthesia, is preferred by addicted operating room personnel (and is undetectable by conventional urine screen). An intermittent heroin user may not develop dependence, but with regular use physical addiction is almost universal. It has been estimated that the average time from first use to physical dependence is 2 years.[73] All opiates cross the placenta and the fetus also becomes addicted. Intermittent users are at a higher risk of lethal overdose because of their low tolerance and the variable potency of drugs sold on the street.[74]

Heroin is used intravenously, by skin popping, by snorting, or by smoking. Smoking opium has again become popular because of the risk of HIV.[12] Heroin is frequently sold in 100 mg bags, which contain 40–50 mg of heroin plus an inert base of sugar, starch, quinine, lidocaine, and/or powdered milk. Street heroin is often adulterated by other synthetic narcotics and psychoactive substances, and the strength and composition are often not known by the user. Many addicts use 3–5 bags/day.

Heroin addiction threatens the woman, fetus, and infant in several ways. The risk of an overdose, the serious effects of withdrawal, and the high risk of HIV are all potentially fatal. The rates of prematurity, stillbirth, fetal growth retardation, and neonatal mortality are 3 to 7 times higher than the general population,[75] and the rate of SIDS is increased.[76,77]

Many of the adverse affects of heroin (Tables 13-6, 13-7) are not from the drug itself but are environmental and lifestyle related. Prostitution is common. Addicts are often malnourished. Infections are common with organisms including staphylococci, streptococci, bacteroids, candida, and clostridium sepsis. Skin popping is associated with infections with clostridium tetani. HIV and hepatitis are common, with approximately 50% of heroin addicts testing positive for HIV.[51] The addict cycles between intoxication and

Table 13-6. Complications of Heroin Use in Pregnancy (Maternal)

Spontaneous abortion (SAB)
Stillbirth
Intrauterine growth restriction (IUGR)
Premature labor
Affects of solvents and talc
  obstructive pulmonary vascular disease
  hyperglobulinemia
False positive serologic test for syphilis
Malnutrition
Infections (contaminated syringes, prostitution):
  —HIV
  —STD
  —UTI
  —chorioamnionitis
  —hepatitis (types B, C)
  —tetanus,
  —cutaneous abscesses
  —cellulitis,
  —thrombophlebitis
  —endocarditis (right-sided)
  —pulmonary abscesses (metastatic to bone, cartilage)
  —septic pulmonary emboli
  —septic emboli to placenta
    leading to fibrosis
    inflammation
    placental insufficiency

withdrawal with all the associated effects on her and the fetus.

Withdrawal is rarely fatal to the mother, but can be for the fetus. It can cause late spontaneous abortion (from contractions, arteriolar

Table 13-7. Complications of Heroin Use in Pregnancy (Fetal)

Small for gestational age (SGA)
Aspiration pneumonia
Meconium aspiration
Asphyxia
Transient tachypnea
Abstinence syndrome
Infections
  Conjunctivitis
  Septicemia
  Pneumonia
  Hepatitis
  STDs
  HIV
Sequelae: child abuse, neglect
    long-term learning/behavioral sequelae

spasm), late pregnancy intrauterine fetal demise, fetal hyperactivity, and meconium passage.[78] Deliberate attempts to withdraw, or inadvertent withdrawal from the administration of an antagonist should be avoided. Signs of withdrawal are agitation, sweating, vomiting, chills, muscle spasms, abdominal pains, myalgias, uterine cramps, and diarrhea.[72,79] The infant of a heroin addict, or of a mother on methadone maintenance, is also addicted and can undergo withdrawal that requires treatment and is potentially fatal.

Maternal signs and symptoms of heroin use are miosis, euphoria, drowsiness, constipation, abscesses, infections, tracks, and healed scars (from injection) and nasal hyperemia (from snorting). Overdose results in respiratory depression, cardiac arrhythmias, cyanosis, convulsions, hypothermia, coma, and cerebral edema. Symptoms are reversed by naloxone, thus aiding the diagnosis. Naloxone should be used with extreme caution in pregnancy because of the effects of withdrawal on the fetus.

The teratogenicity of opiates is not clear since many users also use other street drugs, and the effect of the drug can not be separated from the substance with which it is cut. Heroin is frequently cut with quinine, a known teratogen. There are case reports of fetal anomalies but these are anecdotal and many mothers were poly-drug users.

Treatment

Diagnosis is the first step in treatment. Unexplained endocarditis, episodes of cellulitus, pneumonia, previous usage, and a history of drug seeking may be clues to use.

Withdrawal of the addicted patient is not desirable during pregnancy. The casual or infrequent user may undergo careful withdrawal, with addition of methadone if needed. In the dependent user, instituting methadone maintenance avoids many of the complications of heroin addiction, especially those related to the drug scene. Methadone maintenance should be continued at least until after delivery.

Methadone is a long-acting synthetic opiate

which is well absorbed, blocks heroin-induced euphoria and prevents abstinence symptoms. Typical required methadone doses are 20 to 40 mg/day administered in the context of a methadone maintenance program. Pregnancy sometimes increases the required maintenance dose to avoid withdrawal, particularly in the third trimester when the half-life of methadone decreases. This may require twice-a-day dosing interval or increased dose. Addicts may tend to supplement inadequate methadone dosing with street drugs, and positive urine screens for nonmethadone opiates may mean methadone dosing should be increased.

The risk of IUGR is still present with methadone but perinatal mortality is reduced.[56,78] Respiratory distress syndrome may occur with less frequency in prematurely delivered infants.[80] Adequate nutrition, vitamins, and calories are an important part of treatment. An early ultrasound to establish dates and repeated evaluations to assess possible IUGR are useful. NSTs should be done weekly in the latter part of pregnancy. Infections should be screened for frequently and cultures taken because of the increased risk of unusual organisms. All febrile intravenous drug using patients should be admitted to rule out pneumonia and endocarditis.[81] A significant number of addicts are depressed, and a higher than average number have personality disorders. This aspect of care should be addressed.

Fifty percent of addicts present for the first time in labor,[82–84] so those with no previous care should be screened on presentation to identify and treat neonates at risk for withdrawal.

Stadol (butorphanol) and Nubain (nalbophine) are both commonly used analgesics in labor. They are partial antagonist of opium receptors and their use can precipitate withdrawal. They should be avoided in opiate dependent patients. The usual daily dose of methadone should be given orally on the day of delivery. It can be given IM also.

Methadone's half-life is prolonged in the newborn because of the immaturity of enzymatic systems. Neonatal abstinence syndrome (NAS) generally occurs with doses of methadone of greater than 20 mg/d. Neonatal withdrawal appears 3–5 days from the mother's last dose of heroin. Withdrawal may not occur for up to 10 days with methadone. The infant may be discharged before the onset of withdrawal, so arrangements should be made to identify and treat the neonate experiencing late withdrawal. Taking into account the issue of consent, blood testing on neonates of all known and suspected maternal users is desirable to confirm opiate use, and to identify HIV risk.

Most addicted neonates show withdrawal symptoms, some severe, but only half need treatment.[78,85,86] The severity, onset, and duration of neonatal withdrawal is correlated with daily opiate (heroin or methadone) intake, serum drug levels and total intake for 12 weeks prior to delivery.[83,86-88] Heroin stimulates sweat glands and sweating in the newborn may be a subtle clue to withdrawal. Other short term neonatal effects are hyperbilirubinemia,[89] hyperthyroidism, anoxia, hypoglycemia, hypocalcemia, sepsis, hyperviscosity, intracranial hemorrhage[72] and thrombocytosis in the second week of life.[90] Long-term effects are difficult to measure and separate from the child's environment.

The treatment for overdose is naloxone hydrochloride (this also aids in the diagnosis) 0.4–2 mg IV (IM, SQ, or endotracheally if IV access is not available) with repeated doses of 2 mg up to 10 mg. The half-life is short (60 min) so a patient needs to be observed for 24 hours and given repeated doses as needed. Naloxone should be used only in crisis situations because of the fetal risk of precipitous withdrawal. After crisis intervention, methadone maintenance should be initiated. Pulmonary edema, while uncommon, can occur up to 48 hours after use.

Breast-Feeding

Methadone levels peak 2–4 hours after an oral dose so the optimal time to breast-feed is just before a dose. It is generally felt breast-feeding is compatible with a methadone dose of <20 mg/day. A higher dose actually helps prevent neonatal withdrawal, and in the past this

was thought to be beneficial. Today, with the risk of HIV in this population, it is generally recommended that breast-feeding be avoided for active heroin users because of the risk of HIV transmittal via breast milk.

HALLUCINOGENS

PCP

Phencyclidine (PCP) or "angel dust" is a CNS stimulant or depressant, depending on dose, that can be smoked or ingested. It has potent sympathomimetic properties and is a dissociative anesthetic. It causes behavioral disturbances, agitation, psychosis, catatonic, violent, and bizarre behavior. Ingestion results in a higher dose (>30 ng/ml serum) and can cause stupor, coma, and broncospasm. Massive overdose can result in hypotension, apnea, status epileptics, and renal failure. Specific fetal effects are unknown. Morbidity and mortality to mother and fetus are from behavioral effects. Trauma, accidental or self-inflicted injury, are the primary risks to the fetus.

Treatment in pregnancy is generally supportive and includes protection of the patient and provision of a quiet, nonstimulatory environment. Diazepam can be used for seizures, phenytoin for recurrent seizures, aminophylline for broncospasm and diphenhydramine for dystonic reactions.

LSD

Lysergic acid diethylamide, like PCP, causes bizarre behaviors. Chromosomal anomalies have been suggested but this has never been confirmed. No other fetal effects have been demonstrated. There is a risk to mother and fetus from trauma.

Marijuana

Marijuana, the dried leaves and flowers of the cannabis sativa plant, is most commonly smoked in our culture. The primary active agent is tetrahydrocanibinol, a mild psychotropic drug that produces euphoria and sensory enhancement. It is the most common illegal drug used in the United States, but "heavy" use is much less common. While 56% of women aged 18 to 25 reported that they had used marijuana, 6% reported use of marijuana at least once a week.[91] Marijuana smoke includes hundreds of substances in addition to the active agent, including carbon monoxide. While it is like tobacco smoke in this way, the average daily volume of marijuana smoke inhaled is clearly minor compared to the average daily volume of tobacco smoke inhaled by regular users.

Marijuana smoking has been associated with tachycardia, exercise intolerance, bronchitis, sinusitis, and pharyngitis. Chronic consumption leads to anovulation and decreased sperm count and motility.[92] The studies of its maternal and fetal effects provide ambiguous results, with no area of risk being clearly demonstrated.[72] It may well be that the level of use required to produce clinically significant detrimental effects is higher than that included in most studies, and higher than that used by a large majority of marijuana smoking patients.

Marijuana smoking is often associated with other substance abuse, which should be identified and treated. Users should be advised that the risks, especially for chronic, heavy use, remain unknown in pregnancy and advised to quit or decrease consumption.

BARBITURATES

Barbiturates can be divided into long-acting (phenobarbital, barbital), which are cleared by the kidney, and short-acting (amobarbital, secobarbital, pentobarbital) which are metabolized by the liver. Barbiturates are used legitimately for control of seizures. Illegally, barbiturates are usually used in combination with other drug use, especially to mitigate the "crash" following use of amphetamines and cocaine. Acute intoxication can cause CNS depression, ataxia, nystagmus, miosis, respiratory depression, hypotension, coma, hypothermia, and rhabdomyolysis.

Use of prescribed barbiturates for seizure control in patients who are not abusing other substances does not impair fetal growth and development, but illegal use does. Dependence, and the accompanying problems of maternal, fetal, and neonatal withdrawal can be produced by both illegal use and long-term therapeutic use.[93]

Maternal withdrawal causes restlessness, irritability, insomnia, and autonomic stimulation. Delirium, psychosis and seizures can occur and can be fatal if untreated (this is in contrast to narcotic withdrawal). Abrupt fetal withdrawal can have the same serious consequences as opiate withdrawal (spontaneous abortion, fetal hyperactivity, meconium passage, fetal distress, and fetal demise). In epileptics on phenobarbital, the risk of delivering a child with congenital defects is 2 to 3 times higher[94] but it is not clear if this finding is from the underlying disease, the medication, or a combination of both.

Treatment

Treatment of the chronic user includes hospitalization, regulation, and controlled decrease in dose, maintenance of nutrition, treatment of infections, and psychosocial support. For nonprescribed use, attempts should be made to determine if cocaine or amphetamines are also used and treat for this. For acute overdose activated charcoal is given orally or by NG tube. Some advocate forced alkaline diuresis, which aides in the excretion of long-acting, but not short-acting, drugs. Dopamine is used for hypotension.

Blood and urine screens can be useful to predict the likelihood of maternal or neonatal withdrawal. The average onset of withdrawal is 6 days (3–14 range) in the newborn.[94] Controlled maternal and neonatal withdrawal can be managed with incrementally decreasing doses of phenobarbital and can avoid the serious consequences of abrupt withdrawal.

Breast-Feeding

Barbiturates may accumulate in the infant because of slower elimination, and blood levels may exceed those of the mother. This may result in sedation. In general breast-feeding is not encouraged in barbiturate dependent women. An exception is secobarbital which the American Academy of Pediatrics considers compatible with breast-feeding.

TRANQUILIZERS (BENZODIAZEPINES)

There are no proven teratogenic fetal effects of benzodiazepines[12] and their toxic effect is difficult to assess. Most illicit use is in combination with other drugs to blunt abstinence and undesirable effects of alcohol, cocaine and amphetamines. Their use produces tolerance and withdrawal syndrome in the mother and fetus/neonate. They are used legally for seizures, and such use does not cause IUGR. Signs of overdose are coma, prolonged hypoxia, and death. Their effects are potentiated by alcohol.

Withdrawal symptoms of benzodiazepines are similar to but not as severe as barbiturates. The risk of intrauterine death is low. The drugs accumulate in the fetus, especially in the third trimester, and can result in severe neonatal depression.[12] Antenatal withdrawal is desirable. Neonatal withdrawal can occur from mothers using these drugs legitimately for seizure disorder.

Treatment is controlled withdrawal, identification, and treatment for other drug use and supportive measures such as counseling and nutritional supplementation. Withdrawal should occur before delivery to minimize the problems of neonatal depression.

INHALANTS

Children and adolescents are the primary users of a variety of inhalants which produce some desired ''high.'' The inhalants include glue, paint thinner, gasoline, toluene, solvents, and a variety of aerosols and gases. The user is often experimenting, trying anything that is rumored to have an effect. These substances can be fatal, producing arrhythmias leading to sudden death, or serious harm to the user, including bone marrow toxicity, liver damage, renal failure, peripheral neuropathy, atrophy, cerebellar signs, and organic brain syndrome.[92] IUGR, preterm delivery, and fetal demise have been reported for inhalant users.[95] The effects of inhalant use on the fetus and infant have not been well studied, and would be difficult to assess since abusers use a variety of inhalants and other drugs.

The adolescent patient is at risk for inhalant use, especially if there is a history of tobacco, alcohol, or illegal drug use. Efforts should be made to identify users and support termination of this practice, including counseling on the risks of inhalant use. Beta-mimetic tocolysis should not be used since renal tubular acidosis, pulmonary injury, and cardiac arrhythmias are exacerbated by beta-agonists.[12]

REFERENCES

1. Abel EL. *Marijuana, Tobacco, Alcohol and Reproduction.* Boca Raton, FL: CRC Press, 1983.

2. Harlap S, Shiono PH. Alcohol, smoking and incidence of spontaneous abortions in the first and second trimester. *Lancet.* 1980;26:173–176.

3. Russel M, Biggler LR. Screening for alcohol related problems in an outpatient obstetric-gynecological clinic. *Am J Obstet Gynecol.* 1979; 34:4–12.

4. Jones KL, Smith DW, Uelland CN, Streissguth AP. Patterns of malformation in offspring of chronic alcoholic mothers. *Lancet.* 1973;1: 1267–1271.

5. Sokol RJ, Ager J, Martier S. Significant determinants of susceptibility to alcohol teratogenicity. *Annals NY Acad of Sciences.* 1986;477: 87–102.

6. Emhart CB, Socol RJ, Martier S, et al. Alcohol teratogenicity in the human: a detailed assessment of specificity, critical period, and threshold. *Am J Obstet Gynec.* 1987;156:33–39.

7. Mills JL, Graubard BI, Harley EE, Rhoads GG, Berendes H. Maternal alcohol consumption and birth weight: how much drinking during pregnancy is safe? *JAMA* 1984;252:1875–1879.

8.   Pietrantoni M, Knuppel RA. Alcohol use in pregnancy. *Cl Perinat*. 1991;18:93–111.

9.   Abel EL, Sokol RJ. Fetal alcohol syndrome is now leading cause of mental retardation. *Lancet*. 1986;1:222.

10. Sokol RJ, Martier SS, Ager JW. The T-ACE questions: practical prenatal detection of risk-drinking. *Am J Obstet Gynecol*. 1989;160: 863–870.

11. Halmesmaki E. Alcohol counselling of 85 pregnant problem drinkers: effect on drinking and fetal outcome. *Br J Obstet Gynaecol* 1988;95: 243–247.

12. Lee RV. Drug Abuse. In: *Medical Complications During Pregnancy*, 4th Ed. Burrow GN, Ferris TF, eds. Philadelphia; WB Saunders: 579–596.

13. Briggs GG, Freeman RK, Yaffe SJ, eds. *Drugs in Pregnancy*, 3rd Ed. Baltimore: Williams & Wilkins, 251–252.

14. American College of Obstetricians and Gynecologists. Smoking and reproductive health. *ACOG Technical Bulletin 180*. Washington, DC: ACOG, 1993.

15. Werler MM, Pober BR, Holmes LB. Smoking in pregnancy. *Teratology* 1985;32:473–481.

16. Longo LD. The biological effects of carbon monoxide on the pregnant woman, fetus and newborn. *Am J Obstet Gynecol*. 1977;129:69–103.

17. Bureau MA, Shapcott D, Berthiaume Y et al. Maternal cigarette smoking and fetal oxygen transport; A study of P50, 2,3-diphosphoglycerate, total hemoglobin, hematocrit and type F hemoglobin in fetal blood. *Pediatrics* 1983;72: 22–26.

18. Rotmensch ST, Nores JA, Hobbins JC. Tobacco smoking. In: *Principles and Practice of Medical Therapy in Pregnancy*, 2nd Ed. 1992, Gleicher N, ed. 86–88.

19. Kuhnert BR, Kuhnert PM, Debanne S, Williams TG. The relationship between cadmium, zinc, and birth weight in pregnant women who smoke. *Am J Obstet Gynecol* 1987;157:1247–1251.

20. Kelly J, Mathews KA, O'Conor M. Smoking in pregnancy. Effects on mother and fetus. *Br J Obstet Gynecol*. 1984;91:111–117.

21. Phelan JP. Diminished fetal reactivity with smoking. *Am J Obstet Gynecol*. 1980;136: 230–233.

22. Barrett JM, Vanhooydonk JE, Boehm FH. Acute effect of cigarette smoking in the fetal heart rate nonstress test. *Obstet Gynecol*. 1981; 57:422–425.

23. Thaler I, Goodman JDS, Bawes GS. Effects of maternal cigarette smoking on fetal breathing and fetal movement. *Am J Obstet Gynecol*. 1980;138:282–287.

24. Cnattingius S, Haglund B, Meirik O. Cigarette smoking as risk factor for late fetal and early neonatal death. *Br Med J*. 1988;297:258–261.

25. Kleinman JC, Pierre MB, Madans JH, Land GH, Schramm WF. The effects of maternal smoking on fetal and infant mortality. *Am J Epidemiology*. 1988;127:274–282.

26. Meyer MB, Jonas BS, Tonascia JA. Perinatal events associated with maternal smoking during pregnancy. *Am J Epidermiol*. 1976;103:464–476.

27. Harrison GG, Branson RS, Vaucher YE. Association of maternal smoking with body composition of the newborn. *Am J Cl Nutrition*. 1983;38:757–762.

28. Martin TR, Bracken MB. Association of low birth weight with passive smoke exposure in pregnancy. *Am J Epidemiol*. 1986;124:633–642.

29. Beaulac-Baillargeon L, Desrosiers C. Caffeine-cigarette interaction on fetal growth. *Am J Obstet Gynecol*. 1987;157:1236–1240.

30. Alberman E, Creasy M, Elliot M. Maternal factors associated with fetal chromosomal anomalies in spontaneous abortions. *Br Obstet Gynaecol*. 1976;83:621–627.

31. Fedrick J, Anderson ABM. Factors associated with spontaneous pre-term birth. *Br J Obstet Gynaecol*. 1976;83:342–350.

32. Curet LB, Rao AV, Zachman RD, et al. and The Collaborative Group on Antenatal Steroid Therapy. Maternal smoking and respiratory distress syndrome. *Am J Obstet Gynecol*. 1983;147: 446–450.

33. White E, Shy KK, Daling JR, Guthrie RD. Maternal smoking and infant respiratory distress syndrome. *Obstet Gynecol*. 1986;67:365–370.

34. Fielding JE. Smoking and pregnancy. *N Engl J Med*. 1978;298:337–339.

35. Lewak N, VandenBerg BJ, Beckwith BJ. Sud-

den infant death syndrome risk factors. *Clin. Ped.* 1979;18:404–411.

36. Rantakallio P. A follow-up study to the age of 14 of children whose mothers smoked during pregnancy. *Acta Paediatr Scand.* 1983;72:747–753.

37. Slotkin TA, Orband-Miller L, Queen KL. Development of (3H) nicotine binding sites in brain regions of rats exposed to nicotine prenatally via maternal injections of infusions. *J Pharmacol Exp Ther.* 1987;242:232–237.

38. Taylor B, Wadsworth J. Maternal smoking during pregnancy and lower respiratory tract illness in early life. *Arch Dis Child.* 1987;62:786–791.

39. Weitzman M, Gortmaker S, Walker DK, Sobol A. Maternal smoking and childhood asthma. *Pediatrics.* 1990;85:505–511.

40. Stjernfeldt M, Berglund K, Lindsten J, et al. Maternal smoking during pregnancy and risk of childhood cancer. *Lancet.* 1986;1:1350–1352.

41. Andres RL, Jones KL. Social and illicit drug use in pregnancy. In: *Maternal-Fetal Medicine Principles and Practice*, Creasy RK, Resnik R, eds. Philadelphia: WB Saunders, 1994, 182–198.

42. Vio F, Salazar G, Infante C. Smoking during pregnancy and lactation and its effects on breast-milk volume. *Am J Clin Nutr.* 1991;54:1011–1016.

43. Martin RT, Bracken MB. The association between low birth weight and caffeine consumption during pregnancy. *Am J Epidemiol.* 1987;126:813–821.

44. Ritchie J, Green N. Local anesthetics. In: *The Pharmacological Basis of Therapeutics*, 7th Ed. Goodman A, Gillman L, Rall T, Murad F, eds. New York: Macmillan, 1985, 309–310.

45. Cherukuri R, Minkoff H, Hansen RL, et al. A cohort study of alkaloidal cocaine (''crack'') in pregnancy. *Obstet Gynecol.* 1988;72:147–151.

46. Dombrowski MP, Wolfe HM, Welch RA, Evans MI. Cocaine abuse is associated with abruptio placentae and decreased birth weight, but not shorter labor. *Obstet Gynecol* 1991;77:139–141.

47. Bingol N, Fuchs M, Diaz S, et al. Teratogenicity of cocaine in humans. *J Pediatr* 1987;110:93–96.

48. Chasnoff I, Griffith D, MacGregor S, et al.

Temporal patterns of cocaine use in pregnancy. *JAMA* 1989;261:1741–1744.

49. MacGregor SN, Keith LG, Chasnoff IJ, et al. Cocaine use during pregnancy; adverse perinatal outcome. *Am J Obstet Gynecol.* 1987;157:686–690.

50. Neerhof MG, MacGregor SN, Retzky SS, et al. Cocaine abuse during pregnancy: peripartum prevalence and perinatal outcome. *Am J Obstet Gynecol.* 1989;161:633–638.

51. Hadeed AJ, Siegel SR. Maternal cocaine use during pregnancy: effect on the newborn infant. *Pediatrics.* 1989;84:205–210.

52. American College of Obstetricians and Gynecologists. Substance abuse in pregnancy. *ACOG Technical Bulletin 195*. Washington, DC: ACOG, 1994.

53. Cherukuri R, Minkoff H, Hansen RL, et al. A cohort study of alkaloidal cocaine (''crack'') in pregnancy. *Obstet Gynecol.* 1988;72:147–151.

54. Keith L, MacGregor S, Friedell S, et al. Substance abuse in pregnant women: recent experience at the Perinatal Center for Chemical Dependence of Northwestern Memorial Hospital. *Obstet Gynecol.* 1989;73:715–720.

55. Little BB, Snell LM, Klein VR, et al. Cocaine abuse during pregnancy: Maternal and fetal implications. *Obstet Gynecol.* 1989;73:157–161.

56. Gillogley KM, Evans AT, Hansen RL, et al. The perinatal impact of cocaine, amphetamine and opiate use detected by universal intrapartum screening. *Am J Obstet Gynecol.* 1990;163:1535–1542.

57. Oro AS, Dixon SD. Perinatal cocaine and methamphetamine exposure: Maternal and neonatal correlates. *J Pediatr.* 1987;111:571–578.

58. Little BB, Snell LM: Brain growth among fetuses exposed to cocaine in utero: Asymmetrical growth retardation. *Obstet Gynecol.* 1991;77:361–364.

59. Dixon SD, Bejar R. Echoencephalographic findings in neonates associated with maternal cocaine and methamphetamine use: Incidence and clinical correlates. *J Pediatr.* 1989;115:770–778.

60. Tenorio GM, Navzi M, Bichers GH, et al. Intrauterine stroke and maternal polydrug abuse. *Clin Pediatr.* 1988;27:565–567.

61. Doberczak TM, Shanzer S, Senie RT, et al. Neonatal neurologic and electroencephalographic

effects of intrauterine cocaine exposure. *J Pediatr.* 1988;113:354–358.

62. Kramer LD, Locke GE, Ogunyemi A, et al. Neonatal cocaine related seizures. *J Child Neural.* 1990;5:60–64.

63. Lipshultz S, Frassica J, Ora J. Cardiovascular abnormalities in infants prenatally exposed to cocaine. *J Pediatr.* 1991;118:44–51.

64. Rosenstein BJ, Wheeler JS, Heid PL. Congenital renal abnormalities in infants with in utero cocaine exposure. *J Urol.* 1990;144:110–112.

65. Bauchner H, Zuckerman B, McClain M, et al. Risk of sudden infant death syndrome among infants with in utero exposure to cocaine. *J Pediatr.* 1988;113:881–884.

66. Durand DJ, Espinoza AM, Nickerson BG. Association between prenatal cocaine exposure and sudden infant death syndrome. *J Pediatr.* 1990;117:909–911.

67. Griffith DR, Chasnoff IJ, Freier MC. Developmental follow-up of cocaine exposed infants through three years. *Infant Behav Dev.* 1990;13:126.

68. MacGregor S, Keith L, Bachicha J, et al. Cocaine abuse during pregnancy: correlation between prenatal care and perinatal outcome. *Obstet Gynecol.* 1989;74:882–885.

69. Racine A, Joyce T, Anderson R. The association between prenatal care and birth weight among women exposed to cocaine in New York City. *JAMA.* 1985;270:1581–1586.

70. Thorp JM. Management of drug dependency, overdose and withdrawal in the obstetrical patient. *Obstet Gynecol Cl NA.* 1995;22:131–142.

71. Little BB, Snell LM, Gilstrap LC III. Methamphetamine abuse during pregnancy: outcome and fetal effects. *Obstet Gynecol.* 1988;72:541–544.

72. Hoegerman G, Schnoll S. Narcotic use in pregnancy. In: *Clinics in Perinatology.* 1991;18(1):53–76.

73. Selwyn PA, Hartel D, Wasserman W, et al. Impact of the AIDS epidemic on mortality and morbidity among intravenous drug users in a New York City methadone maintenance program. *A J Pub Health.* 1969;79:1358–1362.

74. Perlmutter JF. Heroin addiction and pregnancy. *Obstet Gynecol Surv.* 1974;29:439–446.

75. Fricher HS, Segal S. Narcotic addiction, pregnancy and the newborn. *Am J Dis Child.* 1978;132:360–366.

76. Pierson PS, Howard P, Klaber HD. Sudden deaths in infants born to methadone-maintained addicts. *JAMA* 1972;220:1733–1734.

77. Chavez CJ, Ostrea EM Jr, Stryker JC, Smialek Z. Sudden infant death syndrome among infants of drug-dependent mothers. *J Pediatr.* 1979;95:407–409.

78. Blinick G, Wallach RC, Jerez E, Akerman BD. Drug addiction in pregnancy and the neonate. *Am J Obstet Gynecol.* 1976;125:135–142.

79. Naeye RL, Blanc W, LeBlanc W, et al. Fetal complications of maternal heroin addiction: Abnormal growth, infections and episodes of stress. *J Pediatr.* 1973;83:1055–1061.

80. Glass L, Rajegowda BK, Evans HE. Absence of respiratory distress syndrome in premature infants of heroin-addicted mothers. *Lancet.* 1971;2:685–686.

81. Marantz PR, Linzer M, Feiner CJ, et al. Inability to predict diagnosis in febrile intravenous drug abusers. *An Intern Med.* 1987;106:823–828.

82. Connaughton JF, Reeser D, Schut J, et al. Perinatal addiction: Outcome and management. *Am J Obstet Gynecol.* 1977;129:679–686.

83. Green M, Silverman I, Suffet F et al. Outcomes of pregnancy for addicts receiving comprehensive care. *Am J Drug Alcohol Abuse.* 1979;6:413–429.

84. Wilson G. Clinical studies of infants and children exposed prenatally to heroin. *Ann NY Acad Sci.* 1989;562:183–194.

85. Newman RG, Bashlow S, Calko D. Results of 313 consecutive live births of infants delivered to patients in the New York City methadone maintenance program. *Am J Obstet Gynecol.* 1975;121:233–237.

86. Harper RG, Solish G, Feingold E, et al. Maternal ingested methadone, body fluid methadone, and the neonatal withdrawal syndrome. *Am J Obstet Gynecol.* 1977;129:417–424.

87. Ostrea EM, Chavez CJ, Strauss ME. A study of factors that influence the severity of neonatal narcotic withdrawal. *J Pediatr.* 1976;88:642–645.

88. Strauss ME, Andresko M, Stryker JC, et al. Relationship of neonatal withdrawal to maternal

methadone dose. *Am J Drug Alcohol Abuse.* 1976;3:339–345.

89. Zelson C, Lee SJ, Casalino M. Neonatal narcotic addiction. *N Engl J Med.* 1973;298: 1216–1220.

90. Burstein Y, Giarclina PJV, Ramsen A, et al. Thrombocytosis and increased circulation platelet aggregates in newborn infants of polydrug users. *J Pediatr.* 1979;94:895–899.

91. National Institute on Drug Abuse. U.S. Dept. of Health and Human Services, *National Household Survey on Drug Abuse 1988 Population Estimates.* Washington DC: 1989.

92. American College of Obstetricians and Gynecologists. Substance abuse. *ACOG Technical Bulletin 194.* Washington, DC: ACOG, 1994.

93. Desmond MM, Schwanecke RP, Wilson GS, et al. Maternal barbiturate utilization and neonatal withdrawal symptomatology. *J Pediatr.* 1972;80:190–197.

94. Briggs GG, Freeman RK, Yaffe SJ. *Drugs in Pregnancy and Lactation* 3rd Ed. Baltimore: Williams & Wilkins, 1990, 494–496.

95. Wilkins-Hang L, Cabow PA. Toluene abuse during pregnancy: obstetrical complications and perinatal outcomes. *Obstet Gynecol.* 1991;77: 504–509.

96. Crabbe SG, Niebyl JR. *Obstetrics, Normal and Problem Pregnancies.* 2nd ed. New York: Churchill Livingstone 1991.

QUESTIONS

1. Criteria for fetal alcohol syndrome can include all of the following *except*:
   a. growth retardation
   b. microcephaly
   c. retarded midfacial development
   d. cerebral palsy
   e. mental retardation

2. The following may have adverse effects when given to heroin or methadone dependent patients
   a. Nubain (nalbophine)
   b. terbutaline
   c. demerol
   d. general anesthesia

3. Neonatal withdrawal:
   a. occurs sooner with methadone than with heroin-dependent neonates
   b. is frequently fatal
   c. requires treatment in the majority of cases
   d. may not occur for up to 10 days with methadone dependent infants

4. Methadone dosing __ in late pregnancy:
   a. may need to be increased
   b. may need to be decreased
   c. usually remains the same

5. All the following are complications of tobacco use except:
   a. spontaneous abortions
   b. placenta abruption
   c. fetal growth retardation
   d. SIDS
   e. neonatal neurobehavorial abnormalities

14

Renal Complications of Pregnancy

Alice S. Petrulis

INTRODUCTION

The care of the pregnant women with renal disease or hypertension has changed over the decades. Historically, women with either of these diseases were discouraged from conceiving and, once pregnant, were discouraged from continuing the pregnancy. The basis of these views was the experience of some investigators suggesting that renal disease worsened with pregnancy.

However, this perspective has been challenged. There has been a reevaluation of this accumulated data as a result of the reality that many women with renal disease and hypertension were becoming pregnant and wished to continue the pregnancy. In addition, many women who have undergone renal transplantation have also become pregnant. It is the responsibility of the health care providers for these women to be aware of the growing literature in these areas.

This chapter will review the causes of acute renal failure in pregnancy, the risks to pregnant women with renal disease, and the risks to the hypertensive pregnant woman. The last segment will deal with prepregnancy counseling and includes a discussion of pregnancy in the renal transplant patient.

RENAL DISEASE AND PREGNANCY

Glomerular Disease and Pregnancy

There are very few series examining pregnancy in patients with chronic renal failure, primarily due to the fact that fertility decreases with creatinine clearances less than 50 cc per min. However, Katz reviewed 121 patients who had chronic renal disease with levels of serum creatinine less than 1.4 mg/dl.[1] The data suggests that there is deterioration of all renal parameters. Glomerular filtration rate decreased in 16%. One-half of patients with moderate ($\geq$150/100 mm hg) to severe hypertension ($\geq$170/110 mm hg) had normal blood pressures prepregnancy. It could not be predicted prepregnancy which patients would develop severe hypertension. Twenty-four-hour excretion of protein increased commonly and was seen in at least half of the patients. Sixty-eight percent of those patients with increased proteinuria had >3 grams of protein excreted per 24 hours. However, postpartum there was a reversal in these parameters back to the prepregnancy levels. In this study mild proteinuria was <1 g per day. Normal urinary protein excretion is less than 150 mg/day.

Hou examined 25 women during pregnancy with serum creatinine levels of 1.7–2.7 mg/dl and described more severe compromises in renal function. Seven patients had decrements in glomerular filtration rate (GFR) which did not reverse postpartum. More than half developed worsening hypertension.[2]

The outlook for the fetus in women who become pregnant despite the presence of renal disease appears to be favorable as long as significant maternal hypertension is absent and renal function is not severely reduced.

Diabetic Nephropathy and Pregnancy

An increase in 24-hour excretion of protein throughout pregnancy is common in diabetic patients known to have proteinuria prior to pregnancy. However, most patients have decrements in the degree of proteinuria postpartum. Hypertension is common and becomes an important determinant of outcome of pregnancy. In most patients renal function remains unchanged.

The outlook for the fetus is good if hypertension and significant renal impairment are absent at the onset. Risks to the fetus include preterm delivery and an increased incidence of growth retardation.

Some data exists that head-out water immersion may be effective in decreasing the edema of diabetic nephropathy and renal diseases. Changes in splanchnic blood flow occur resulting in an increase in increases in salt and water excretion. This maneuver, combined with sodium restriction may be effective in limiting the edema during pregnancy without using diuretics. If diuretics are necessary, loop diuretics are more beneficial, remembering that since the albumin in the urinary lumen binds the loop diuretic, then greater doses than initially assumed are usually required.

There is currently no data to suggest that protein restriction may be beneficial to the diabetic with proteinuria. It is clear however, that high-protein diets will worsen the proteinuria.

Diabetics should be evaluated throughout pregnancy for retinopathy. This allows early detection of proliferative changes and expectant laser therapy to prevent retinal hemorrhage.

Systemic Lupus Erythematosus and the Antiphospholipid Syndrome

Systemic lupus erythematosus (SLE) occurs in one in every 1660 pregnancies. Despite the abundance of clinical data there seems to be little consensus as to whether pregnancy adversely affects the course of the disease or whether the maternal and fetal outcome of pregnancy is compromised.

It appears that fertility is normal in the absence of significant renal impairment and proteinuria. Furthermore, it is the impression that active disease does have an adverse effect on fertility.

The effect of pregnancy on the natural history of SLE may be summarized by stating that equal thirds improve, become worse, or remain the same.

Most series report an increased incidence of abortions, stillbirths, prematurity, and babies that are small for gestational age.

One-third of patients with SLE have the antiphospholipid syndrome (APS). This syndrome may also be found in patients who do not meet the criteria for SLE. It is characterized by the presence of antiphospholipid antibodies (anticardiolipin and the lupus anticoagulant), and the occurrence of arterial or venous thrombosis, recurrent fetal loss, thrombocytopenia, or neurologic disorders.[3]

It is not cost-effective to routinely screen for the antiphospholipid antibodies, but it may be useful if the patient has SLE, recurrent fetal losses, or a history of thromboembolic disease.[4]

Treatment is empiric as data is lacking. Low-dose aspirin appears to be effective if the patient has SLE or APS. Heparin likewise appears to have value if the patient has a history of thrombosis. Prednisone is not routinely recommended for prophylaxis of SLE flares or for treatment of APS. Immunosuppressives may have a role if systemic disease is present.

ACUTE RENAL FAILURE IN PREGNANCY

The occurrence of renal failure in pregnancy is an unusual complication. It occurs in less than 1% of all pregnancies. Over time, the incidence of acute renal failure in pregnancy has decreased. In the 1950s, it was thought to be at least 22%.[5]

When evaluating a pregnant patient with acute renal failure, it may be easiest to view potential etiologies as being (1) prerenal; (2) obstructive; (3) intrinsic; and (4) causes unique to pregnancy.[6] (See Table 14-1.)

Prerenal Azotemia

Prerenal causes of acute renal failure relate to a decrease in the true or effective vascular volume of the patient. A clue to the presence of prerenal azotemia is a BUN/creatinine ratio that exceeds the normal of 10 to 1. One of the major causes of prerenal azotemia in pregnancy is hyperemesis gravidarum.

Obstruction

Obstructive uropathy may be another cause of acute renal failure in pregnancy. Despite the

Table 14-1. Causes of Acute Renal Failure During Pregnancy

Prerenal azotemia
  Volume depletion
  Edema-forming states
Obstruction
  Gravid uterus
  Hydramnios
  Bilateral nephrolithiasis
Intrinsic renal failure
  Acute glomerulonephritis
  Acute interstitial nephritis
  Bilateral renal cortical necrosis
  Acute tubular necrosis
  Infection
Causes unique to pregnancy
  Preeclampsia
  HELLP syndrome
  Acute fatty liver of pregnancy
  Postpartum acute renal failure

size of the gravid uterus, however, it is unusual for uterine compression to be a cause of renal failure. Polyhydramnios is another possible, though uncommon, cause of renal failure due to obstruction. The most common cause of obstructive nephropathy, however, is nephrolithiasis. It must be remembered that the normal physiology of pregnancy includes dilatation of the calyceal system, renal pelvis, and ureters. This phenomena may persist up to 16 weeks after delivery. This normal "hydronephrosis" of pregnancy, however, does not affect renal function.

Intrinsic Renal Failure

Acute glomerulonephritis secondary to viral diseases or acute allergic interstitial nephritis from antibiotics may occur during pregnancy and lead to changes in kidney function. Likewise, pyelonephritis, if bilateral, may also cause acute renal failure. The pregnant woman is at increased risk of pyelonephritis due to the increased incidence of urinary tract infections during pregnancy (2%).

Bilateral renal cortical necrosis (BRCN) is not an uncommon cause of acute renal failure in pregnancy. It is extremely uncommon in the nonpregnant state. Ten to forty percent of cases of renal failure in pregnancy are related to bilateral renal cortical necrosis. The causes of BRCN include preeclampsia, septic abortion, abruption, and uterine hemorrhage. The exact etiology of the cortical necrosis is unclear and it is speculated that it may be related to the hypercoagulable state of pregnancy. Although the diagnosis may be made by arteriogram, renal biopsy, or CT scan, the simplest way to make the diagnosis is clinically. Acute renal failure due to acute tubular necrosis usually resolves within 10–14 days. For the patient who is dialysis dependent for greater than 6–8 weeks with minimal or no urine output, the clinical diagnosis of BRCN is usually assigned. Management consists of continued dialysis.

Acute tubular necrosis (ATN) is probably the most common diagnosis among the causes of acute renal failure secondary to intrinsic factors.

The etiology of ATN in pregnancy for the most part is the same as those of the nonpregnant state and includes nephrotoxins and sepsis. Pregnancy-related causes of ATN include abruption, intrauterine fetal demise, and amniotic fluid embolism.

Causes Unique to Pregnancy

There are several causes of acute renal failure that are unique to pregnancy. Preeclampsia is the most common cause of acute renal failure in pregnancy. Preeclampsia occurs in approximately 5–8% of all pregnancies. Ten to twenty percent of patients with preeclampsia will develop acute renal failure. The diagnosis is heralded by the occurrence of hypertension or proteinuria and edema in a pregnancy greater than 20 weeks gestation. The abnormal renal presentation reverses postpartum. It is extremely uncommon for a patient to require dialysis for acute renal failure related to even severe preeclampsia.

The HELLP syndrome is probably a manifestation of severe preeclampsia. The letters stand for Hemolysis, Elevated Liver enzymes, and Low Platelets. Coagulation parameters are usually normal. Renal dysfunction may also occur, but returns to normal after delivery.

Acute fatty liver of pregnancy usually presents in a woman after 35 weeks of gestation and is associated with nausea, vomiting, jaundice, and may progress to hepatic encephalopathy. Acute renal failure occurs in almost all cases. In addition, disseminated intravascular coagulation may also be seen. The aspartate amino transferase (AST) and alanine amino transferase (ALT) levels are frequently only mildly elevated. Death is a common occurrence with this entity. The incidence is less than 1 in 13,000 pregnancies. Liver biopsy reveals the presence of microvesicular fat in swollen hepatocytes. Treatment for this disorder is delivery.

Postpartum acute renal failure is a disease associated with microangiopathic hemolytic anemia, hypertension, seizures, thrombocytopenia, and acute renal failure. It may occur 48 hours to one month after a seemingly normal delivery. Pathologically there is fibrinoid necrosis and thrombosis on renal biopsy. It has been suggested that bacterial endotoxin may stimulate the coagulation cascade or initiate thrombosis by causing endothelial damage. Some strains of E. Coli have been associated with this disease. Because it shares many similar features of the hemolytic uremic syndrome and also thrombotic thrombocytopenia purpura, it is felt by many authors to represent part of a spectrum of the same disease. This disease has a high morbidity and mortality rate. Attempts at treatment modalities have included intravenous infusions of prostacyclin, plasma exchanges, and antiplatelet therapy.

HYPERTENSION IN PREGNANCY

Hemodynamic Changes of Normal Pregnancy

Normal pregnancy is associated with a number of hemodynamic effects. By the eighth week of pregnancy both systolic and diastolic blood pressures have begun to decline and reach their nadir at twenty weeks. Associated increases in heart rate are seen.

By definition, hypertension exists when the blood pressure exceeds 140/90 mm Hg.

Renal blood flow increases during the first trimester and GFR increases by at least 50%. This is reflected in both the BUN and creatinine levels. The values for BUN are frequently less than 10 mg/dl. Serum creatinine is usually 0.6 ± 0.2 mg/dl.

The renin-angiotensin system is likewise affected. Plasma renin substrate, renin, and aldosterone levels increase. Yet, despite these increases, systemic blood pressures are decreased. The explanation lies in the apparent resistance of the vasculature to the pressor effects of angiotensin II. This resistance to the hypertensive effects of angiotensin II is felt to be absent in women destined to develop preeclampsia and is the basis for the angiotensin infusion test.

Classification

The classification of the hypertensive disorders in pregnancy includes: (1) preeclampsia; (2) chronic hypertension; (3) superimposed preeclampsia; and (4) transient hypertension.

Confusion frequently lies in the use of the term "pregnancy-induced-hypertension" (PIH). This term encompasses a range of disorders collectively known as toxemia of pregnancy and includes isolated hypertension (nonproteinuric hypertension), preeclampsia (proteinuric hypertension), and eclampsia.

Differential Diagnosis of Hypertension

The thrust of the clinical evaluation of the patient is to address the issue of whether the hypertension is primary (essential) or secondary. Therefore the history, physical, and laboratory testing should be directed at excluding the secondary causes of hypertension. Secondary causes of hypertension include renovascular hypertension (renal artery stenosis), chronic renal failure, hyperaldosteronism, aortic coarctation, Cushing's disease, pheochromocytoma, and cocaine (See Table 14-2).

Evaluation of the Hypertensive Patient (See Table 14-3)

The medical history should include an assessment of target organ damage (heart, brain, and kidneys). A history of the extent and treatment of prior hypertension should also be obtained. In addition, it is important to learn previous side effects of therapy or known resistance

Table 14-2. Differential Diagnosis of Hypertension

Essential
Renovascular hypertension
Chronic renal failure
Primary hyperaldosteronism
Coarctation of the aorta
Cushing's disease
Pheochromocytoma
Cocaine

Table 14-3. Evaluation of Hypertension

History
  Past history/treatment
  Family history
  Medications
  Comorbid disease
  Diet/lifestyle
  Alcohol/drugs
Physical exam
  Blood pressure with pulse
    bilateral/leg
  Cardiopulmonary evaluation
  Bruits
  Edema
  Cushingoid features
Laboratory
  Potassium, blood urea nitrogen, creatinine
  Uric acid, serum glutamic oxaloacetic transaminase
  Dipstick urine
  Toxicology screen
    (when appropriate)

to therapy. The history should include acknowledgement of other coexisting disease which may be associated with hypertension such as polycystic kidney disease or long-standing diabetes.

A family history of hypertension, cerebral vascular disease, coronary artery disease, or diabetes should also be obtained.

Recent literature suggests that over-the-counter decongestant medications containing phenylpropanolamine (Dimetapp) do not affect blood pressure control.[7] Nasal sprays and other cold remedies may worsen underlying hypertension.

A history of ethanol use, smoking, excessive sodium ingestion, caffeine use, and "street drugs" should be obtained. Cocaine is being increasingly recognized as a cause of accelerated hypertension. Proteinuria may also be seen in accelerated hypertension. Since cocaine may also cause placental abruption and intrauterine fetal demise, the occurrence of all these signs in a pregnant woman may result in mistakenly diagnosing preeclampsia.

In the history it is also important to note the occurrence of headaches, palpitations, flushing or diaphoresis. These may help in one's suspicion regarding a diagnosis of pheochromocytoma. Since the incidence of pheochromocytoma is less than 1:1000 in a hypertensive population, a patient complaining of many of these symptoms may well be describing an anxiety syndrome or panic attack.

The physical exam is primarily directed at the vascular system. Tachycardia associated with hypertension is a hint about catecholamine excess, that is, pain, vomiting, drug withdrawal, anxiety, cocaine use, or volume depletion.

The fundoscopic exam should be done to note the presence of arteriolar narrowing, arteriovenous compression, hemorrhages, exudates, or papilledema. The neck should be evaluated for distended neck veins, carotid bruits, and thyromegaly. The cardiopulmonary exam may give evidence regarding the presence of left ventricular enlargement or congestive heart failure. An abdominal exam may reveal the presence of renal artery bruits or polycystic kidneys.

The presence of edema gives information regarding the volume status of the patient. Violaceous striae, moon facies, and a buffalo hump may suggest Cushing's syndrome.

It is particularly important in this young population to evaluate the patient for the presence of coarctation of the aorta as reversibility of the hypertension following surgery may occur if diagnosed by the early twenties. Delayed or absent femoral pulses with leg pressures which are lower than arm pressures are seen in this disease.

Laboratory evaluation should include measurements of renal function (BUN and creatinine), and potassium with the additional testing being done if preeclampsia is suspected in the differential.

The absence of proteinuria exceeding 3 g per 24 hours directs one away from the diagnosis of glomerular disease as the etiology of the hypertension. Essential hypertension is usually associated with less than 1 g of protein excretion per 24 hours. An exception to this, however, is in the case of accelerated or malignant hypertension where nephrotic range proteinuria may be associated. This will dissipate when the hypertension is controlled.

Treatment of Hypertension

Only a limited number of antihypertensive agents are acceptable for use in pregnancy. Still unanswered is the question of timing for initiation of therapy. The National High Blood Pressure Education Program Working Group Report on High Blood Pressure in Pregnancy[8] recommends initiating therapy when the diastolic blood pressure exceeds 100 mm Hg.

Drugs which are acceptable for use in pregnancy include alphamethyldopa and hydralazine. There is growing use of beta-blockers, the combined alpha/beta blocker labetalol and calcium channel blockers.

Angiotension-converting enzyme inhibitors are contraindicated in pregnancy because of case reports describing oligohydramnios and acute renal failure in the neonate.

PRECONCEPTUAL COUNSELING

Counseling in Patients with Hypertension

There is no data that demonstrates that preconceptual control of hypertension prevents preeclampsia. However, good judgment dictates that a normotensive state should be obtained prior to pregnancy if possible.

Control of hypertension during pregnancy likewise does not guarantee that preeclampsia will be prevented. Hypertension should be controlled, though, to prevent maternal cerebrovascular complications. In addition, the hypertensive state is associated with an increased incidence of placental abruption.

Counseling in Patients with Glomerular Disease

The woman who desires pregnancy and has underlying glomerula renal disease must be apprised of the decrease in fertility as the glomerular filtration rate decrease. If pregnancy occurs, there is an increased risk of developing deterioration in renal function which may result in dialysis, worsening of hypertension and increases in the degree of proteinuria. There will be an increased risk of developing preeclampsia and this may result in the potential for preterm delivery. For patients with a serum creatinine of less than 1.4 mg/dl it is likely that, even though these renal changes may occur, there will be a postpartum reversal of these parameters. This is not true for serum creatinine levels greater than this and the patient must be apprised of a greater potential for worsening disease resulting in an earlier likelihood of requiring dialysis.

Counseling for Renal Transplant Patients

Over the last two decades, there has been enough experience of pregnancy after renal transplantation that appropriate recommendations may be made. It appears that conceptual plans can be made at a minimum of two years posttransplant.[9] Immunosuppressives including cyclosporin A, azothioprine, and steroids can be continued throughout pregnancy. Control of hypertension is mandatory. Graft function is not adversely affected if renal function is stable and well preserved at the time of conception.[10]

Review of Prophylaxis for Preeclampsia

Several studies suggest that low-dose aspirin (60–150 mg) may be effective in preventing preeclampsia in high-risk populations such as prior severe preeclampsia, hypertension, lupus erythematosus, multiple births, and renal disease.[11] Not all studies are in agreement with this.[12] Most investigators will agree that the risk/benefit ratio for low dose aspirin in low risk groups does not warrant its use.[13] Most recently, results from the Maternal Fetal Network trial do not warrant its use in high risk pregnancies.

High doses of calcium (2 g per day) during pregnancy may prevent preeclampsia.[14] The results of the multicenter NIH trial, however, do not support this.

CONCLUSIONS

The care of the pregnant woman with renal disease or hypertension involves close management by both the obstetrician/perinatologist and the internist/nephrologist. Often times large series or prospective randomized trials do not exist to help guide care and management is empiric.

Counseling of the patient is imperative, requiring that the pregnant woman participate in the decision-making process. Frequently, premature delivery of the fetus with all its associated risks is the outcome with a return to baseline status for the mother. However, complications for these women are not uncommonly seen and include sepsis, stroke, intrauterine fetal demise, dialysis, and death.

Indications for acute dialysis are several and include hyperkalemia, volume overload, severe azotemia, uncontrolled acidosis, hypermagnesemia, and hyponatremia. Fortunately, it is uncommon that a severely preeclamptic woman requires dialysis. However, this is a greater possibility for the pregnant woman with severely compromised renal function.

Prepregnancy counseling is vital, though most commonly the obstetrician is faced with a high-risk woman who is already pregnant. Discussion of the potential complications is more often the scenario, however.

REFERENCES

1. Katz AI, Davison JM, Hayslett JP, et al. Pregnancy in women with chronic renal disease. Kid Int. 1980;18:192–206.

2. Hou SM, Grossman SD, Madias NE. Pregnancy in women with renal disease and moderate renal insufficiency. *Am J Med.* 1985;78:185–194.

3. Arnout J, Spitz B, Van Assche A, et al. Antiphospholipid Syndrome. *Hypertension in Pregnancy.* 1995;14:147–178.

4. Boumpas DT, Austin HA, Fessler BJ, et al. Systemic lupus erythematosus: emerging concepts. *Ann Int Med.* 1995;122:940–950.

5. National High Blood Pressure Education Program Working Group. Report on High Blood Pressure in Pregnancy. *Am J Obstet Gynecol.* 1990;163:1689–1712.

6. Grunfeld JP and Pertuiset N. Acute renal failure in pregnancy. *Am J Kid Dis.* 1987;9:359–362.

7. Petrulis AS, Imperiale TF, and Speroff T. The acute effects of phenylpropanolamine and brompheniramine on blood pressure in controlled hypertension: a randomized double-blind crossover trial. *J Gen Intern Med.* 1991; 6:503–506.

8. Krane NK. Acute renal failure in pregnancy. *Arch Int Med.* 1988;148:2347–2357.

9. Bung P and Molitor D. Pregnancy and postpartum after kidney transplantation and cyclosporin therapy-review of the literature and a new case. *J Perinat. Med.* 1991;19:397–401.

10. Rizzoni G, Ehrich JHH, Broyer M, et al. Successful pregnancies in women on renal replacement therapy: report from the EDTA registry. *Nephrol Dial Transplant.* 1992;7:279–287.

11. Imperiale TF and Petrulis AS. A meta-analysis of low-dose aspirin for the prevention of pregnancy-induced hypertensive disease. *JAMA* 1991;266:260–264.

12. CLASP Collaborative Group. CLASP: a randomized trial of low-dose aspirin for the prevention and treatment of preeclampsia. *Lancet.* 1994;343:619–629.

13. Sibai BM, Caritis SN, Thom E, et al. Prevention of preeclampsia with low dose aspirin in healthy nulliparous pregnant women. *N Engl J Med.* 1993;329:1213–1218.

14. Belizan JM, Villar J, Gonzalez L, et al. Calcium supplementation to prevent hypertensive disorders of pregnancy. *N Engl J Med.* 1991;325: 1399–1405.

QUESTIONS

1. Fetal outcome in pregnancies complicated by renal disease is affected by:
   a. Hypertension
   b. Renal impairment
   c. Proteinuria
   d. All of the above
2. Antiphospholipid antibodies include:
   a. Anticardiolipin antibodies and the lupus anticoagulant
   b. Sedimentation rate
   c. Rheumatoid factor
   d. All of the above
3. Pregnant women with diabetic nephropathy should
   a. Achieve glycemic control
   b. Have controlled blood pressure
   c. Undergo ophthalmologic evaluation
   d. All of the above

True or false

4. In the absence of active disease, fertility in patients with SLE appears to be normal.
5. Diabetics with proteinuria will usually have increases in the degree of proteinuria during pregnancy.

Part IV

INFERTILITY AND ONCOLOGIC PROBLEMS OF PREGNANCY

15

Is Pregnancy Following Infertility at High Risk?

Khalid M. Ataya

INTRODUCTION

Infertility, which affects approximately 15% of couples, has generated a lot of interest among investigators worldwide. A pregnancy after a period of infertility is naturally considered to be more precious than otherwise by both the patient and her attending obstetrician. Infertile women who conceive have pregnancies that have been reported to be *high risk*. With new advances in assisted reproductive technologies, obstetricians are having to deal with increasing numbers of multiple gestations. Moreover, oocyte donation and embryo transfer have challenged the obstetricians to more commonly deal with women getting pregnant in their 40s, 50s, and beyond. While some studies have suggested that the obstetrical complication rate is higher in the infertile group in general, it is helpful to relate specific pregnancy problems to the etiology of infertility in the first place.

For the sake of discussion in this chapter, the potential risks to pregnancies occurring in infertile women will be divided into those complications that commonly occur in the first, second, or third trimesters. Multifetal pregnancy and oocyte donation issues will be discussed under separate subheadings.

FIRST-TRIMESTER COMPLICATIONS

As infertility patients tend to be older, it is wise to discuss genetic factors and their implications on these pregnancies. Depending on the etiology of infertility, different patient subgroups may be at risk of specific complications. Figure 15-1 summarizes an approach to this group of patients.

Ectopic Pregnancy

An increased incidence of ectopic pregnancy in infertile women has been reported.[1-3] Ghazi et al.[4] reported a 2.6-fold increase in ectopic pregnancy, whereas Bhalla et al.[5] reported a 5-fold increase in ectopic pregnancy. Kalby et al.[6] also studied 290 patients with primary and secondary infertility and found an increased incidence of ectopic pregnancy in the tuboperitoneal factor subgroup.

First Trimester Bleeding/Abortion

Kalby et al.[6] found an increased incidence of spontaneous abortion in the ovulation factor subgroup of infertile patients. Early pregnancy loss (including ectopic pregnancy) in infertile

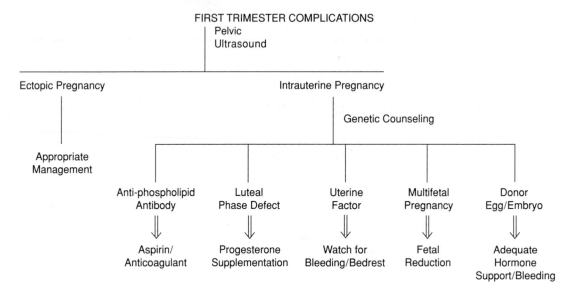

Figure 15-1. Complications during the first trimester in pregnant women with history of infertility.

women is likely to be increased.[1,2,7-9] The magnitude of this increase has been reported to be 3-fold.[9] The rate of first-trimester bleeding is also significantly higher.[5]

Antiphospholipid Antibodies

Abnormal lupus anticoagulant (LA) was initially associated with pregnancy wastage.[10,11] LA and autoantibodies to phospholipid, histone, and polynucleotide antigens have been associated with endometriosis,[12] unexplained infertility,[13] in vitro fertilization (IVF) failure[14] and the presence of sperm antibodies.[15] The correlation between LA and broadly based autoantibody abnormalities has therefore assumed importance for the diagnosis of a broad spectrum of reproductive failure. LA is also associated with IUGR and poor obstetrical performance.

Infertility with Uterine Factor

Patients with infertility related to uterine factors may be at risk for poor obstetrical performance. In this subgroup of patients, the combination of infertility and reduced ability to carry the pregnancy to term can join to further limit the ability of a couple to have a living child. The impediment to successful pregnancy

outcome can vary from difficulty in implantation, to first- or second-trimester abortion or premature labor later.

Intrauterine Adhesions

Intrauterine adhesions can occur following overzealous curetting, or infection with endometrial tissue destruction such as in tuberculosis. Treatment of tuberculous endometrial pathology is rarely followed by subsequent pregnancy. Intrauterine adhesions can result in spontaneous abortion of pre- and postimplantation embryos. Surgical excision of mild-moderate post-traumatic adhesions commonly results in establishment of ensuing pregnancy.

Uterine Leiomyomas

Egwautu[16] studied 141 women with leiomyomas. The preoperative spontaneous abortion and fetal loss rates were 62% and 21% respectively (compared to the control of 5% and 4%). Postoperatively, the spontaneous abortion and fetal loss rates dropped down to 11% and 6% respectively.

Congenital Uterine Malformations

Patients with reproductive tract anomalies can present with infertility and/or poor obstetrical performance. The anomalies can include uterus didelphis, unicornuate, bicornuate, septate, subseptate, and arcuate uterus[17] and the T-shaped uterus associated with DES exposure.[18] All types of uterine anomalies have been associated with poor pregnancy outcome. High abortion rates, second-trimester abortion, and premature labor have been reported in these patients. The physician should be aware of the possibility of incompetent cervix in this subset of patients.

SECOND-TRIMESTER COMPLICATIONS

Complications in the second trimester occur less commonly than in the first or third trimesters. These include detection and management of congenital anomalies following chorionic villus sampling, amniocentesis, and/or ultrasound. Because of the higher age of this population, these women are at increased risk of fetal anomalies. Moreover, women with uterine malformation are also at risk of cervical incompetence. These patients should be followed very closely and may benefit from cerclage procedures.

THIRD-TRIMESTER COMPLICATIONS

For the sake of this discussion, these will be divided into maternal antenatal, labor and deliv-ery, and fetal complications. An approach to complications in this subset of patients is summarized in Figure 15-2.

Maternal Antenatal Complications

A higher incidence of hypertensive disease of pregnancy has been recorded[2,3] in patients with history of infertility. A significant increase in the proportion of women with preexisting hypertension and gestational diabetes has also been reported.[2] The subfertile group also contained a significantly higher proportion both of women of age ≥36 and of primigravida. It is possible that these two factors may account for the different obstetric and neonatal outcomes in these two groups (see section on confounding variables below). Pregnant women with history of anovulatory infertility related to polycystic ovaries should be checked for diabetes since insulin resistance is common in this subgroup.

Labor and Delivery Complications

A significantly higher rate of induction of labor in infertile patients has been reported.[1-3] These and other authors[5,6] also found a higher rate of caesarean section. Increased forceps/operative delivery rates in those with a history of infertility has been recorded.[1,2] The rate of preterm deliveries (28.1%) was higher in one study,[5] whereas the studies by others[1,2] found no

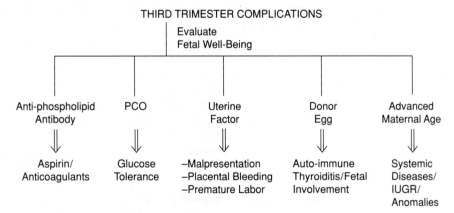

THIRD TRIMESTER COMPLICATIONS

Figure 15-2. Complications during the third trimester in pregnant women with history of infertility. PCO = polycystic ovarium syndrome; IUGR = intrauterine growth restriction.

such difference. The difference could be related to the rate of multiple gestation. This in turn related to the type of infertility treatments.

The reported more than doubling of the caesarean section rate[19,20] cannot be explained on the basis of either age or parity. It may be that an obstetrician's response to certain events, such as delay in progress and suspected fetal distress, are influenced, whether consciously or subconsciously, by a history of infertility. The diagnosis of fetal distress in labor was not significantly more common in the subfertile than in the control group.[20] Tuck et al.[21] reported that elective section was twice as common in the older ($\geq$35) primigravida with a history of infertility (21%) than in those without such a history (11%), but the emergency section rate was similar in both groups (18% and 16% respectively).

Pregnancies occurring in uteri with history of intrauterine adhesions seem to be at risk of developing placenta increta, uterine sacculation and a paper-thin uterine fundus. Therefore these patients should be considered at high risk.[22] Premature labor, abnormal presentation, excessive bleeding from the placentation site and poor early neonatal outcome is associated with uterine leiomyomata, bicornuate, arcuate, subseptate, and septate uterus.[23,24] Postmyomectomy scar rupture has been reported.[25] If a patient had undergone myomectomy, information needs to be obtained as to the depth of the myoma and as to whether caesarean section would be needed in future pregnancies. This judgement is best provided by an experienced reproductive surgeon. Clearly, subserosal myomectomy does not necessitate abdominal delivery. Entry into the uterine cavity at abdominal myomectomy usually requires subsequent caesarean section. Pregnancies following infertility treatment are more likely to be multiple with increased risk of premature labor (see section on multifetal pregnancy below).

Fetal Complications

All pregnancies occurring in infertile women warrant genetic counselling, ultrasonography, and appropriate testing for fetal growth retar-

dation and hypoxia in late pregnancy. The overall rate of malformations is not increased in the total infertile group. An increased incidence of intrauterine growth retardation and stillbirths in infertile patients has been reported.[1,2] The rate of stillbirth (28.1%) was higher in one study[5] but other studies[1,2] found no such difference. A significant increase in fetal distress, low Apgar score, and low birthweight in women with a history of infertility compared with the general obstetric population[2] has been reported.

Women with premature ovarian failure undergoing oocyte donation should be tested for autoimmune disease. An association of autoimmune phenomena with premature ovarian failure has been documented.[26–28] Children born to women with autoimmune thyroid gland disorders are at risk of developing passive thyroid autoimmune hyperthyroidism[29] or hypothyroidism.[30]

Confounding Variables of Age and Parity

Tuck et al.[22] compared 196 primigravida aged $\geq$35 years with 196 matched primigravida aged 20–25 years and reported a significantly higher proportion of preterm labor, caesarean section, vaginal operative delivery, and chronic hypertension in the former group. Within their older primigravid group (35 years or more) these differences were not sustained when previously fertile and infertile women were compared. It is probable that infertile women are more likely to be older and nulliparous,[2] (or of significantly lower gravidity[20]) than the average obstetric population. It is therefore likely that some previous findings of pregnancy outcomes in subfertile women[2] could be explained in part by the age and parity factors.

The findings of at least one study,[21] indicate that, once singleton pregnancy is established beyond 16 weeks, women with a history of infertility may be considered to have an obstetric and neonatal outcome no different to that of women without such a history, except for an increased likelihood of being delivered by caesarean section. This conclusion obviously excludes first-trimester complications which are clearly increased in different subsets of patients with infertility. The fact that a higher proportion of infertility patients is older and of less parity should always be kept in mind as these can influence maternal and fetal wellbeing. Multiple gestations, which occur more commonly in patients receiving ovulation induction regimens, clearly increases morbidity and mortality. Egg and embryo donation also pose a special circumstance where recipients with premature ovarian failure may have associated autoimmune thyroiditis with its fetal transmission sequelae.

EGG DONATION

With recent advances in assisted reproductive technology, it is now possible to transfer embryos into the preprimed uterus of postmenopausal women in their 50s and beyond. This clearly raises some medical concerns, let alone social and ethical dilemmas. Some clinicians have thus questioned whether oocyte donation to older women endanger the health and life of the mother and fetus. Pregnancy is a time of considerable cardiovascular stress. Thus, older women with decreased cardiovascular reserve may be expected to be at higher risk of adapting insufficiently to the stress and demands of pregnancy. Retrospective population studies have generally demonstrated an age-related increase in the incidence of pregnancy-induced hypertension, diabetes, stillbirths, and small-for-gestational-age babies in women delivering after their 35th birthday.[31] It should be noted that the association between age and chromosomal anomalies is, in all likelihood, obviated by the use of oocytes donated by younger women. Rochat et al.,[32] summarizing results from the Maternal Mortality Collaborative, reported an overall maternal mortality ratio of 14.1 per 100,000 births for 1980–1985. The maternal mortality rates for women over the age of 40 were estimated at approximately 60 per 100,000 for whites and over 200 per 100,000 for nonwhites. Younger individuals with cardiovascular disease such as pulmonary hypertension or prior myocardial in-

farction, who are too ill to carry a pregnancy are often advised to terminate an ongoing pregnancy. Clearly, such individuals should not be offered oocyte donation, regardless of age. Emphasis should be centered on education, counseling, and testing, with the matter of reproductive choice reserved for the well-informed patient.

Cornet et al.[33] reported that the obstetric profiles of eight pregnancies after oocyte donation to women with primary ovarian failure were normal while Sauer et al.[34] reported a high rate of vaginal bleeding in the first trimester. A maternal death due to subarachnoid hemorrhage in a twin pregnancy after oocyte donation complicated by hypertension was reported.[35] Antinori et al.[36] reported only one case of severe hypertension (4.8%) among 21 term pregnancies after oocyte donation to menopausal women, and a low incidence of complications during oocyte donation pregnancies in a limited series was reported by Sauer et al.[37] Pados et al.[38] studied the obstetrical performance of 69 clinical pregnancies, 53 of which reached term following transfer of donated embryos. There was a high incidence of uterine bleeding during the first trimester of pregnancy (34.6%), as well as preeclampsia (32.7%) and intrauterine growth retardation (11.5%) especially in twin pregnancies (37.5%). The high incidence of IUGR in this study, apart from the contribution of the great proportion of twin pregnancies (15.4%) might be attributed to the advancing age of patients.[39,40] Bleeding was more frequent among patients with ovarian failure than among those with functional ovaries (38.2% and 27.8%, respectively). Maternal mortality, perinatal morbidity, and mortality remained at very low levels and this obviously reflects the quality of obstetrics care, as well as the lack of multifetal gestations and preterm deliveries in this study.

MULTIFETAL PREGNANCY: REDUCTION

Births resulting from in-vitro fertilization (IVF) or gamete intrafallopian transfer (GIFT) have a significantly higher proportion of preterm births. The maternal risks of multifetal gestation include an increased incidence of preterm labor requiring medical treatment, preterm delivery, preeclampsia, pregnancy-induced hypertension, gestational diabetes mellitus, anemia, postpartum hemorrhage, and thrombophlebitis. In addition, there is an increased incidence of fetal complications, including preterm birth and all of its potential accompanying problems, intrauterine growth restriction (IUGR), malpresentation, cord accidents, and congenital anomalies. Reducing short-term and long-term maternal and neonatal morbidity is a major consideration for patients who choose multifetal pregnancy reduction. In addition, patients who elect reduction have usually been through a series of infertility treatments and are especially concerned with the chance that they could lose the entire pregnancy. This is a particular problem for those who are considering a reduction from triplets to twins, in light of recent research indicating that this choice may not significantly reduce the risks. A mean gestation age similar to that published for nonreduced twins (35.3 weeks) and triplets (35.7 weeks) can be achieved.[41] The incidence of congenital anomalies is not increased compared to other multifetal pregnancies specially with twins. Patients should be counseled extensively about the importance of obtaining prenatal care from a physician with experience in managing multifetal gestations. Women who choose multifetal pregnancy reduction are highly motivated to have a successful pregnancy outcome. They tend to be compliant with the medical plan for their care and, consistent with their financial ability to afford infertility treatment, they usually have the monetary resources to discontinue working and obtain assistance at home.[41]

Multifetal pregnancy reduction is a relatively safe procedure, having a pregnancy loss rate of 7–33%. The most widely accepted technique is first-trimester intrathoracic injection of KCl under ultrasound guidance. Even though acceptable outcomes usually can be achieved even starting with high fetal numbers, there is still a price to be paid in increased fetal loss rate and

an increased risk of prematurity. Thus, overzealous infertility treatment does have deleterious effects even if fetal reduction can be performed by trained physicians.

REFERENCES

1. Newton J, Round L, Curson R. The outcome of pregnancy in previously infertile women. *Acta Europ Fert.* 1978;8:161–167.

2. Varma TR, Patel RH. Outcome of pregnancy following investigation and treatment of infertility. *Int J Gynaecol Obstet.* 1987;25:113–120.

3. Varma TR, Patel RH, Bhatena RK. Outcome of pregnancy after infertility. *J Obstet Gynaecol India.* 1987;367–374.

4. Ghazi HA, Spielberger C, Källén B. Delivery outcome after infertility—registry study. *Fert Steril.* 1991;55:726–732.

5. Bhalla AK, Sarala G, Dhaliwal L. Pregnancy following infertility. *Aust NZ J Obstet Gynaecol.* 1992;32:249–251.

6. Kalby A, Gallardo V, Moctezuma J, Garza Rios P, Karchmer K. Course of pregnancy in patients with known infertility. *Gineco Obstetr De Mexico.* 1992;60:105–109.

7. Liu HC, Jones HW Jr, Rosenwaks Z. The efficiency of human reproduction after in vitro fertilization and embryo transfer. *Fertil Steril.* 1988;49:649–653.

8. Hack M, Brish M, Serr DM, Insler V, Lunenfeld B. Outcome of pregnancy after induced ovulation. *JAMA.* 1970;211:791–797.

9. Caspi E, Ronen J, Schreyer P, Goldberg MD. The outcome of pregnancy after gonadotrophin therapy. *Br J Obstet Gynaecol.* 1976;83:967–973.

10. Lubbe WF, Butler WS, Palmer SJ, Lippins GC. Lupus anticoagulant in pregnancy. *Br J Obstet Gynaecol.* 1984;91:357–363.

11. Lubbe WF, Butler WS, Palmer SJ. Fetal survival after prednisone suppression of maternal lupus anticoagulant. *Lancet.* 1983;1:1361–1363.

12. Gleicher N, El Roeiy A, Confino E, Friberg J. Is endometriosis an autoimmune disease? *Obstet Gynecol.* 1987;70:115–122.

13. Gleicher N, El Roeiy A, Confino E, Friberg J.

Reproductive failure because of autoantibodies: unexplained infertility and pregnancy wastage. *Am J Obstet Gynecol.* 1989;160:1376–1385.

14. El-Roeiy A, Gleicher N, Confino E, Friberg J, Dudkiewicz AB. Correlation between peripheral blood and follicular fluid: autoantibodies and impact on in vitro fertilization. *Obstet Gynecol.* 1987;70:163–170.

15. El-Roeiy A, Valesini G, Friberg J, et al. Autoantibodies and common idiotypes in men and women with sperm antibodies. *Am J Obstet Gynecol.* 1988;158:596–603.

16. Harris WJ. Uterine dehiscence following laparoscopic myomectomy. *Obstet Gynecol.* 1992; 80:545–546.

17. Egwuatu VE. Fertility and fetal salvage among women with uterine leiomyomas in a Nigerian teaching hospital. *Int J Fert.* 1989;34:341–346.

18. Ludmir J, Samuels P, Brooks S, Mennuti MT. Pregnancy outcome of patients with uncorrected uterine anomalies managed in a high-risk obstetric setting. *Obstet Gynecol.* 1990;76: 906–910.

19. Thorp JM Jr, Fowler WC, Donehoo R, Sawicki C, Bowes WA Jr. Antepartum and intrapartum events in women exposed in utero to diethylstilbestrol. *Obstet Gynecol.* 1990;76:828–832.

20. Hill GA, Bryan S, Herbert CM, Ahah DM, Wentz AC. Complications of pregnancy in infertility couples: routine treatment versus assisted reproduction. *Obstet Gynecol.* 1990;75: 790–794.

21. Li TC, MacLeod I, Singhal V, Duncan SL. The obstetric and neonatal outcome of pregnancy in women with a previous history of infertility: A prospective study. *Brit J Obstet Gynaecol.* 1991;98:1087–1092.

22. Tuck SM, Yudkin PL, Turnbull AC. Pregnancy outcome in elderly primigravida with and without a history of infertility. *Br J Obstet Gynaecol.* 1988;95:230–237.

23. Friedman A, DeFazio J, DeCherney A. Severe obstetric complications after aggressive treatment of Asherman Syndrome. *Obstet Gynecol.* 1986;67:864–867.

24. Maneschi M, Maneschi F, Fuca G. Reproductive impairment of women with unicornuate uterus. *Acta Europaea Fertilitatis.* 1988;19: 273–275.

25. Acien P. Reproductive performance of women with uterine malformations. *Human Reprod.* 1993;8:122–126.

26. Irvine W, Chan M, Scarth L, et al. Immunological aspects of premature ovarian failure associated with idiopathic Addison's disease. *Lancet.* 2;1968:883–886.

27. Coulam C. The prevalence of autoimmune disorders among patients with primary ovarian failure. *Am J Reprod Immunol.* 1983;4:63–66.

28. Alper M, Garner P. Premature ovarian failure; its relationship to autoimmune disease. *Obstet Gynecol.* 1985;66:27–30.

29. Zakarija M, McKenzie J. Pregnancy associated changes in the thyroid-stimulating antibody of Grave's disease and the relationship to neonatal hyperthyroidism. *J Clin Endocrinol Metab.* 1983;47:1036–1040.

30. Takasu N, Mori T, Koizumi Y, Takeuch S, Yamada T. Transient neonatal hypothyroidism due to maternal immunoglobulins that inhibit thyrotropin-binding and post-receptor processes. *J Clin Endocrinol Metab.* 1984;59:142–146.

31. Hansen JP. Older maternal age and pregnancy outcome: A review of the literature. *Obstet Gynecol Surv.* 1986;41:726–742.

32. Rochat RW, Koonin LM, Atrach HK, Jewett JF. Maternal mortality in the United States: Report from the maternal mortality collaborative. *Obstet Gynecol.* 1988;72:91–97.

33. Cornet D, Alvarez S, Antoine J, et al. Pregnancies following ovum donation in gonadal dysgenesis. *Human Reprod.* 1990;5:291–293.

34. Sauer M, Paulson R, Macoso T, Francis M, Lobo R. Oocyte and pre-embryo donation to women with ovarian failure; an extended clinical trial. *Fertil Steril.* 1991;55:39–43.

35. Beweley S, Wright J. Maternal death associated with ovum donation twin pregnancy. *Human Reprod.* 1991;6:898–899.

36. Antinori S, Versaci C, Hossein Gholami G, Panci C, Caffa B. Oocyte donation in menopausal women. *Human Reprod.* 1993;8:1487–1499.

37. Sauer M, Paulson R, Lobo R. Pregnancy after age 50: Application after oocyte donation to women after natural menopause. *Lancet.* 1993; 341:321–323.

38. Pados G, et al. The evolution and outcome of oregnancies from oocyte donation. *Human Reprod.* 1994;9:538–542.

39. Kujansuu E, Kivinen S, Tuimala R. Pregnancy and delivery at the age of forty and over. *Int J Gynaecol Obstet.* 1981;19:341–345.
40. Forman M, Meirik O, Berendes H. Delayed childbearing in Sweden. *JAMA.* 1984;252:3135–3139.
41. Tabsh K. A report of 131 cases of multifetal pregnancy reduction. *Obstet Gynecol.* 1993;82:57–60.

QUESTIONS

1. Pregnancies following donor oocyte/embryo replacement are associated with a high incidence of:
   a. third-trimester bleeding
   b. second-trimester bleeding
   c. first-trimester bleeding
   d. congenital anomalies
2. Pregnancies in women over 50 following donor egg/embryo replacement:
   a. invariably result in hypertension or preeclampsia
   b. have a high incidence of congenital anomalies
   c. invariably result in cardiovascular complications
   d. should have a preconception consult with a perinatologist
3. Pregnancies following infertility related to polycystic ovarian disease are associated with:
   a. third-trimester bleeding
   b. second-trimester bleeding
   c. abnormalities of glucose metabolism
   d. ectopic pregnancy
4. Pregnancies following infertility related to tubal disease are associated with:
   a. ectopic pregnancy
   b. severe preeclampsia
   c. premature labor
   d. postpartum sepsis
5. Complications of pregnancies in women with uterine anatomic abnormalities include the following except:
   a. premature labor
   b. habitual abortion
   c. preeclampsia
   d. abnormal presentation
   e. excessive postpartum bleeding

16

Genital Tract Malignancies in Pregnancy

M. A. Selim and A. D. Shalodi

INTRODUCTION

Genital tract malignancies occurring with pregnancy are rare. When they occur they create a dilemma for the patient and physician. They raise many ethical, moral, and medical questions concerning the fetus and the mother. Gynecologic malignancies are the second most common cancer after breast cancer occurring during pregnancy.[1]

The physiologic changes of pregnancy such as increased vascularity, lymphatic drainage, and immunological change may contribute to early dissemination of these malignant processes.[2]

CANCER OF THE CERVIX

Cancer of the cervix is the most common gynecologic malignancy occurring with pregnancy. However, the incidence in the literature is very variable and most authorities from large cancer centers feel that 1% of women who have carcinoma of the cervix are pregnant at the time. The most common symptom is bleeding. Therefore, whenever bleeding occurs during pregnancy, it has to be investigated by pelvic ex-

amination, pap smear, and colposcopic-directed biopsies. During the third trimester such procedures should be done as double setup procedure in the operating room. The pap smear is very helpful in the diagnosis of abnormal lesions on the cervix; however, it has a false negative rate of about 20–30%.[3] Colposcopically directed cervical biopsies are extremely accurate during pregnancy as all patients will have satisfactory colposcopy (Selim et al.[4]). This will alleviate the need for cone biopsies with complications during pregnancy (except if biopsies showed microinvasion) to rule out frank invasion.[4]

Gravidity and parity are important factors in cancer of the cervix. Although early intercourse appears to be the most important etiologic factor, multiple parity usually goes hand in hand (2). In addition, multiple pregnancies (>2) have a poorer prognosis.[5]

Treatment

Premalignant Lesions

Pregnant patients with an abnormal pap smear, unexplained bleeding or discharge, and/ or abnormal growth or lesions on the cervix should have colposcopic-directed biopsies. Colposcopies in pregnancy are always satisfactory

221

due to physiologic changes at the cervix which allow the transformation zone and endocervical canal to be adequately visualized.[4] Adding to this, if the biopsies correlate with the pap smear and diagnosis is intraepithelial neoplasia, the patient can be followed and continue with her pregnancy without further treatment. During the pregnancy the patient needs to be followed by pap smears and repeat colposcopy at least once at 28–32 weeks of the pregnancy. There is no contraindication for vaginal deliveries unless there is obstetrical contraindication.[4] Postpartum, patients need to be evaluated colposcopically and then the method of treatment and follow-up must be decided.

Cone biopsy in pregnancy for microinvasion carries several risks: severe blood loss, blood transfusion, and a high rate of abortion or premature labor. For this reason cone biopsy should be avoided if possible. In our experience at this institution with the large number of high-risk obstetric patients and the high incidence of abnormal paps, we have avoided cone biopsies in pregnancy from 1973 to the present. Whenever we found microinvasion on colposcopic-directed biopsy, we repeated biopsies generously, or we did excisional biopsies with cold knife or lately by the loop electrosurgical excision procedure (LEEP). LEEP during pregnancy is reported in 40 patients with very successful results.[6]

Malignant Lesions

With microinvasion, Stage IA (i.e., stromal invasion less than 3 mm without vascular or lymphatic invasion and margins of resection are free) the patient can continue with her pregnancy to term. There are no contraindications for vaginal delivery unless there is an obstetrical reason. Postpartum, the patient needs to be examined colposcopically and endocervical curettings need to be done. If colposcopy is satisfactory, endocervical curettings are negative and if the patient has completed her family, the patient can be treated by total abdominal hysterectomy. However, if the patient desires more children, the patient is advised to complete her family and then definitive treatment is to be

done as in carcinoma in situ. However, if the colposcopy is unsatisfactory and/or endocervical curettings are abnormal (less than invasion), cone biopsy is recommended before the final decision of treatment or follow-up (Figure 16-1).

Invasive Carcinoma

The decision about the treatment of carcinoma of the cervix in pregnancy depends on the stage of the disease, trimester, and the desire of the patient (Figure 16-2).

Studies showed clearly that stage for stage carcinoma of the cervix in pregnancy behaves equally in nonpregnant young patients, i.e., pregnancy has no influence on the prognosis.[7] However, more advanced stages are found in the third trimester and postpartum.[7] This emphasizes the need for early diagnosis. In addition, patients treated by surgery or irradiation for the same stages have equal results.[2,7,8] However, due to the young age of the patients, radical surgery would be preferable in early stages to preserve the ovaries and the vagina and because patients with negative nodes and margins have very good prognosis and do not require further treatment. If those patients were treated by radiation originally, the longer they survive the possibility of radiation complications increases, including fistulas and other malignancies which are difficult to treat.

In patients with Stage IA_2, IB, or IIA and pregnant less than 24 weeks, the best treatment would be radical hysterectomy, para-aortic lymph node biopsy, and pelvic lymphadenectomy. If the lymph nodes and margins are free of malignancy, no further treatment would be needed. However, about 15% of the patients will have positive nodes[8] and will require chemotherapy and irradiation.

Patients with advanced stages (more than Stage IIA) should be treated by total pelvic irradiation followed by intracavitary irradiation. Spontaneous abortion will occur during or after the total pelvic irradiation.[7] If abortion did not occur spontaneously by the completion of the total pelvic irradiation, a modified radical hysterectomy should be considered.[2]

Patients with early stages (IA_2, IB, IIA) and

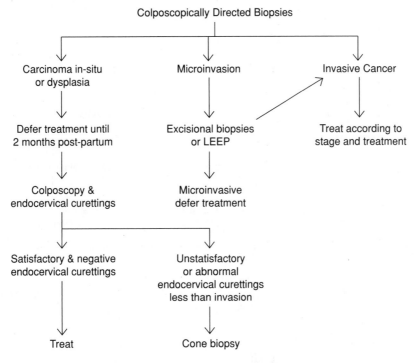

Figure 16-1. Colposcopically Directed Biopsies.

pregnant more than 24 weeks can be followed until the fetus reaches maturity, then the patient would have a cesarean section with radical hysterectomy, para-aortic lymph node biopsy, and pelvic lymphadenectomy for the same reasons mentioned above.

Patients with advanced stages can have a cesarean section at term followed by total pelvic irradiation and intracavitary irradiation.

The reason for advising abdominal delivery is the fear of severe bleeding from the malignant cervix which would tear very easily during dilatation. Studies available in the literature show that the method of delivery has no influence on prognosis of the cancer.[2,7]

UTERINE CANCER

Adenocarcinoma of the endometrium is very rare in pregnancy. In 1994, there were 12 cases reported in the literature.[10]

The age range is 21 to 43 years of age, parity ranged between 0 to 10. The common symptom is vaginal bleeding, but 2 patients presented for elective abortion. In our institute 2 cases were discovered postpartum due to persistent vaginal bleeding. One of them had a history of hyperplasia treated conservatively before pregnancy. Most of the patients have well-differentiated adenocarcinoma and Stage I but one patient (Suzuki et al.[11]) had moderately differentiated and another case was Stage II and died from recurrence. Two patients had concurrent endometrial carcinoma of the ovaries.[13,14]

The rarity of endometrial carcinoma during pregnancy is understandable due to the protection of the progesterone, however, when it occurs during pregnancy it is difficult to explain. The best possible explanation is that some areas in the endometrium lack progesterone receptors. For this reason, they will have continuous estrogen stimulation and eventually progress into cancer.[10,15]

The treatment in patients with Stage I who have completed their families, is total abdominal hysterectomy, bilateral salpingo-oophorectomy, and surgical staging. State II is best

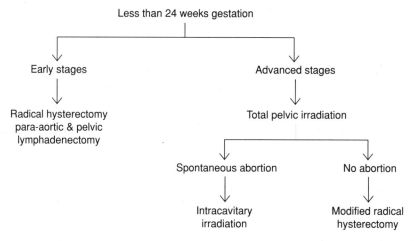

Figure 16-2a. Management of carcinoma of the cervix in pregnancy (less than 24 weeks gestation).

treated by radical hysterectomy. Advanced stages are treated by irradiation and hysterectomy. Patients with early stages of well-differentiated adenocarcinoma who desire further pregnancy, can be treated by progestational agents and close follow-up.[10]

Leiomyosarcoma and carcinosarcoma are very rare. Lau and Wong[16] in 1993 reported two cases of leiomyosarcoma and collected 5 previous cases of leiomyosarcoma that were previously reported in the literature. All cases were found incidentally at cesarean hysterectomy or postpartum. The management of sarcoma in pregnancy should be aggressive as these malignancies are more virulent than adenocarcinoma. For this reason, hysterectomy and lymphadenectomy are the treatment of choice with supplementation of chemotherapy.

OVARIAN AND FALLOPIAN TUBE CARCINOMA

Ovarian malignancy with pregnancy is very rare and the incidence ranges from 1 in 81 to 1 in 2500.[17] However, adnexal masses with pregnancy are more common. Most of the masses are functional and resolve spontaneously. Therefore a unilateral, noncomplex mass less than 5 cm in the first trimester can be followed by ultrasound through the second trimester. If the mass persists or increases in size, elective surgical exploration would be indicated. Adnexal masses persisting after the first trimester will be pathologically confirmed to be malignant in about 2%–3% of the cases.[17]

Most of the masses present without symptoms are discovered by pelvic exam in early

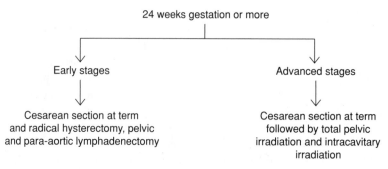

Figure 16-2b. Management of carcinoma of the cervix in pregnancy (24 weeks gestation or greater).

pregnancy or abdominal palpation in late pregnancy. Ultrasound has been of great help in detecting and following these masses. Unfortunately, 15%–18% can present in early pregnancy with acute abdomen due to torsion or hemoperitoneum. In these cases emergency surgery will be necessary.

Tumor markers such as CA-125 are not helpful in pregnancy due to high false positive results. The same can be said about other markers such as alpha-fetoprotein (AFP), lactate dehydrogenase (LDH), and beta human chorionic gonadotropin (BhCG).

Management

As we mentioned previously, if the lesion is small and appears to be benign on ultrasound and asymptomatic, the patient can be followed closely until the second trimester. If it persists or increases in size, the best time for exploration is about 18 weeks as the incidence of abortion is nearly zero and also before the uterus becomes very large and impedes exploration.

Before exploration, if there is peritoneal fluid it should be collected for cytology. If there is no fluid, peritoneal washings should be done. The cyst is then removed and frozen section is performed. If the cyst is benign, no further treatment is needed. However, if it is malignant adequate surgical staging is to be performed, including biopsy of the para-aortic and ipsilateral pelvic lymph nodes, and debulking all masses.

The most common malignancy is the germ cell tumors, especially dysgerminoma. They are usually unilateral and if they are surgically Stage IA, surgery usually is more than enough. However germ cell tumors such as endodermal sinus tumor and embryonal tumors, combined chemotherapy is essential even in early stages. This poses a big dilemma to the physician and the patient as data concerning the effect of the chemotherapy on the fetus is inadequate. Therefore, this has to be discussed thoroughly with the patient. It is very important to avoid chemotherapy in the first trimester and to time the chemotherapy in later trimester so as not to coincide with delivery, as chemotherapy can transfer through the placenta, affecting the bone marrow of the fetus. In addition, since the mother will be on chemotherapy postpartum, breastfeeding is prohibited.[2]

Epithelial neoplasms are rarer than germ cell tumors. They also are discovered in early stages and lower grades during pregnancy. In most of the cases unilateral oophorectomy and adequate surgical staging are more than adequate. However, advanced stages and/or high-grade tumors will need supplementary chemotherapy. The roles of chemotherapy applied to the germ cell tumors would apply to epithelial tumors.

Fallopian Tube Malignancy

Fallopian tube malignancy is usually an adenocarcinoma and is very very rare in pregnancy. In most instances the diagnosis is established at laparotomy or incidental finding in tubal ligation specimens. The treatment, if it is an early stage, is unilateral salpingectomy and adequate surgical staging.[18] In advanced stages the treatment is total abdominal hysterectomy, bilateral salpingo-oophorectomy and chemotherapy.

VAGINAL CARCINOMA

Cancer of the vagina occurs mostly in patients older than 50 years of age; therefore carcinoma of the vagina is very rare in pregnancy. The most common cancer of the vagina reported in recent years is the clear cell adenocarcinoma in patients exposed to diethylstilbestrol (DES) in utero. However, rare cases are reported of squamous cell carcinoma and sarcoma botryoids.

The treatment depends on the stage of the disease and the trimester of pregnancy. If the lesion is early stage and early pregnancy, the best treatment is radical hysterectomy, vaginectomy, and lymphadenectomy. However, if they are advanced lesions the best treatment is radiotherapy. If the lesion is discovered in late pregnancy, wait for maturity of the fetus and then institute the treatment according to the stage of the disease. It appears that pregnancy has no influence on the prognosis of the disease.[19]

VULVAR CARCINOMA

Vulvar carcinoma is primarily a disease of the sixth and seventh decade, however 15% of vulvar cancers occur in women 40 years of age or younger.[20] Still, carcinoma of the vulva is rarely diagnosed during pregnancy. The most important factor in treatment is whether it is diagnosed as precancerous or invasive. If it is intraepithelial, conservative management during pregnancy is acceptable.

If it is invasive and it is a small lesion (T_1), it should be treated by radical local excision with ipsilateral inguino-femoral lymphadenectomy (if the depth of invasion is less than 1 mm).[21] More advanced lesions require modified radical or radical vulvectomy and bilateral inguino-femoral lymphadenectomy. If there are multiple positive nodes or macroscopically positive node, delivery should be considered as soon as fetal viability has been achieved[21] so that postoperative radiotherapy and/or chemotherapy could be instituted.

The method of delivery after vulvectomy has to be individualized. If the vagina is stenosed, cesarean section is preferable. However, if the vagina is supple, there is no contraindication for vaginal delivery.

REFERENCES

1. Allen HH, Nisker HA, eds. *Cancer in Pregnancy Therapeutic Guidelines.* Mt. Kisco, NY: Futura, 1986.

2. DiSaia PJ, Creasman WT, eds. *Clinical Gynecologic Oncology*, 4th Ed. St. Louis, MO: Mosby Yearbook Inc., 1992.

3. Selim MA, So-Bosita JL, Blair O, and Little BA. Cervical biopsy versus conization. *Obstet Gynecol.* 1973;41:177–182.

4. Selim MA, Vasquez HH, and Masri R. Indications and experience in colposcopy in management of cervical neoplasia. *Surg Gynec Obstet.* 1977;145:529–532.

5. Selim MA and Kurohara SS. Significance of gravidity in cancer of the cervix uteri. *Am J Obstet Gynec.* 1970;106:731–735.

6. Blomfield PI, Buxton J, Dunn J, and Luesley DM. Pregnancy outcome after large loop excision of the cervical transformation zone. *Am J Obstet Gynec.* 1993;169:620–625.

7. Graham JB, Sotto LS J, and Paloucek FP. *Carcinoma of the Cervix.* Philadelphia: W.B. Saunders, 1962.

8. Selim MA, Kurohara SS, and Webster JH. Surgical or radiation therapy for cancer of the cervix Stage I. *Obstet Gynec.* 1971;38:251–254.

9. Selim MA and Shalodi AD. Treatment of cervical Stage IB. *J. of Islamic Med Association of N AM.* 1991;23:103–106.

10. Schneller JA and Nicastri AD. Intrauterine pregnancy coincident with endometrial carcinoma: a case study and review of the literature. *Gynecol Oncol.* 1994;54:87–90.

11. Suzuki A, Kanishi I, Okamura H, and Nakashima N. Adenocarcinoma of endometrium associated with intrauterine pregnancy. *Gynecol Oncol.* 1984;18:261–269.

12. Wall JA and Lucci JA. Adenocarcinoma of the corpus uteri and pelvic tuberculosis complicating pregnancy. *Obstet Gynec.* 1953;2:629–635.

13. Pulitzer DR, Collins PC, and Gold RG. Embryonic implantation in carcinoma of the endometrium. *Arch Pathol Lab Med.* 1985;109:1089–1092.

14. Hoffman MS, Cavanagh D, Walter TS, Ionata F, and Ruffals EH. Adenocarcinoma of the endometrium and endometrioid carcinoma of the ovary associated with pregnancy. *Gynecol Oncol.* 1989;32:82–85.

15. Pai UL, Razi A, Selim MA, and Petrelli M. Endometrial adenocarcinoma arising in secretory endometrium. *Gynecol Oncol.* 1993;49:268–270.

16. Lau TK and Wong WSF. Uterine leiomyosarcoma associated with pregnancy: a report of two cases. *Gynecol Oncol.* 1994;53:245–247.

17. Grendys, Jr EC and Barnes WA. Ovarian cancer in pregnancy. *Surg Clin North Am* 1995;75:1–14.

18. Gatto VW, Selim MA, and Lankerani M. Pri-

mary carcinoma of the fallopian tube in an adolescent. *J Surg Oncol.* 1986;33:212–214.

19. Selim MA. Cancer of the vagina and vulva. *Primary Care of Cancer, 1987.* Recommendations for screening, diagnosis and management. Regional Cancer Research Center of Northeast Ohio. Office of Community Health, Case Western Reserve University School of Medicine. Library of Congress Catalog Card Number 86-73119.

20. Henson D and Tarone R. An epidemiologic study of cancer of the cervix, vagina and vulva based on the third national cancer survey in the United States. *Am J Obstet Gynec.* 1977;129: 525–532.

21. Gitsch A, van Eijkeren M, and Hacker NF. Surgical therapy of vulvar cancer in pregnancy. *Gynecol Oncol.* 1995;56:312–315.

QUESTIONS

For each of the following multiple choice questions, choose the one most appropriate answer.

1. The incidence of false negative pap smear is:
   a. 5–10%
   b. 20–30%
   c. 30–40%
   d. all of the above
   e. none of the above
2. The treatment of intraepithelial carcinoma of the cervix depends on:
   a. age
   b. parity
   c. the desire for more children
   d. all of the above
   e. none of the above
3. The most important factor in the prognosis of cervical carcinoma in pregnancy is:
   a. trimester
   b. stage
   c. grading
   d. all of the above
   e. none of the above
4. The incidence of pelvic lymph node involvement in Stage I of the cervix is:
   a. 10%
   b. 15%
   c. 25%
   d. 30%
5. The treatment of invasive carcinoma of the cervix in pregnancy depends on:
   a. stage
   b. trimester
   c. age
   d. both a and b
   e. all of the above
6. The reason(s) for performing radical hysterectomy for early stages of carcinoma of the cervix in pregnancy is (are):
   a. to conserve of the ovary
   b. to save the vagina
   c. to prevent complications of radiation
   d. all of the above
   e. none of the above
7. Invasive cervical carcinoma in the last trimester necessitates delivery of viable fetus by cesarean section to:
   a. prevent spread of disease
   b. prevent severe hemorrhage and laceration
   c. prevent fetal infection
   d. all of the above
   e. none of the above
8. The best times for laparotomy for ovarian mass during pregnancy is:
   a. first trimester
   b. second trimester
   c. third trimester
   d. all of the above
   e. none of the above
9. The best timing for chemotherapy during pregnancy is (are):
   a. first trimester
   b. second trimester
   c. third trimester
   d. all of the above
10. Vaginal deliveries are contraindicated after radical vulvectomy:
    a. stenosed introitus
    b. at any time
    c. both a and b
    d. all of the above
    e. none of the above

17

Gestational Trophoblastic Neoplasia

M. A. Selim and A. D. Shalodi

INTRODUCTION

The term *gestational trophoblastic neoplasia* (GTN) is applied to include hydatidiform mole, invasive mole, and choriocarcinoma. They are biologically and morphologically interrelated tumors which arise during gestation and have the ability to produce human chorionic gonadotropin (hCG). They are the first tumors to be successfully treated by chemotherapy (Methotrexate) with very high cure rate.[1]

HYDATIDIFORM MOLE

The incidence of hydatidiform mole varies from one geographic area to another. In the United States, the incidence is 1 in 1200 pregnancies. In the far east, the incidence is reported in 1 in 120 pregnancies. A significant increase in the incidence of moles is found in women 15 years of age or younger and 40 years of age or older.[2] Berkowitz et al.[3] suggested that nutritional factors such as deficiency of animal fat-soluble vitamins may contribute to this disease.

A patient with molar pregnancy has an increased risk of trophoblastic recurrence in later pregnancies of 0.6% to 2.0%.[1] With recurrent molar pregnancy, there is an increased risk of malignant transformation; however, the patient may also have subsequent normal pregnancies.[4]

Symptoms

Over 90% of the patients with molar pregnancy will present with vaginal bleeding in the first trimester. The bleeding can be prolonged and heavy to the degree that the patient would require a blood transfusion. Nausea and vomiting occur in about one-third of the patients. These symptoms and preeclampsia in the first trimester should raise the suspicion for molar pregnancy. A small number of patients may present with hyperthyroidism or bronchial asthma. Clinically in 50% of the patients, the uterine size will be larger than the gestational age with bilateral thecal luteal cysts.[1] However in a recent study by Soto-Wright et al.[5] they suggest that there are fewer current patients with complete mole present with the traditional symptoms of excessive uterine size, anemia, preeclampsia, hyperthyroidism, or hyperemesis.

Diagnosis

A patient in the first trimester with vaginal bleeding, a more enlarged uterus than dates, ovarian cysts, and preeclampsia would raise the suspicion for a hydatidiform mole. However, the best methods for diagnosis of a mole are high levels of hCG and ultrasound.

A quantitative pregnancy test greater than 1,000.000 Iu/L is suggestive but not conclusive as such a level can occur in multiple normal pregnancy. The presence of a fetal heart does not exclude a mole, as a mole can be associated with twin fetuses.[6] Also, a normal hCG titer for gestational age cannot exclude a mole.

Classically, characteristic multiple sonographic echoes without a fetus is a typical diagnostic picture on ultrasound. However, recently Soto-Wright et al.[5] suggested that nonspecific appearance of first-trimester molar pregnancy as chorionic villi may be too small to produce the characteristic vesicular pattern. In a series of 69 patients, ultrasound suggested that diagnosis in only 71% of the patients. Because complete mole may be diagnosed earlier in gestation now than it used to be, clinicians should be aware that ultrasound may not be as reliable in early pregnancy.

Pathology

Complete mole is characterized histologically by trophoblastic proliferation, hydropic degeneration, absence of central vessels and absence of the fetus. Karyotype is usually 46XX but rarely 46XY. The histologic grade has no prognostic significance.[7]

On the other hand, the trophoblastic changes of a partial mole are fetal and affect the syncytial layer only. The fetus is present and usually dies in the first trimester. A rare, living infant is born in the second or third trimester. Partial moles are usually triploid in karyotype.

Treatment

The best treatment for complete and partial mole is evacuation of the uterus usually by suction dilatation and curettage. Eighty percent of patients will have a normal hCG level within two months of evacuation.[8] Therefore, a careful monitoring of the patient with serial quantitative hCG should be ordered at one- to two-week intervals until two successive normal values are obtained. The patient and the values are followed every month for six months, then every two months for another six months. During this interval the patient should be on reliable contraception.

Most of the authors are against prophylactic chemotherapy because the majority of patients will have spontaneous cure, there is a marginal decrease in the rate of postmolar neoplasm and an increase of mortality rate due to chemotherapy toxicity.[9] Therefore the best approach is to monitor the patient. As long as the titer of hCG is decreasing, there is no evidence of the metastasis and uterus is involuting, then no further treatment is required. However any rise or plateau of the hCG level, evidence of metastasis, and/or noninvoluting uterus, the patient would need to be reevaluated. Metastatic work-up is performed and the patient is treated by chemotherapy.[10]

Histologic confirmation is not essential as repeat curettage does not add to cure and may lead to perforation.[11] Hysterectomy is only indicated in treatment of mole whenever the patient desires sterilization (Figure 17-1).

GESTATIONAL TROPHOBLASTIC NEOPLASIA

About 20% of patients with hydatidiform mole will develop malignant sequelae of choriocarcinoma or invasive mole. Malignant transformation is preceded by hydatidiform mole in 50% of the cases, abortion in 25%, full-term pregnancy in 22.5%, and ectopic pregnancy in 2.5%.[12]

Pathology

Invasive mole is characterized by the presence of chorionic villi with hydropic degeneration, trophoblastic proliferation, and invasion of the myometrium.

Choriocarcinoma, on the other hand, characterized by absence of the villi, is a pure sheet

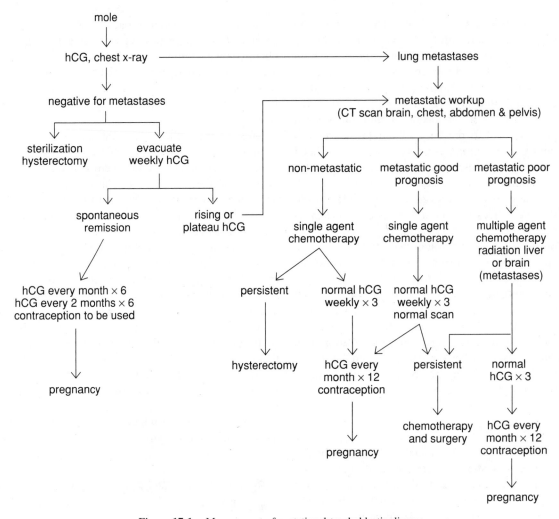

Figure 17-1. Management of gestational trophoblastic disease.

of epithelial neoplasia derived from syncytiotrophoblast and cytotrophoblast. These sheets of cells have a high affinity for vascular invasion, and therefore, systematic metastases.[13]

Placental site trophoblastic neoplasm is characterized by the absence of the villi, proliferation of only the intermediate cytotrophoblast cells and rarely metastasis.[13]

Diagnosis

As previously discussed under treatment of molar pregnancy, whenever the hCG titer rises or plateaus, evidence of metastases and/or non-

involuting uterus, a diagnosis of malignant trophoblast should be considered. The patient should have a metastatic work-up, be staged (see below) and then treated accordingly (Figure 17-1).

Malignant trophoblastic disease occurring following abortion or term pregnancies, even though the majority report abnormal bleeding, is rarely diagnosed early. For this reason, any bleeding or abnormal symptoms postpartum should arouse suspicion for trophoblastic disease. Physical examination, determination of hCG titer, ultrasound of pelvis, endometrial biopsies, and CT scan of the chest or brain depending on symptoms should be considered.

Table 17-1. International Federation of Gynecologists and Obstetricians Staging System

Stage	Description
0	Molar pregnancy
I	Confined to the uterus
II	Metastases to the pelvis and vigina
III	Metastases to the lung
IV	Metastases to the brain, liver, etc.

Metastases from choriocarcinoma are more to the lungs (80%), vagina (30%), pelvis (20%), liver (10%), brain (10%), bowel, kidney, and spleen (5%).[14] Such metastases, especially the CNS metastases, can present with bizarre symptoms including seizure and coma. For these reasons, these patients should be investigated thoroughly to rule out metastatic choriocarcinoma.

Classification

Several staging systems have been proposed but the most widely used are The International Federation of Gynecologists and Obstetricians (FIGO) and The World Health Organization (WHO) (Tables 17-1 & 17-2), respectively.

FIGO staging uses only the anatomic distribution and does not take in account other very important factors such as the level of hCG, du-

ration of the disease, site of metastases, etc. For these reasons, it is very deficient. The WHO system corrects that but is complicated and difficult to remember.

A simple and practical classification based on the experience of the National Institutes of Health[15] easily allows identification of high-risk patients so that they can be treated aggressively. This system divides the patients into nonmetastatic and metastatic. The metastatic patients are subdivided into those with good prognosis and those with poor prognosis (Table 17-3). Non-metastatic patients and who have good prognosis metastatic disease can be treated successfully by single-agent chemotherapy with a low toxicity. Patients with poor prognosis metastatic disease require aggressive treatment of triple chemotherapy.

Management

Nonmetastatic gestational trophoblastic neoplasia is the most common of the spectrum of GTN. By definition, it is limited to the uterus. As shown in Figure 17-1, this disease can be treated by a single-agent chemotherapy which is usually Methotrexate or Dactinomycin. To reduce the toxicity, folinic acid rescue is usually used with methotrexate with a very good cure rate.[12,16] The therapy should be repeated every 7–10 days until a normal level of beta hCG is

Table 17-2. World Health Organization Staging System

Prognostic Factor	Score[a]			
	0	1	2	4
Age (year)	≤39	>39		
Antecedent pregnancy	hyd. mole	abortion	term	
Interval (months)[b]	<4	4–6	7–12	>12
hCG (IU/l)	$<10^3$	$10^3 - 10^4$	$10^4 - 10^5$	$>10^5$
ABO groups		O × A or A × O	B or AB	
Largest tumor	<3 cm	3–5 cm	>5 cm	
Site of metastases	lung	spleen, kidney	GI, liver	brain
Number of metastases	1–3	4–8	7–8	
Prior chemotherapy			one drug	two or more drugs

[a] The total score for a patient is obtained by adding the individual score for each factor 4 = low risk, 5–7 = intermediate, >7 = high risk.

[b] Time between end of antecedent of pregnancy and start of chemotherapy.

Table 17-3. Malignant GTD

A. Nonmetastatic GTD
B. Metastatic GTD
  1. Good prognosis
    a. Duration <4 months
    b. Pretherapy serum beta hCG <40,000 IU/ml
    c. Lung metastases
  2. Poor prognosis—any of the following risk factors
    a. Duration >4 months
    b. Prior term pregnancy
    c. Pretherapy serum beta hCG >40,000 IU/ml
    d. Brain or liver metastases
    e. Failed prior chemotherapy

reached in 2–3 successive weeks. The patient should be followed monthly in the first six months, then bimonthly in the following six months. In addition, the patient should be on effective contraception during this period. If the disease persists, reevaluation of the patient for metastatic disease is essential and the patient should be treated by multiple agents as in high-risk groups (see below). However if the patient does not desire further fertility, hysterectomy should be considered.

Metastatic Gestational Trophoblastic Neoplasia

Good prognosis metastatic neoplasia patients are characterized by metastases only to the lungs, the duration of the disease is less than four months, and pretherapy serum beta hCG level is less than 40,000 IU/ml (Table 17-3). The treatment for these patients is similar to non-metastatic GTN (Figure 17-1).[1]

Poor prognosis metastatic trophoblastic neoplasia patients will have liver or brain metastases, pretherapy beta hCG > 40,000 IU/ml, duration of disease more than 4 months or preceded by full-term pregnancy and/or failed prior chemotherapy (Table 17-3). These patients require intensive treatment with multiple agents and multiple modalities which lead to multiple toxicities and morbidities (Figure 17-1).[14] The most effective combination of chemotherapy is using Etoposide, Dactinomycin, Methotrexate, and Folinic acid on days one and two, and Vin-

cristine and Cyclophormide on day eight (EMA-CO).[17] Radiation to brain metastases plus the chemotherapy is essential. Surgery may be necessary to reduce intracranial pressure and can be life-saving. Brain and liver metastases carry poor prognosis, however, brain metastases fair better than liver metastases.[1]

PLACENTAL SITE TROPHOBLASTIC NEOPLASIA

Placental site trophoblastic neoplasia is a very rare tumor which carries poor prognosis. Vaginal bleeding is the common symptom after abortion, mole, or normal pregnancy. hCG level is often low even with metastases. This tumor is chemoresistant. The best treatment in nonmetastatic disease is hysterectomy.[1,13]

REFERENCES

1. DiSaia PJ, Creasman WT, eds. *Clinical Gynecologic Oncology*, 4th Ed. St. Louis, MO: Mosby Yearbook Inc., 1992.

2. Bandy LC, Clarke-Pearson LD, Hammond CB. Malignant potential of gestational trophoblastic disease at the extreme age of reproductive life. *Obstet Gynec.* 1984;64:395–399.

3. Berkowitz RS, Cramer DW, Bernstein MR. Evolving concepts of molar pregnancy. *J Reprod Med.* 1991;36:40–44.

4. Berkowitz RS, Goldstein DP, Bernstein MR. Reproductive experience after complete and partial molar pregnancy and gestational trophoblastic tumors. *J Reprod Med.* 1991;36:3–8.

5. Soto-Wright Y, Bernstein M, Goldstein DP, Berkowitz RS. The changing clinical presentation of complete molar pregnancy. *Obstet Gynec.* 1995;86:775–779.

6. Suzuki M, Matsunalu A, Waketa K, Nishijima M, Asanai K. Hydatidiform mole with a surviving coexisting fetus. *Obstet Gynec.* 1980;56:384–388.

7. Genest DR, Laborde O, Berkowitz RS, Goldstein DP, Bernstein MR, Lage J. A clinicopathologic study of 153 cases of complete hydatidiform mole (1980–1990): histologic grade

lacks prognostic significance. *Obstet Gynec.* 1991;78:402–409.

8. Lurain JR, Brewer JI, Torok EE, et al. The natural history of hydatidiform mole after primary evacuation. *Am J Obstet Gynec.* 1981;145: 591–595.

9. Ratnam SS, Teoli ES, Dawood MY. Methotrexate for prophylaxis of choriocarcinoma. *Am J Obstet Gynec.* 1971;111:1021–1027.

10. Curry SL, Hammond CB, Tyrey L, et al. Hydatidiform mole: diagnosis, management and long-term follow-up in 347 patients. *Obstet Gynec.* 1975;45:1–8.

11. Schlaerth JB, Morram CP, Rodriguez M. Diagnostic and therapeutic curettage in gestational trophoblastic disease. *Am J Obstet Gynec.* 1990;162:1465–1471.

12. Goldstein DP. Gestational trophoblastic neoplasia. In: Kistner RW (ed). *Gynecology Principles & Practice*, 3rd Ed. Chicago: Yearbook Medical Publishers, Inc., 1979.

13. Mazur MT, Kurman RJ. Choriocarcinoma and placental site tumor. In: Szulman AI, Buckobaum HJ, eds. *Gestational Trophoblastic Disease.* New York: Springer-Verlag, 1987.

14. Berkowitz RS, Goldstein DP, Bernstein MR. Modified triple chemotherapy in the management of high risk metastatic gestational trophoblastic tumors. *Gynec Oncol.* 1984;19:173–181.

15. Soper JT, Clarke-Pearson DL, Hammond CB. Metastatic gestational trophoblastic disease: prognostic factors in previously untreated patients. *Obstet Gynec.* 1988;72:338–343.

16. Lurain JR, Elfstrand E. Single agent methotrexate chemotherapy for treatment of nonmetastatic gestational trophoblastic tumors. *Am J Obstet Gynec.* 1995;172:574–579.

17. Bagshawe KD. Treatment of high risk choriocarcinoma. *J Reprod Med.* 1984;29:813–820.

QUESTIONS

For each of the following multiple choice questions, choose the most appropriate answer.

1. Molar pregnancy is more commonly found in:
   a. blacks
   b. caucasians
   c. orientals
   d. all of the above

2. All of the following are usually found in molar pregnancies except:
   a. eclampsia
   b. hyperthyroidism
   c. proteinuria
   d. fetal heart tones
   e. high HCG

3. The diagnosis of invasive mole is made by:
   a. D&C
   b. endometrial biopsy
   c. HCG assays
   d. hysterectomy
   e. none of the above

4. Elevated beta HCG level, declining 4 weeks after evacuation of a molar pregnancy is managed by:
   a. D&C
   b. hysterectomy
   c. chest x-ray and D&C
   d. chemotherapy
   e. none of the above

5. Plateau level of beta HCG after evacuation of a molar pregnancy is managed by:
   a. D&C
   b. hysterectomy
   c. hysterotomy
   d. chemotherapy
   e. none of the above

6. The most commonly used chemotherapeutic agent in treatment of gestational trophoblastic neoplasia (GTN) is:
   a. Cis-Platinum
   b. Etoposide (VP-16)
   c. Methotrexate
   d. Bleomycin
   e. none of the above

7. Which of the following is (are) characteristic(s) of good prognosis metastatic GTN:
   a. lung metastases
   b. pretherapy serum beta HCG <40,000 IU/ml
   c. duration of disease <4 months
   d. all of the above
   e. none of the above

8. Which of the following is (are) characteristic(s) of poor prognosis metastatic GTN:
   a. liver and brain metastases
   b. pretherapy serum beta HCG >40,000 IU/ml
   c. duration of disease >4 months or term pregnancy
   d. failed chemotherapy
   e. all of the above

Part V

LABOR, DELIVERY, NEONATAL MANAGEMENT AND PATHOLOGY

18

Labor and Delivery

Stephen P. Emery

INTRODUCTION

The purpose of this chapter is to consider events and appropriate interventions during normal and abnormal labor, delivery, and the postpartum period. Labor is presented longitudinally from admission to discharge. Operative delivery, breech delivery, and fetal surveillance are addressed.

NORMAL LABOR

This chapter discusses commonly encountered events of the intrapartum period. The following topics will suggest to the resident the need for vigilance in management of the obstetric patient. Most complications are preventable or easily managed when they are anticipated. Anticipation requires knowledge and experience, both of which will come with study and time.

Triage in Screening Room

Upon arrival to labor and delivery, the pregnant patient should be placed into an examination room where she can be readily evaluated for possible admission. Equipment for rapid assessment should be on hand and in working order. Access to prenatal records and computerized lab data is mandatory. Not only is the screening room visit an important part of normal labor assessment, but it also serves as an additional source of prenatal contact for many patients. Some patients may have no additional prenatal care other than what they receive through the screening room. It is prudent to carefully evaluate each patient and to document physical and laboratory findings for future reference.

Triage is oriented toward the patient's presenting complaint. A thorough history and physical exam, in conjunction with prenatal chart review, are performed. Often the need for admission is obvious (labor, pyelonephritis, pneumonia). Occasionally, consultation with other services (surgery, neurology) will be necessary.[1]

A pregnant woman may be admitted to the hospital for multiple reasons: she may have a normal pregnancy and be in labor at term. She may have a complication of pregnancy (preterm labor, preeclampsia, abnormal fetal testing results). She may have a medical or surgical condition requiring care in association with a normal or abnormal pregnancy (appendicitis, pulmonary embolism). According to the patient's risk status, she should be admitted to either the labor hall, the high-risk obstetric unit, or the antepartum floor. In any event, a careful and thorough evaluation of the patient's total risk status will help to avoid unexpected complications during her hospitalization.

In the event of labor, an accurate diagnosis is sometimes difficult but always very important. If the correct diagnosis of labor is missed, the patient and fetus may be exposed to the risks of delivering remote from a medical facility. If labor is falsely diagnosed, the temptation to intervene and induce or augment labor is difficult to resist. Labor is typically diagnosed as cervical dilation and effacement in association with painful, rhythmic uterine contractions. A patient may have painful contractions without cervical changes, or may be dilated to 4 cm without appreciable uterine contractions. If in doubt, the patient may be observed on labor and delivery for an additional hour and then reexamined. If a change in exam is appreciated, the diagnosis of labor is made. In any event, documentation of fetal status by a nonstress test (NST) in any patient with obstetric complaints is a good policy. Nonreassuring testing may clarify the need for admission.[2]

Admission History and Physical (H+P)

Ideally, a complete history and physical were performed by the admitting physician when the patient was triaged, and now needs to be documented. It is important that the history and physical be done as soon as possible since emergent decisions are sometimes required upon admission. The history and physical are of course obstetric oriented but should not be limited to obstetric issues. Bear in mind the myriad of medical conditions that impact upon pregnancy and are impacted by pregnancy. Important features to be included into the initial assessment are outlined below.

Presenting Complaint

The presenting complaint in obstetrics is often straightforward ("I broke my water" or "I'm contracting"). Occasionally, patients may present in labor with a symptom such as headache or nausea and vomiting that may lead to an important and potentially overlooked diag-

nosis (preeclampsia, HELLP syndrome). The message is to pay attention to the patient's presenting complaint: What brought her to the hospital? It will often lead to the appropriate diagnosis and intervention.

Dating Parameters

Accurate dating is fundamental to adequate prenatal care. Having the patient's prenatal chart available often precludes debate over gestational age. Still, dating parameters should be reviewed on all patients as initial errors in dating may have been carried over through gestation. Often, however, dating is uncertain or ambiguous. Several methods are available to assess gestational age on labor and delivery. First is a careful history that would include menstrual history, last menstrual period, previously assigned due dates, sexual contact, quickening, etc. If prenatal records are available, one could use uterine size at first visit, first auscultation of fetal heart tones, and serial fundal heights as rough guidelines. Previous ultrasound reports from other institutions (done for first-trimester bleeding or to rule out an ectopic) are often very helpful and should be sought. A rule-of-thumb is that a first-trimester ultrasound is accurate +/− one week, a second-trimester ultrasound +/− two weeks, and a third-trimester ultrasound +/− three weeks. Often, however, the above dating parameters are inaccurate or unavailable. In these cases an ultrasound performed on labor and delivery will give some idea of gestation and will also assess amniotic fluid volume and placental grade. If all parameters are inadequate and intervention is being considered, an amniocentesis for the presence of phosphatidylglycerol (PG) and the lecithin/sphingomyelin (L:S) ratio is prudent. The presence of PG or an L:S ratio greater than 2.0 is consistent with maturity in most instances. A notable exception is in maternal diabetes mellitus, where fetal lung maturation may lag.[3]

Obstetric History

A gravid patient's obstetric history provides valuable information for predicting outcome and complications. The absence of a history (primigravida or nullipara) is in and of itself significant. Important information includes number of pregnancies, number of deliveries, gestational age at delivery, type of delivery, type of uterine scar if a previous cesarean section, fetal weight, medical or obstetric complications, type of and reason for intervention, postpartum complications, and neonatal outcome.

Antenatal Course

A wealth of information is contained in an appropriately recorded prenatal chart. With early screening and proper follow-up, most prenatal problems can be properly addressed, thus minimizing antenatal complications. Important prenatal information to note on the admission history and physical are gestational age at presentation, number of prenatal visits, testing results (alpha-fetoprotein, 1-hour oral glucose tolerance test, vaginal and cervical cultures, blood type, and antibody screen), ultrasound results, etc. Also important to note are any complications that developed in the course of pregnancy (first-trimester bleeding, abnormal triple screen, hospitalizations, etc.).

Past Medical and Surgical History

A myriad of medical and surgical conditions impact upon pregnancy. The admission H+P should note significant past and present medical and surgical conditions (rheumatic heart disease, Marfan's Syndrome, repaired intracranial berry aneurysm, etc.). It is to be hoped that many of these issues were addressed in the prenatal course and a concise plan outlined in the prenatal chart. Document in the admission H+P any postpartum plans for follow-up (isoniazid for positive PPD, colposcopy for abnormal pap).

Social History

Pertinent social history includes use of tobacco, alcohol, and illicit drugs (quantity, frequency of use, and route of administration). Also important is a sense of the patient's disposition. This confidential and often sensitive information is not sought out of curiosity and should not be used to pass judgment. The social history adds insight into the patient's obstetric risk status. It points toward the need for additional evaluation and intervention (HIV testing, Social Services consult, drug screen).

Prenatal Laboratory Tests

Important prenatal lab results to record on admission are blood type and antibody screen, rubella immune status, VDRL, diabetes screen, hepatitis screen, triple check, group B Strep, gonorrhea and Chlamydia culture status, and cervical cytology. Other tests can be obtained as needed.

Obstetric Examination

Important to obstetric management is a complete obstetric examination. It begins with an abdominal exam to determine lie (longitudinal versus transverse), presentation, fundal height, fetal number, estimated fetal weight, engagement of the presenting part, and palpation for soft tissue abnormalities (uterine fibroids, adnexal enlargement). Unusual contours of the abdomen and uterus should be noted. Surgical scars should prompt investigation.

Before a digital vaginal exam is performed, the possibility of ruptured membranes should be explored. Membrane rupture should be ruled out at triage because the issue is central to further decision-making. A history of leaking fluid usually serves as adequate screening. If the response is positive or equivocal, a sterile speculum exam needs to be performed to document membrane rupture. Briefly, a sterile speculum is inserted into the vagina and the cervix and posterior fornix is inspected for evidence of pooled amniotic fluid, vernix, or meconium. If doubt still exists, vaginal fluid can be collected using a cotton-tipped swab. Fluid can be placed on a microscope slide to look for ferning, or a nitrazine test may be performed. Ferning of amniotic fluid is the result of high solute content. The nitrazine test takes advantage of the higher pH of amniotic fluid (pH 7.0 to 7.5) as compared to the vagina (pH 4.5 to 5.5). Nitrazine paper turns bright blue in the presence of amniotic fluid. As can be expected, none of these tests are foolproof and documentation of ruptured membranes may prove to be arduous.[4] An ultrasound examination is sometimes helpful to assess fluid volume. Finally, in situations where documenting membrane status is crucial, such as in the case of prematurity, amniocentesis with instillation of indigocarmine dye, followed by a period of observation, may be indicated.[5]

Painless vaginal bleeding in the third trimester should be considered to be from a placenta previa until proven otherwise. Before a sterile speculum or digital vaginal exam is performed in this situation, documentation of the placental position by review of prenatal records or by prompt obstetric ultrasound is mandatory.[6]

Next, clinical circumstances permitting, a digital vaginal exam is performed to evaluate the cervix, the pelvis, and the presenting part. The initial cervical exam establishes the benchmark for progress in labor. Dilation, station, and effacement are assessed. Notation of cervical position (posterior, anterior, or mid) and consistency (firm or soft) is helpful as a baseline.

Adequacy of the pelvis can be digitally assessed by clinical pelvimetry. Main points to note are anterior-posterior diameter, subpubic angle, prominence of spines, and convergence of sidewalls. This should be correlated with the estimated fetal weight in order to anticipate dystocia.

Position of the presenting part is established by palpating for the fetal occiput (vertex presenting) or sacrum (breech presenting) in relation to the maternal pelvis (right, left, anterior, posterior). Thus "right occiput anterior" implies that the occiput of the fetal vertex is in the anterior position and rotated less than 45 degrees to the right. Asynclitism applies to the anterior or posterior rotation of the fetal parietal bone with the cranium in the transverse position ("anterior" or "posterior" asynclitic). If unsure of presenting part (ear, nose, scrotum), do not hesitate to obtain a second opinion or confirm by ultrasound.

Conduct of Normal Labor

Stages of Labor

Labor is traditionally separated into two phases: latent and active.[7] Briefly, the active phase of labor is divided into first, second, and third stages. The *first stage* of labor can be illustrated using the familiar Friedman curve (Figure 18-1). The curve demonstrates the concept of progressive cervical dilation and effacement in association with descent of the presenting part. The maximum slope of the curve for dilation is generally a minimum of 1.2 centimeters per hour in nulliparas and 1.5 centimeters per hour in multiparas. Nulliparous women tend to descend and efface before dilating while multiparous women tend to dilate before effacement and descent, but this varies widely. The *second stage* of labor begins with complete cervical dilation and effacement and ends with expulsion of the fetus. The length of the second stage is quite variable with the median being 50 minutes in nulliparas and 20 minutes in multiparas. A nullipara may take up to two hours to complete the second stage. An additional hour may be granted with regional anesthesia. The *third stage* of labor begins after delivery of the fetus and ends with expulsion of the placenta.

Management practices for the first stage of labor vary considerably. General principles include monitoring for maternal well-being, pain control, observing for at least the minimally accepted rate of progress in labor, and fetal surveillance.[8]

Maternal monitoring refers to frequent assessment of physical findings such as temperature, pulse, and blood pressure, as well as contraction frequency and degree of maternal discomfort. It also serves as an opportunity to provide contact in the form of reassurance and encouragement. It is helpful to make oneself available to family members to answer questions and provide reassurance. Oral intake should be withheld during active phase due to slow gut motility and the increased risk of aspiration. Intravenous access is appropriate in the event of an obstetric emergency or to provide IV hydration in cases of prolonged labor. It also serves as a route for medications such as sedation or oxytocin if needed. Bladder care involves frequent emptying to avoid overdistention, which may lead to an increased chance of hypotonia and infection as well as labor abnormalities from obstruction. Amniotomy may be

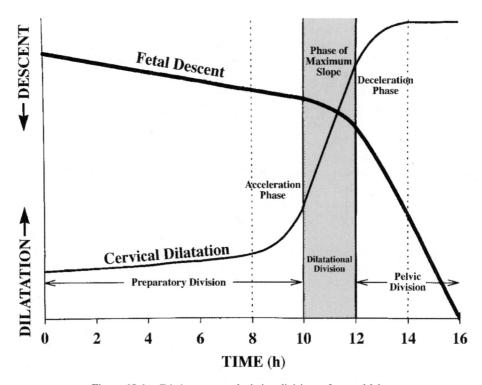

Figure 18-1.   Friedman curve depicting divisions of normal labor.

performed once active labor is well established to rule out meconium-stained fluid. Many practitioners feel that amniotomy significantly shortens the active phase, though evidence is lacking.[9,17] Risks associated with amniotomy are cord prolapse if performed at too high a station, and risk of an ascending infection if done prematurely. Amniotomy may be necessary to place internal monitors or may be used as a form of induction. In the case of overt chorioamnionitis, infected amniotic fluid should probably be drained when the diagnosis is made. A uterus overdistended by polyhydramnios will probably contract more effectively after careful drainage of excess amniotic fluid by needle amniotomy or amniocentesis. Needle amniotomy involves transcervical puncturing of small holes in the exposed membranes. The goal is to drain excess amniotic fluid without prolapsing the umbilical cord or causing rapid collapse of the uterus.

Progress in labor is gauged by the rate of cervical dilation and effacement in association with descent of the presenting part.[10] This is determined by repeated vaginal examinations, preferably by the same examiner. Frequency of exams may vary considerably depending on the course of labor. In general it is prudent to minimize exams in the presence of ruptured membranes in latent phase labor. Otherwise, q2 hour exam in active phase labor is reasonable. Patients progressing rapidly may require more frequent exams. A sudden change in fetal or maternal status, such as a prolonged fetal heart rate (FHR) deceleration or a sudden increase in maternal discomfort, should prompt immediate examination.

Adequate progress in labor is generally defined as cervical dilation of at least 1.2 cm/hr in nulliparas and 1.5 cm/hr in multiparas, in association with descent of the presenting part. If labor is progressing normally, there is no indication for intervention and the best policy is support and careful observation. Slower progress is referred to as protraction. A cessation of progress is an arrest. As mentioned above, the diagnosis of labor is not always straightforward and may require a period of observation. Typically, a cervix dilated to 3–4 cm with contractions in a nulliparous patient is taken as active phase, as is a 4-cm dilated cervix in a multipara. Progress should be measured after active phase is established to avoid misdiagnosing a prolonged latent phase as a protraction or arrest disorder.[11] In other words, the accurate diagnosis of true labor is essential to proper management.

The *second stage of labor* begins with complete dilation of the cervix and ends with expulsion of the fetus (Figure 18-2). It involves descent of the presenting part in association with maternal voluntary expulsive efforts. Its length is highly variable depending on parity, fetal weight, pelvic size, type of anesthesia, and efficacy of maternal effort. It lasts approximately 50 minutes in nulliparas and 20 minutes in multiparas. Up to three hours may be allowed for a nulliparous patient with a well-functioning epidural.

Expulsion of the fetus begins with a bulging of the perineum and separation of the labia. With each push, the labia are further spread and the presenting part becomes visible. (In the interest of space, we will limit the discussion to vertex presentation.) As the perineum distends and is stretched tight, a decision on whether to perform an episiotomy is made. If the perineum appears to stretch adequately and does not threaten to rupture, an episiotomy may not be necessary.[12] Episiotomy is beneficial in cases that require added room at the outlet such as shoulder dystocia, operative deliveries, and prematurity.

As the head extends through the introitus, care is taken to control its rate of delivery. This can be achieved in several ways including the modified Ritgen maneuver, which allows control of the fetal head by upward displacement of the chin.[13] Another is simply to rest the operator's hand on the fetal head to assess the speed of delivery while adding a slight squeeze to the perineum to prevent perineal rupture. This method works well with the cooperative parturient who demonstrates well-controlled expulsive efforts.

Once the head is delivered, the patient is instructed to refrain from pushing until the mouth and nares can be suctioned clear of secretions. Before pushing is resumed, the nuchal region is inspected for a loop of cord. If present, the cord should be either reduced around the head or clamped and cut on the perineum.

Next, the shoulders, now rotated to the anteroposterior plane, are delivered either spontaneously or with mild nuchal traction along the long axis of the fetus; first the anterior, then the posterior (Figure 18-3). Finally, the body passes through the introitus, usually with a gush of amniotic fluid. Once delivered, the mouth and nose are further suctioned if necessary, the umbilical cord is clamped and cut, and the infant is handed to either the mother or to a caregiver.

The *third stage of labor* involves spontaneous or manual delivery of the placenta. Spontaneous expulsion is almost always preferable and usually follows shortly after delivery. Signs of placental separation from the uterine wall include a sudden gush of blood, lengthening of the cord and a firm, globular uterus that rises into the abdomen as the placenta passes down into the lower uterine segment and vagina. Maternal expulsive efforts are usually enough to deliver the placenta. If not, the placenta can be expressed by upward abdominal pressure on the fundus while keeping mild tension on the cord. Once delivered into the vagina, the placenta is lifted from the introitus by the cord. Trailing membranes are removed with ring forceps. The cord must not be used to apply traction on the placenta, especially before separation. What can result is uterine inversion, often with catastrophic consequences.

Once delivered, the placenta must be inspected for completeness. The maternal surface is viewed and the membranes accounted for. If portions of the placenta or membranes are missing, or if the placenta fails to separate, then manual removal is indicated. Manual removal involves transcervical intrauterine extraction under sterile technique along with sedation and antibiotic coverage. Briefly, a gloved hand is placed into the uterine cavity while an abdominal hand grasps and holds the fundus firmly. A

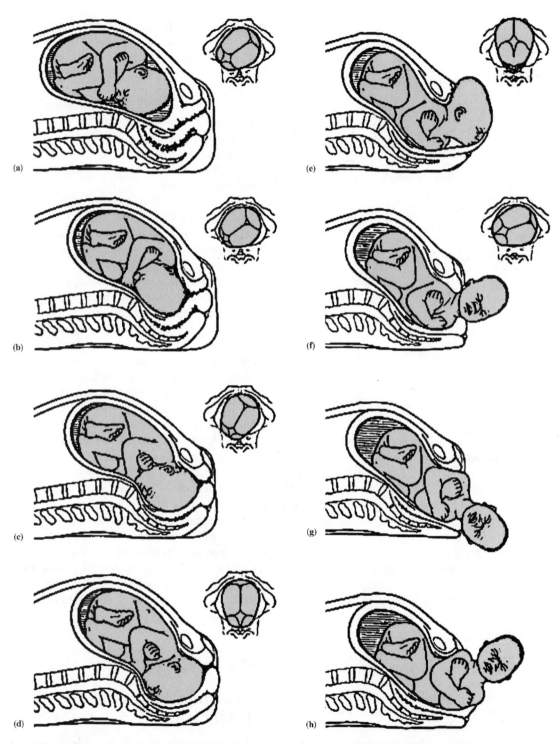

Figure 18-2. Cardinal movements of labor in occiput presentation. Adapted from Moore and Persaud, The Placenta and Fetal Membranes in *The Developing Human*, 5th edition. Philadelphia: W.B. Saunders, 1993.

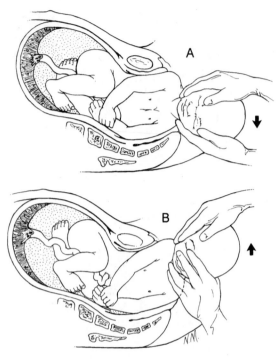

Figure 18-3. Delivery of anterior and posterior shoulders. (Courtesy of Cunningham FG et al. *Williams Obstetrics*, 20th ed. Norwalk, CT: Appleton & Lange, 1997.)

plane of separation is developed and continued between placenta and decidua until the entire placenta is separated. Manual extraction follows. A similar procedure applies for retained placental cotyledons or membranes. Draping the hand with a wet sterile sponge tape improves membrane removal.

Finally, the birth canal must be inspected for evidence of trauma. Any lacerations of the cervix, vagina, or vulva, or an episiotomy, needs to be repaired. In the interest of space, please refer to a more detailed text for appropriate techniques.[58,59]

Postpartum Management

Immediate postpartum care is oriented toward monitoring for hemorrhage and restoring the mother to normal physiologic function as soon as is safely possible. In the case of vaginal delivery, either spontaneous or operative, attention is turned to observing for uterine atony by frequent vital signs and fundal palpation. Typically, 20 mu oxytocin are infused in 1 L IV fluids to maintain uterine tone.[14] Increased vaginal bleeding is usually the result of uterine atony but may be from unappreciated lacerations. An expanding fundus may signal uterine bleeding confined to the endometrial cavity. A change in vital signs without obvious bleeding may signify hematoma formation. In any event, increased bleeding or a change in status warrants immediate attention.

Other issues to be addressed in the recovery period are early ambulation, vulvar and perineal care, bladder surveillance to avoid overdistention (especially after regional anesthesia) and maternal-neonatal bonding. In the case of cesarean section, the same issues apply plus the additional considerations of anesthesia, a surgical wound, and postoperative pain. Typical postpartum stays are 24 hours for a vaginal delivery and two days for an uncomplicated cesarean section. In this time, patients are encouraged to resume normal activity as soon as possible including diet, ambulation, bathing, and nursing. This time serves as an opportunity for additional maternal and fetal surveillance. It also serves as an opportunity for patient education regarding contraception, immunization, and follow-up. Upon discharge, all patients should have an established means of contraception and appointments for follow-up for herself and her baby. Anti-D immunoglobulin should be administered to Rh-negative women with Rh-positive newborns. Iron and prenatal vitamins are continued for one month. A prescription for postoperative pain relief is often indicated. Otherwise, a nonsteroidal anti-inflammatory preparation is sufficient for most women.

ABNORMAL LABOR

Abnormalities of the Latent Phase

The *latent phase of labor*, or Phase 1 of parturition, involves uterine and cervical preparedness for labor (Figure 18-4). These changes oc-

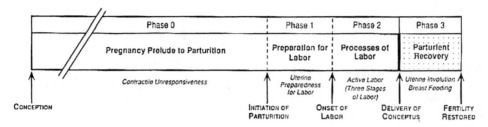

Figure 18-4. Phases of parturition.

cur normally at around 38 weeks gestation and include cervical ripening, development of the lower uterine segment, and increased myometrial contractility. Abnormalities of this phase include premature initiation of labor (premature labor), failure of initiation of labor (postterm pregnancy), hypertonic uterine dysfunction, and prolonged latent phase.

Preterm labor is discussed in detail in Chapter 7. Postdate pregnancies are defined as those beyond 42 completed weeks of gestation. The incidence is low and usually the result of dating error. Certain fetal anomalies such as anencephaly, fetal adrenal hypoplasia, intraabdominal pregnancy, absence of the fetal pituitary, and placental sulfatase deficiency are associated with postmaturity. These pregnancies, which all have in common decreased estrogen concentrations, have stimulated interest in research models for labor initiation. Clinically, postterm pregnancy is managed by increased antenatal surveillance, pharmacologic cervical ripening, and labor induction after 42 completed weeks unless other complications arise. Postterm pregnancies are at an increased risk for oligohydramnios with cord compression, labor abnormalities, meconium aspiration, macrosomia, shoulder dystocia, congenital anomalies, and cesarean section.[15,16]

Hypertonic uterine dysfunction involves the initiation of painful uterine contractions without progressive cervical dilation. It often leads to multiple visits to the labor and delivery unit for false labor, maternal exhaustion and dehydration from pain, and considerable anxiety on the part of the patient and family members. The etiology is felt to be irritable uterine contractions that are not fundal-dominant and therefore inefficient.

They cause pain like labor but do no work toward expulsion of the pregnancy. Dysfunctional latent phase labor is best treated with sedation and IV hydration in the form of a "morphine sleep." Twelve to fifteen milligrams of morphine sulfate are given IM, which suppresses irritable uterine contractions and allows the patient (and her family) to rest. Often, the patient awakens with a fundal-dominant and progressive labor pattern.[17]

Prolonged latent phase is defined as regular uterine contractions and slow but progressive cervical dilation for greater than 20 hours in the nullipara and more than 14 hours in the parous woman. These are statistically derived numbers from epidemiologic data that includes wide variation. On it's own, prolonged latent phase has little bearing on maternal or neonatal outcome. It is problematic in that it clouds the diagnosis of true labor, and invites meddlesome intervention such as amniotomy, augmentation, or even cesarean section. As with hypertonic dysfunction, sedation usually arrests dysfunctional contractions and establishes an active labor pattern.

Abnormalities of the Active Phase

Abnormalities of the First Stage

Latent phase labor (Phase 1) begins with the mother's perception of regular uterine contractions, progresses slowly, and ends with the *first stage of the active phase* (Phase 2) (Figure 18-1). This stage is defined by Friedman as the point in labor at which the cervix begins to dilate rapidly.[18] The first stage of the active phase is further divided into three phases: acceleration phase, phase of maximum slope, and deceleration phase. Typically, the cervix begins to dilate rapidly at between 3 and 5 cm. Thus, the active phase begins at around 4-cm dilation, which is also the acceleratory phase of the first stage. Latent phase can last up to 44 hours, whereas active phase typically lasts less than ten. The phase of maximum slope follows the acceleration phase. It is in this phase that the cervix is expected to dilate at a minimum rate of 1.2 cm/hr for nulliparas and 1.5 cm/hr for parous women. These numbers are derived from epidemiologic data and are the low ends of normal. Faster progress is not a problem; slower progress may be. At the end of the phase of maximum slope is the deceleration phase, where cervical dilation slows and descent of the presenting part quickens.

Abnormalities of the *first stage of labor* are either protraction or arrest of cervical dilation, or in descent of the presenting part. According to Friedman's work, protraction of dilation refers to progress less than 1.2 cm/hr in nulliparas and less than 1.5 cm/hr in parous women. Protraction of descent refers to less than 1 cm/hr in nulliparas and less than 2 cm/hr in parous women. Arrest of dilatation is no cervical change in 2 hours. Arrest of descent is 1 hour without descent of the presenting part.

When protraction or arrest disorders are encountered, they should alert the clinician of potential adverse outcome and stimulate a thorough investigation for a cause. Protraction and arrest are both associated with increased maternal and neonatal morbidity and mortality in the form of uterine rupture, chorioamnionitis, and fetal death, to name a few. They elevate the pregnancy to a high-risk status.

The first step in the investigation of an etiology includes reassessing the course of labor to confirm active phase. A 4-cm dilated and effaced cervix in the presence of regular, painful uterine contractions is good evidence of labor beyond the latent phase. Investigation also includes the assessment of frequency, intensity, and duration of uterine contractions by placement of an intrauterine pressure catheter (IUPC).[19] Fetal size, lie, presentation, and po-

sition should be reassessed and a second opinion sought if necessary. Reinspection of the pelvic architecture for evidence of contracture is indicated. Contracture is unlikely if the diagonal conjugate is normal, the sidewalls are not convergent, the spines are not prominent, the sacrum is not J-shaped, and the subpubic angle is not narrow. A high station in association with excessive caput and molding may signify an inlet disproportion, especially in the nullipara. Finally, assessment of the fetal heart rate tracing with a fetal scalp electrode may identify changes in fetal status.

Dystocia, or *difficult labor*, has a number of causes, both fetal and maternal. Fetal etiologies include fetal size as in macrosomia, or size of the presenting part as in hydrocephalus. Fetal lie may be abnormal as in transverse or oblique lie. Presentation may be abnormal as in breech, compound, or face. Position may be abnormal as in occiput posterior. Finally, fetal anomalies such as soft tissue tumors can cause dystocia. Maternal etiologies can be considered in terms of bony or soft tissue abnormalities. Examples of bony abnormalities are pelvic contractures of the inlet, midpelvis, or outlet. Maternal soft tissue abnormalities are widely varied and may involve any organ of the genitourinary tract. Examples include uterine leiomyomata; ovarian tumors; cervical, vaginal, and vulvar masses; and bladder overdistention. Therefore, when dystocia is encountered, the experienced clinician knows to look closely for a potentially overlooked etiology.

With the IUPC in place, inspection of the contraction pattern will demonstrate the adequacy of uterine contractions. Contractions occurring every 2 to 3 minutes, lasting approximately 60 seconds, and approximately 50 mm Hg intensity above baseline, or a total of 200 mm Hg in 10 minutes (or Montevideo units), are considered adequate for progressive cervical dilation, effacement, and descent. Additional augmentation will unlikely effect an improved outcome.

Contractions occurring less frequently and with less intensity are a sign of hypotonic uterine dysfunction. Hypotonic uterine dysfunction

Table 18-1. Diagnosis and Treatment of Abnormal Labor Patterns (Courtesy of Cunningham FG et al. *Williams Obstetrics*, 20th ed. Norwalk, CT: Appleton & Lange, 1997.)

Labor Pattern	Diagnostic Criterion		Preferred Treatment	Exceptional Treatment
	Nulliparas	*Multiparas*		
Prolongation Disorder				
(Prolonged latent phase)	> 20 hr	> 14 hr	Therapeutic rest	Oxytocin or cesarean delivery for urgent problems
Protraction Disorders				
1. Protracted active phase dilatation	< 1.2 cm/hr	< 1.5 cm/hr		
2. Protracted descent	< 1.0 cm/hr	< 2 cm/hr	Expectant and support	Cesarean delivery for CPD[a]
Arrest Disorders				
1. Prolonged deceleration phase	> 3 hr	> 1 hr	Without CPD[a]: Oxytocin	Rest if exhausted
2. Secondary arrest of dilatation	> 2 hr	> 2 hr		
3. Arrest of descent	> 1 hr	> 1 hr	With CPD[a]: Cesarean delivery	Cesarean delivery
4. Failure of descent	No descent in deceleration phase or second stage of labor			

[a] CPD: Cephalopelvic disproportion.
Modified from Cohen and Friedman (1983).

is associated with obstructed labor for whatever cause, and may be a protective mechanism from uterine rupture. Therefore, proceed with caution. If fetal and pelvic reassessment does not indicate cephalopelvic disproportion, then a trial of oxytocin augmentation may be warranted. Protraction and arrest disorders often respond to oxytocin stimulation in these circumstances (Table 18-1). Oxytocin is not without risks and should be used judiciously. Recent concern in the United States and elsewhere about the high rate of cesarean section has led to interest in aggressive oxytocin augmentation of labor. Reports in the literature are mixed, but the overall assessment appears to be that the cesarean section rate can be significantly lowered with the judicious use of oxytocin augmentation.[21-23] However, after a point maternal and neonatal complications begin to rise to preclusive levels. Oxytocin should be used in hypotonic dysfunction without apparent cephalopelvic disproportion, but not without careful consideration.

Once in an adequate contraction pattern, cervical change must be assessed closely. If no change is noted in two hours, then additional augmentation is unlikely to be beneficial. Cesarean section is at this point the only reasonable alternative.

Abnormalities of the Second Stage

The *second stage of labor* begins with complete cervical dilation. At this point, the patient often senses a strong desire to bear down as if to defecate. With adequate expulsive efforts, the median length of the second stage is 50 minutes for nulliparas and 20 minutes for multiparas. Protraction in a nullipara is a second stage of two hours, extended to three with the use of conduction analgesia. In a multiparous patient, the limit is set at one hour, extended to two with conduction analgesia.[20] As above, protraction or arrest of descent should initiate an investigation for a cause, and oxytocin may be used judiciously if no clear etiology other than hypotonic dysfunction is found.

A common cause of second-stage protraction is iatrogenic. Pain relief, in the form of conduction analgesia or intravenous sedation, may remove the patient's ability to push effectively. On the other hand, pain itself may inhibit expulsive efforts. Management involves judicious timing and routes of pain management in the second stage.

Not infrequently, the fetal heart rate tracing will deteriorate in the second stage of labor, presumably from cord compression. The fetal heart tones may show severe variable decelerations or prolonged decelerations with slow recovery to baseline. If delivery is imminent, patient observation is the best approach. If delivery does not appear to be imminent, then fetal scalp pH sampling may be performed to assess acid-base status. If the pH shows fetal acidemia, then delivery by the most expedient route is indicated. If conditions are appropriate (see below), an operative vaginal delivery may be considered. Otherwise, cesarean section is performed.[27]

Occasionally, a patient may not have the ability to effectively bear down, as in the case of patients with spinal cord injuries. Rarely, Valsalva is contraindicated as in the case of certain cardiac, vascular, and CNS disorders. In these cases, an outlet operative delivery is a safe and effective intervention.

Shoulder dystocia is a complication of the second stage that deserves special mention. Like other obstetric emergencies, the management of this condition should be rehearsed in every practitioner's mind. As most cases of shoulder dystocia are not anticipated, the practitioner must be able to respond rapidly and efficiently to maximize outcome.

Shoulder dystocia is the impaction of the fetal anterior shoulder behind the maternal symphysis pubis. The cause appears to be an increased fetal body-to-head size. Predisposing factors in the antepartum period include maternal obesity, diabetes mellitus, and postterm pregnancy. Intrapartum factors include prolonged second stage, use of oxytocin, and midpelvic operative deliveries. All these factors appear to be related to excessive fetal growth with resulting labor abnormalities. Unfortunately, predicting shoulder dystocia is much more difficult and most cases are not associated with the above risk factors.[24–26]

Fetal risks include prolonged hypoxia with resultant acidosis, and trauma related to excessive manipulation. Maternal risks include postpartum hemorrhage from uterine atony and trauma to the birth canal from episiotomy, lacerations, and instrumentation.

Techniques for disimpaction of the anterior shoulder follow in sequential order: (1) Call for help. Enlist the assistance of nursing, anesthesia, and neonatology; (2) cut a generous midline or mediolateral episiotomy to maximize room in the posterior pelvis; (3) apply suprapubic pressure in an attempt to dislodge the anterior shoulder; (4) hyperflex the maternal hips onto the abdomen (McRoberts maneuver) in an attempt to increase the diameter of the pelvic outlet; (5) manually rotate the posterior shoulder 180 degrees (Woods corkscrew maneuver) in an attempt to dislodge the anterior shoulder; (6) attempt to sweep the posterior arm across the fetal thorax and deliver the posterior arm and shoulder; (7) attempt to fracture the anterior fetal clavicle by anterior pressure against the maternal pubis (Internal pressure toward the fetal thorax may result in brachial nerve injury, hemothorax, or pneumothorax. Generally, clavicular fractures on their own heal well.); (8) the Zavanelli maneuver involves rotation of the fetal head into the anteroposterior position and then manual replacement into the pelvis (with the help of a tocolytic), followed by emergent cesarean section. This maneuver may be more difficult to perform than it sounds and should be reserved for when all other efforts fail.

Abnormalities of the Third Stage

The second stage of labor ends with delivery of the fetus. Unfortunately, trouble may not. Problems encountered in the third stage, the immediate postpartum period between delivery of the fetus and delivery of the placenta, include hemorrhage, retained products, and, rarely, uterine inversion.

Postpartum complications, like other obstetric emergencies, can happen quickly and without warning, and can result in rapid deterioration of the patient's status. Therefore, an established plan, well-rehearsed, must be in every caregiver's mind. Often, there is no time for discussion or consultation. This is particularly true for obstetric hemorrhage. Major points in the approach to obstetric hemorrhage are to immediately call for assistance; apply bimanual uterine massage; establish additional IV access; draw blood for coagulation studies; infuse crystalloid, blood products, and uterine tonic agents liberally; and place a Foley catheter to monitor urine output. A soft, boggy uterus points toward uterine atony as the cause of hemorrhage (more common), whereas a firm, contracted uterus suggests laceration somewhere in the birth canal (less common). Quick inspection of the placenta may point toward retained products.

Postpartum hemorrhage can, for simplicity, be broken down into three categories: implantation site bleeding, laceration of the birth canal, and rarely, coagulation defects.

Contraction of the myometrium after delivery ligates the blood supply to the placental implantation site. Therefore, any mechanism that predisposes to uterine atony or to incomplete placental separation will predispose to hemorrhage. Examples include a prolonged labor augmented with oxytocin for a macrosomic infant, a precipitous labor with tetanic contractions from placental abruption, or a retained placental cotyledon or succenturiate lobe. Therapy is aimed at identifying and reversing (if possible) the cause of atony, and stimulating myometrial contractions. Retained placenta must be manually removed. Tocolytics, if in use, should be stopped. Bimanual uterine massage promotes myometrial contraction. Tonic agents, including oxytocin, ergot alkaloids, and prostaglandin derivatives, should be given without delay. Oxytocin is typically given as 20 mu in 1000 cc Ringer's lactate solution (LR), at a rate of 10 ml/min. Rapid, undiluted IV boluses can lead to hypotension and reflex tachycardia.[30] It also has a significant antidiuretic effect that in rare circumstances may lead to water intoxication. A common ergot alkaloid is methylergonovine, 0.2 mg IM or IV. It is associated with occasional episodes of severe hypertension and may worsen hypertension in preeclamptic women.[31] Finally, carboprost tromethamine, a prostaglandin derivative, 0.25 mg IM, is an effective tonic agent. It is associated with typical systemic prostaglandin side effects such as diarrhea, vomiting, fever, and hypertension. It may also cause pulmonary arteriolar and bronchospasm in some women (Figure 18-5).[32]

If the uterine fundus is firm and bleeding persists, the search for a laceration must begin. Lacerations may be uterine, cervical, vaginal, or vulvar. Manual inspection of the uterine cavity may reveal a uterine rupture, especially at the

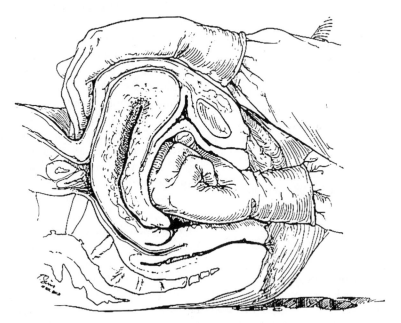

Figure 18-5. Control of postpartum hemorrhage due to uterine atony by bimanual compression and massage. (Courtesy of Cunningham FG, et al. *Williams Obstetrics*, 20th ed. Norwalk, CT: Appleton & Lange, 1997.)

site of a previous uterine scar. The cervix and vagina may be visualized using adequate lighting, retraction, and analgesia. Vulvar bleeding can be controlled using basic principles of episiotomy and laceration repair.

Coagulation defects are not uncommon complications of pregnancy. Predisposing factors include placental abruption, gram negative sepsis, severe intravascular hemolysis, severe pre-eclampsia/eclampsia, massive transfusion, intrauterine fetal demise, and amniotic fluid embolism. Treatment involves reversal of the underlying etiology and aggressive blood component therapy.

Placenta accreta, increta, and percreta refer to abnormal placentation whereby the normal plane of separation between villi and decidua is absent. Predisposing factors are related to poor decidua formation such as with multiparity or previous uterine scars. What results is placental villi attaching to and invading into or through the myometrium. This condition predisposes to uterine rupture in labor as well as postpartum hemorrhage. It also predisposes to uterine inversion if traction is applied to the umbilical cord in attempts to deliver the adherent placenta (Figure 18-6). Significant placenta accreta is best treated with hysterectomy, whereas milder forms can be managed conservatively in the absence of bleeding. The presence of a placenta previa overlying a previous cesarean section scar should raise the suspicion of placenta accreta. Uterine inversion is an obstetric catastrophe that is best managed by prevention. When it occurs, shock may appear out of proportion to blood loss, presumably from an intense vagal response. Treatment revolves around intravascular repletion and manual replacement of the uterus with the assistance of a tocolytic. Laparotomy may be necessary if replacement from below fails (Figure 18-7).[33]

Abnormalities of the Puerperium

A certain degree of relief is typically experienced after delivery of the fetus and placenta. Unfortunately, however, the puerperium is still a time of considerable risk. These risks come in

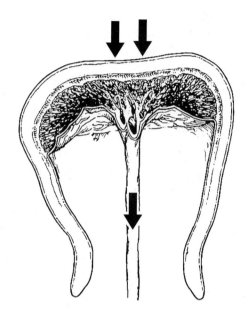

Figure 18-6. Likely mechanism of uterine inversion by traction on the umbilical cord.

the form of infection, thromboembolic disease, breast disease, and hemorrhage.

Infection is a common form of puerperal morbidity, involving the uterus, adnexae, kidneys, bladder, lungs, breasts, IV sites, pelvic blood vessels, and, in the case of cesarean section, the abdominal incision. A sustained maternal temperature of 38.0 degrees centigrade or higher (two or more) in the puerperium, beyond the first 24 hours, should be considered to be of infectious origin and should initiate a search for a cause. Temperatures in the immediate postpartum period (first 24 hours) are less likely to be of infectious nature but should still be approached with caution. Postpartum uterine infections are much more likely to follow cesarean section than vaginal delivery. Other risk factors include prolonged membrane rupture, prolonged labor, multiple vaginal exams, internal monitors, and intrapartum chorioamnionitis. The infection can involve all tissue from the decidua (endometritis) to the myometrium (endomyometritis) to the parametrial tissue (endoparametritis or metritis with pelvic cellulitis). The process may progress to the development of a parametrial phlegmon or a suppurative ab-

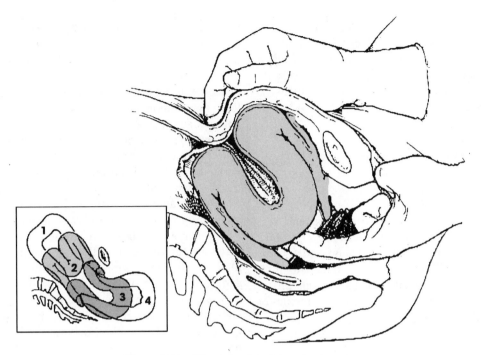

Figure 18-7. Diagnosis of partial uterine inversion.

scess. The bacteriology is that normally found in the bowel and lower genitourinary tract: multiple species of anaerobes and aerobes usually of low virulence. However, in the presence of devitalized tissue, hematomas and serous fluid, they can produce serious infection. Signs and symptoms include fever, tachycardia, leukocytosis, uterine and parametrial tenderness, and possibly foul-smelling lochia. Unfortunately, these findings are common in the postpartum or postoperative period. The clinician's index of suspicion must therefore remain high. Treatment involves empirical, broad-spectrum antimicrobial therapy. Cultures of the lower genital tract are generally not clinically useful. Triple antibiotic therapy of ampicillin, gentamicin, and clindamycin has been the mainstay of treatment. Newer regimens including a penicillin derivative plus a beta lactimase inhibitor have been proven effective in milder infections. Serious life-threatening infections may require additional coverage using imipenim or even chloramphenicol, but the benefits must outweigh the risks. In the event of renal failure from acute

tubular necrosis or other etiologies, aztreonam may be substituted for an aminoglycoside. Metronidazole has good abscess penetration and is useful in the treatment of serious pelvic infections.[34,35]

Other forms of infectious morbidity involving the lower reproductive tract include infected vaginal and vulvar hematomas, infection and breakdown of the episiotomy site or perineal lacerations, and rarely, necrotizing fasciitis. The latter is an infection of deep perineal soft tissue involving myofascial planes, with extension to the thighs, abdomen, and buttocks. Treatment involves emergent operative intervention with wide surgical debridement. Mortality, even with timely intervention, is high.

Due to the combination of stasis, hypercoagulability, and, in the case of operative delivery, endothelial damage, the parturient is at great risk for thrombotic and embolic vascular disease.[36] Early ambulation has been demonstrated to decrease the risk of thrombotic disease. Septic pelvic thrombophlebitis is an extension of a metritis into the pelvic vessels. Its clinical hallmark is a prolonged febrile course marked by temperature spikes, despite the patient's overall improvement on antibiotic therapy. Treatment has traditionally been the addition of intravenous heparin, after which the fever typically abates.

OPERATIVE DELIVERIES

Introduction

Abdominal deliveries include cesarean section using various uterine incisions. *Operative vaginal deliveries* include vacuum and forceps techniques. The focus will be limited to indications and prerequisites for the various procedures. The reader should refer to cited texts for details (58, 59).

Cesarean Section

The history of cesarean section is intriguing. Considering our present aim, suffice it to say that techniques and outcomes have undergone considerable improvement over the last two thousand years. At present, because of technological and scientific advances, the mortality rate is now quite low. Morbidity is also low but still significant and is related to the indication for the operation.

The incidence of cesarean section underwent a dramatic increase over the last three decades, leveling off in the early 1990s at around 23%. Reasons for this increase are various and not all medical. Attention has turned recently to reducing the rate of cesarean section by reevaluating its need in the most frequently cited indications; namely dystocia, previous cesarean section, breech presentation, and fetal distress.[37,38] *Dystocia* and previous section account for two-thirds of all cesarean sections performed. Regarding previous cesarean section, the old adage of "Once a section, always a section" has largely been retired (except in the instance of a classical uterine scar). The concern revolves around the risk of rupture of the uterine scar, resulting in potentially catastrophic results. Currently it is felt that women with a previous low transverse uterine scar may attempt a trial of labor, even for a "repetitive" indication such as previous cephalopelvic disproportion. The incidence of uterine rupture in these cases is quite low. Furthermore, oxytocin augmentation and epidural anesthesia are not contraindicated. Less clear are the issues of labor in women with multiple low transverse uterine scars, previous low vertical uterine incision, multifetal pregnancies, macrosomia, and breech presentation. If a trial of labor is attempted in these patients, careful monitoring with close surveillance is mandatory.

As mentioned above, the most frequent indications for cesarean section are labor abnormalities, previous cesarean section, malposition, and fetal distress. Other less common indications are placenta previa, fetal congenital anomalies where an operative delivery may improve outcome, failed induction, maternal indications for rapid pregnancy termination (severe preeclampsia/eclampsia, cardiovascular collapse) and maternal contraindications to labor (cerebral arteriovenous malformation, Marfan's syndrome with a dilated aortic root, etc.).

The timing of an elective c-section is important as electively delivering a premature infant is indefensible. The American College of Obstetricians and Gynecologists has published guidelines for assessing fetal maturity.[39] In general, documentation of 39 weeks since the last menstrual period assures lung maturity. If dating is in question, amniocentesis for PG and L:S ratio should be performed. Every attempt should be made to have the patient ready for the operating room on the morning of the procedure: she should have been NPO for at least 8 hours, and blood work, history, and physical and operative permits should be on hand.

The type of abdominal incision is primarily predicted on the indication for the procedure. A vertical skin incision is the fastest to perform and gives the best exposure to the adnexa and upper abdomen. It can be easily extended cephalid if needed. It is an appropriate incision for an emergency cesarean section. It is the incision of choice for procedures requiring exposure beyond the lower uterine segment such as an anticipated cesarean hysterectomy or adnexal surgery. Its drawbacks are cosmetic and an increased incidence of dehiscence and ventral hernia. A Pfannenstiel incision is more cosmetic and reportedly stronger, but takes considerably longer to perform (especially repeatedly) and cannot be readily extended to improve exposure.

The type of uterine incision is also dependent upon the clinical picture. A low transverse incision through the lower uterine segment usually provides adequate room for delivery of the fetus. It is also quicker to close and is associated with less blood loss and bladder injury than a vertical incision. However, the uterine vessels are at risk of laceration or damage, especially with large fetuses and deep pelvic arrests. In certain cases such as multiple uterine fibroids with a breech presentation, a low transverse incision may not provide enough exposure for delivery of the aftercoming fetal head. This may necessitate additional manipulation and risk of fetal injury. This is also true with the premature fetus and a poorly developed lower uterine segment. If a low transverse incision was begun, it may be ''T-ed'' vertically into the lower uterine segment. However, in these instances, a vertical incision into the contractile portion of the uterus, or a ''classical'' uterine incision, may be the most appropriate initial incision. The classical incision has the advantages of speed as well as exposure, but at the expense of strength. Vertical uterine scars have a higher incidence of rupture with subsequent pregnancies. Performing this procedure dictates repeat cesarean section for all future deliveries. Other disadvantages of the classical incision are length of time for repair, increased blood loss, and an increased incidence of bowel and omental adhesions to the uterine scar. Still, the vertical uterine incision has a place, albeit well defined, in modern obstetrics. In the appropriate circumstances, one should not hesitate to use it.

The particular techniques of cesarean section vary from institution to institution, but the basic principles remain the same: achieve adequate exposure, handle the fetus delicately, minimize blood loss, minimize tissue trauma, and be prepared for complications.

Achieving adequate exposure is not always easy. Maternal obesity, previous abdominopelvic surgery and pelvic adhesive diseases can complicate the procedure by minimizing the operative field, distorting anatomy and prolonging operative time. This is an important concern when considering operative intervention for fetal distress: do not delay the procedure as it will take time to deliver the fetus. Exposure is essential, however, in assuring a safe procedure for both mother and fetus. It is therefore worth the time to develop tissue planes and to define the anatomy as much as possible. Handling tissue gently decreases tissue injury and may decrease postoperative pain and improve healing.

After the skin incision, the subcutaneous fat is divided to the rectus fascia. Hemostasis is typically achieved using unipolar cautery. Once the fascia is exposed, it is incised on either side of the midline. The fascial incision is then extended bilaterally with Mayo scissors after undermining, taking care to avoid cutting the rectus muscle. Next, the fascial sheath is separated from the rectus bodies superiorly and inferiorly by blunt and sharp dissection. This step is critical for adequate exposure with a Pfannenstiel incision. The rectus and pyramidalis muscle bodies are then divided in the midline by blunt or sharp dissection. Beneath the rectus muscle bodies lies the preperitoneal fat and peritoneum (below the *linea semicircularis*). Care must be taken in opening the peritoneum as intra-abdominal contents may be adherent to the anterior peritoneum. A more cephalid approach minimizes the risk of bladder injury. The peritoneum may be entered by either blunt or sharp dissection, as long as the approach is cautious. Once entered, the peritoneal incision is extended superiorly and inferiorly taking care to avoid underlying structures. Inferiorly, the bladder can be identified by its opaque appearance on transillumination. A careful, layer-by-layer dissection helps to minimize the incidence of accidental cystotomy. At this point some physicians may choose to stretch the incision for added exposure. If done, care must be taken not to lacerate the rectus muscles, fascia or bladder. Next, the uterus may be palpated for excessive rotation, the lower uterine segment inspected for thinness, and the width of the isthmus assessed. A final decision regarding the type of uterine incision must now be made. A thick, poorly developed lower uterine segment with a narrow isthmus in a pregnancy remote from term may preclude a low transverse incision. Multiple uterine fibroids may make the lower segment inaccessible. Assuming a low transverse incision, the bladder is dissected off the lower uterine segment by incising the lower uterine serosa and dissecting inferiorly in the midline between bladder and uterus. Care must be taken not to burrow into the myometrium. The latter may lead to difficult hemostasis after evacuation of the uterus. Finally, the uterus is gently incised transversely to the membranes. The uterine incision is extended bilaterally by blunt or sharp dissection, taking care to avoid the uterine vessels laterally. The incision must be large enough, however, to allow delivery of the presenting part.

A vertical skin incision shares many similarities with the Pfannenstiel: skin is incised to the fascia, fascial incision is performed with undermining, peritoneum is entered cautiously, and hemostasis is performed as needed. A vertical uterine or "classical" incision is created with the scalpel in the lower segment and carried superiorly with bandage scissors. Care must be exercised in ruling out excessive rotation before incising the uterus. Otherwise, injury to the uterine vessels may occur.

Assuming vertex presentation, delivery of the fetal head is achieved by gently placing the operator's caudid hand between the symphysis pubis and the fetal head and applying gradual traction to elevate the head from the pelvis. Care must be taken not to fulcrum against the lower uterine incision margin as deep lacerations are likely to develop. Instead, the hand is gradually introduced until the fetal occiput is palmed. The chin is flexed onto the chest, and the occiput is brought up out of the incision. After this, delivery of the fetus is similar to vaginal delivery. An assistant may supply mild to moderate fundal pressure to aid in delivery. Techniques for delivery of a breech by cesarean section are also

similar to those used in vaginal delivery (discussed below). In fact, it is an excellent opportunity for residents to practice breech extraction techniques. In any event, extraction of the fetus must be performed gently. Remember that cesarean section is usually performed to prevent fetal injury. If the fetal head is wedged deep in the pelvis after a prolonged labor, upward elevation through the vagina may be applied to dislodge the head. If a large fetus is suspected, make a large incision. If the lower uterine segment is poorly developed and the fetus is premature and breech, excessive fetal injury may result from attempting a low transverse incision.

After delivery of the fetus, quickly inspect the uterine incision for brisk bleeding and clamp any identifiable sources. Delivery of the placenta may be hastened by fundal massage and mild to moderate cord traction. The uterus may be externalized for better visualization and ease of repair. However, this is not always possible or preferable and the surgeon should be comfortable managing hemostasis either way. Grasping the apex of the uterine incision with an Allis clamp aids in assuring that the lateral sutures are tied beyond the incision apex. It is prudent to palpate for the uterine arteries at the incision apex before placing the first and last stitch: they are virtually always closer than suspected. The uterine incision may be closed using various sutures, layers, and techniques. Typically, a single layer of running synthetic absorbable or chromic suture is sufficient. A second, imbricating layer may be needed for added hemostasis, as may several figure-of-eight stitches. Chromic suture tends to cut through myometrium less than synthetic absorbable. Classical incisions are repaired in a similar fashion except that the contractile myometrium is much thicker than the lower uterine segment and may require several layers of suture for adequate reapproximation. The serosa should be well apposed to minimize adhesions to bowel or omentum.

Tubal ligation is often combined with cesarean section in patients who require operative delivery and request permanent sterilization. Occasionally, the desire for permanent sterilization may sway the decision over route of delivery toward cesarean section. However, desire for permanent sterilization is not a singular indication for cesarean section. For example, a 39-year-old multipara with two previous cesarean sections for cephalopelvic disproportion, now with a large-for-gestation infant, who desires permanent sterilization, may be better served by an operative delivery with tubal ligation as opposed to an attempted vaginal birth after cesarean section (VBAC). Combined cesarean section and tubal ligation probably carry less risk than two separate procedures. Exposure is usually excellent and the techniques are rather simple; partial salpingectomy being the most common. Unfortunately, these puerperal procedures are associated with slightly higher failure rates. Other procedures, such as those described by Uchita and Irving, reportedly have lower failure rates but require more time and skill.[40-42]

Permanent sterilization is a procedure best performed after thorough discussion of its implications well before the operation. Patients must clearly understand the permanence of the procedure as well as the potential complications. Opening the discussion at the time of cesarean section is not ideal, especially in cases of potentially poor neonatal outcome. Postpartum procedures have a 4:1000 failure rate. With failure, the risk of an ectopic pregnancy ranges from 10 to 50%, depending on the procedure performed. The patient must understand that any symptoms of pregnancy after tubal sterilization must be reported immediately.

The uterine incision should be inspected once the uterus is internalized and off tension. Tagging the suture ends aids in visualization of the incision once the uterus is internalized. After inspection of the incision for hemostasis, the uterus is reperitonealized and the pelvis irrigated free of clot, meconium and vernix. The fascia may be closed in various manners according to operator preference. A common method is a continuous running closure of 0 synthetic absorbable suture. Monofilament delayed synthetic absorbable sutures are advantageous in poorly vascularized or infected wounds. The subcutaneous fat should be irrigated free of clot and debris, and bleeding points cauterized. Subcutaneous sutures have been demonstrated to reduce wound disruption.[43] Skin edges may be approximated by metal clips or by a running subcuticular stitch. After skin closure, the uterus is expressed of clot and blood. The patient is cleaned and transferred to recovery, where postoperative care continues.

Cesarean section is a major abdominal surgical procedure. The surgeon should be prepared to manage complications that arise and be willing to call for assistance when needed. Potential complications include the need for hypogastric artery ligation or hysterectomy for control of hemorrhage, injury to the bowel or urinary tract, extensive adhesive disease that obliterates tissue planes, or the incidental finding of an abdominal or pelvic mass that requires excision. Some complications can be anticipated, allowing an opportunity for preparation. Others, however, are not. A proficient surgical service including experienced personnel and a well-stocked operating suite can do much to affect an optimum outcome.

Unfortunately, space does not permit a discussion of cesarean hysterectomy, hypogastric artery ligation or other operative methods to control hemorrhage. Readers are encouraged to consult an obstetric text for a complete description of current techniques.[57,58]

Operative Vaginal Delivery

Introduction

As with cesarean section and breech extraction, operative vaginal delivery techniques cannot be effectively learned by reading but require direct training under an experienced operator. The following sections will therefore present only an abbreviated discussion of techniques while focusing on background and theoretical considerations. It is hoped that in this way the interested student may be prepared to participate in technical training when the opportunity presents itself.[28,29,44,45]

Forceps Delivery

The main functions of the obstetric forceps are traction and rotation. There are several types of forceps, each with their particular advantages, but the general principles are the same. All forceps are composed of a set of two interlocking branches. Each branch has four components: blade shank, lock, and handle. Blades have a cephalic curve to accommodate the fetal head, and a pelvic curve to accommodate the maternal pelvis. Different styles of forceps have different variations of these components (Figure 18-8). For example, Simpson forceps have a slighter cephalic curve to accommodate a molded fetal head, fenestrated blades, and wide parallel shanks. Tucker-McLane forceps have a more generous cephalic curve, smooth blades, and narrow overriding shanks. Both are useful general-purpose forceps. More specific types are Kielland rotational forceps, Barton forceps, and

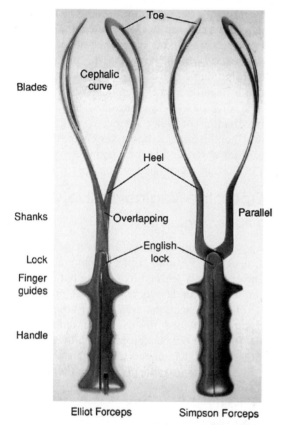

Blades — Cephalic curve — Toe — Heel

Shanks — Overlapping — Parallel

Lock — English lock

Finger guides

Handle

Elliot Forceps   Simpson Forceps

Figure 18-8. Obstetric forceps. With permission from O'Grady, *Modern Instrumental Delivery.* Baltimore: Williams & Wilkins, 1988.

Piper forceps for delivery of the aftercoming head in vaginal breech extraction.

In 1988, the Maternal-Fetal Medicine Committee of the American College of Obstetricians and Gynecologists proposed a classification scheme based on pelvic station in centimeters (0 to +5) instead of the older classification of the lower pelvis divided into thirds.[45] This reclassification was an attempt to clarify and standardize operative procedures (Table 18-2). It has turned out to be a useful prognostic indicator of potential maternal and neonatal risk: outlet forceps pose little or no risk, whereas the risk associated with high forceps is preclusive. A procedure is defined as outlet if the fetal scalp is visible at the introitus, the skull is at the pelvic floor, the sagittal suture is in the anteroposterior diameter (occiput anterior or posterior) with rotation less than 45 degrees, and the fetal head is at or on the perineum. A low forceps procedure is defined as when the presenting part is at or lower than +2 station but not on the pelvic floor and/or with rotation ≤45 degrees from the anteroposterior diameter. Midforcep is defined as when the station is above +2 but the head is engaged. High forceps is not included in the current classification. The name infers application before engagement. As one can imagine, maternal and neonatal morbidity increases with increasing station and degree of rotation. A fundamental prerequisite of forceps application is engagement of the fetal head; the deeper the better. The most common error is incorrect assessment of station (Figure 18-9). An unengaged fetal head with severe caput and molding can be mistaken for an engaged head at +2 station. Application of forceps in this situation can have disastrous consequences (Figure 18-10).

Another prerequisite for safe and proper application of forceps is certainty of position. Position of the fetal skull can be assessed by palpating sagittal suture, anterior (diamond) and posterior (triangular) fontanels, and by sweeping posteriorly to palpate an ear. If position is judged correctly, application will be smooth and the branches should lock easily. Therefore, if difficulty is encountered during application, consider the possibility that position is incor-

Table 18-2.   Classification of Forceps Deliveries[a]

Outlet forceps—the application of forceps when:
  The scalp is visible at the introitus without spreading the labia
  The fetal skull has reached the pelvic floor
  The sagittal suture is in the anterior/posterior diameter or in the right or left occiput anterior or
    posterior position
  The fetal head is at or on the perineum
Low forceps—the application of forceps when the leading point of the skull is at station +2 or more.
    There are two subdivisions[b]:
  Rotation is 45° or less
  Rotation is more than 45°
Midforceps—the application of forceps when the fetal head is engaged but the leading point of the skull
  is above station +2

[a]Adapted from Committee on Obstetrics: Maternal and Fetal Medicine 59: Obstetric Forceps. American College of
Obstetricians and Gynecologists, Washington, DC: 1988.

[b]Station is defined as the distance *in centimeters* between the leading bony portion of the fetal skull and the plane of
the maternal ischial spines.

rectly judged. Do not hesitate to obtain a second opinion.

Important in the preoperative evaluation is a comparison of fetal size to the maternal pelvis. The patient's prenatal course can be reviewed for a fetal growth curve and glucose tolerance test results. Obstetric history can be assessed for previous birthweights. Ultrasound results may document fetal growth and estimated weight. A manual estimated fetal weight should have been performed upon admission; it could be repeated by another examiner. The maternal pelvis can be assessed by clinical pelvimetry. Significant discrepancy between passenger and passageway should lead one to reconsider operative vaginal delivery.

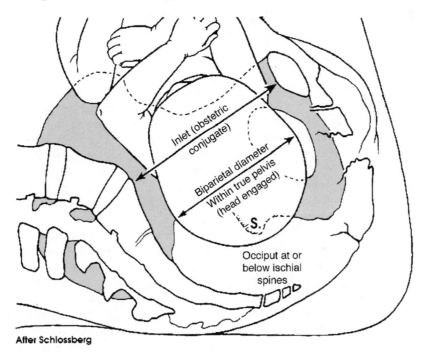

After Schlossberg

Figure 18-9.   Assessing engagement of the fetal head.

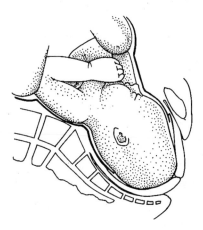

Figure 18-10. Extreme molding of the fetal head disguising high station. (Courtesy of O'Grady JP. *Modern Instrumental Delivery*. Baltimore: Williams & Wilkins, 1988.)

The fetal head should be presenting as vertex or face with mentum (chin) anterior. Face presentation with the mentum posterior cannot deliver vaginally. Also, the cervix must be fully dilated and membranes ruptured before forceps can be placed safely. The maternal bladder should be empty to avoid soft tissue dystocia and bladder injury. Adequate anesthesia is also required before placement. A pudendal block may suffice for an outlet procedure, but will not for higher applications.

Application of the blades to an anteroposterior head is accomplished by gently guiding the blade around the head using a hand in the vagina. The right hand applies the left blade to the maternal left pelvis. The left hand at this time gently supports the branch by the handle as if preventing it from dropping. Force should not be applied to the handle by the left hand if the application is difficult. In a contest between a solid metal object and a soft, malleable fetal skull or maternal myometrium, the metal will usually win. Do not make it a contest! If the application is difficult, stop and reevaluate station and position. The right blade is applied in an identical fashion using opposite hands. If correctly placed, the branches should articulate easily. If minor adjustments are required, they should be done one branch at a time using fingers in the vagina, not by excessive manipulation of the handles.

After the branches are placed and locked, the application should be verified before traction is applied. The shanks and blades should be equidistant from the midline or saggital plane of the skull. Cervical and vaginal tissue cannot intercede between blade and head as it may be lacerated. The operator should be sitting with elbows close to his or her side to avoid using body weight for traction. After appropriate placement is verified, gentle, horizontal traction is applied in conjunction with maternal expulsive effort. The rate of extraction is similar to that of a spontaneous delivery; the operator may rest between contractions. If descent does not occur, the procedure should be terminated in favor of cesarean section. Once the perineum begins to bulge, traction is directed gradually upward until the handles are vertical with delivery of the parietal bones. Episiotomy, if needed, may be cut once the perineum is stretched thin. Branches are removed with the reverse technique of application. Assisted vaginal delivery may then continue as normal. After delivery, the cervix and vaginal walls should be inspected carefully for lacerations.

Vacuum Delivery

Interest in a method of obstetric vacuum extraction dates back to the 1840s. Since then, there have been numerous devices to accomplish the purpose; some with less than desirable outcomes (scalp lacerations, intracranial hemorrhage, retinal hemorrhage). Fortunately, current models using a disposable, plastic cup are associated with much less neonatal and maternal morbidity and may be as safe as or safer than many forceps procedures.

The indications and prerequisites for vacuum delivery are the same as those for forceps. The fetal head must be engaged in the maternal pelvis; preferably deep. The presenting part must be vertex (but not face). The cervix must be completely dilated, the bladder empty, and membranes ruptured. Significant cephalopelvic disproportion must be excluded. The most favorable fetal cranial diameter for vaginal delivery is achieved by placing the vacuum cup over the occiput.

The advantages of the vacuum extractor over forceps are that precise assessment of position and application is less crucial, though still important. An operative vaginal delivery need not be excluded if exact position cannot be agreed upon. The cup can be readjusted and replaced on the fetal head more easily than forceps blades. Also, the vacuum cup is not space-occupying within the pelvis as are metal blades. Therefore, the procedure often requires less anesthesia and is associated with fewer third- and fourth-degree lacerations. Finally, there is a limit to the amount of traction that can be applied. The vacuum will disengage beyond a certain force.

Disadvantages of the vacuum are that it cannot be applied to a face presentation, it may not form an adequate suction grasp on a molded head with significant caput succedaneum, and it should not be used in the case of significant prematurity or fetal coagulopathy.

Another disadvantage of the vacuum is that, since it is technically easier than forceps application, there is a tendency to reach for it without the same sobriety and forethought as with forceps. This, however, is not a flaw in the instrument but rather of our relationship to it.

BREECH DELIVERY

Introduction

Recent attempts to reduce the cesarean section rate in the United States have led to a renewed interest in vaginal breech delivery. Multiple studies have demonstrated the expected results: vaginal delivery of a breech is associated with increased neonatal morbidity and mortality, and that cesarean section is associated with an increased maternal morbidity and mortality. The degree of reported risk varies.[47-54] General opinion is that, in the proper circumstances, the neonatal risk of vaginal breech delivery can be minimized but not eliminated. Re-

gardless of route of delivery, the breech fetus is at greater risk of poor outcome.[46,51]

Diagnosis

Breech presentation is not always clinically obvious. Often, when performing a vaginal exam on a laboring patient, the inexperienced resident will focus on cervical dilation and effacement while overlooking evaluation of presentation. Even the experienced obstetrician can be mislead by abdominal obesity or high station. If in doubt, do not hesitate to check using ultrasound. On abdominal exam, the firm, round, ballotable fetal head can be palpated in the uterine fundus. Fetal heart tones can be auscultated slightly above the umbilicus. On vaginal exam, the sacrum, ischial tuberosities and anus can often be palpated. Sometimes a foot or other small part can be felt that would prompt evaluation.

Types of breech presentation are *frank, complete*, and *incomplete*. The *frank breech* has flexed hips and extended knees. The *complete breech* has flexed hips and one or two flexed knees. The *incomplete breech* has one or both hips extended so that a foot or knee lies below the plane of the breech. This presentation is at particular risk of cord prolapse.

The incidence of breech presentation decreases as pregnancy advances. At term, less than 5% of all pregnancies are in breech presentation. Certain factors are associated with persistent breech presentation. Therefore, the physician should be alerted to these factors when a breech is discovered. Associated factors include prematurity (dating error), multiple gestation, IUGR, uterine anomalies (bicornuate uterus), pelvic tumors (uterine fibroids), anencephaly, polyhydramnios, hydrocephaly (large fetal head occupies the fundus), high parity, placenta previa, and congenital anomalies. When a fetus is found to be in a breech presentation, these complicating factors need to be considered.

Evaluation

The mechanisms of vaginal breech delivery are inherently different from those of a vertex presentation. In a breech delivery, successively larger and less compressible fetal parts pass through the pelvis, ending in an incompressible, nonmolded head. Time is usually not available to await molding as the umbilical cord is most likely compressed against the maternal pelvis. Delay in delivery can result in neonatal asphyxia, and aggressive intervention can result in significant birth trauma.

When considering a trial of vaginal breech delivery, certain fetal and maternal criteria need to be considered. Beginning with fetal considerations, weight and gestational age are primary. Most experts agree that a 1600–3600 gram range is reasonable. Fetal morbidity and mortality increase beyond these parameters. An exception to this is of course the fetus at or below the margins of viability where route of delivery is unlikely to improve outcome. The mortality of footling breeches is preclusive of vaginal delivery, mostly due to cord prolapse. A hyperflexed head on ultrasound or x-ray ("stargazing") is associated with a high incidence of cervical spine injuries. Fetal biparietal diameter should not exceed 9.5 cm. Intrauterine growth restricted fetuses are poor candidates due to the increased head circumference to abdominal circumference ratio and the concomitant risk of head entrapment. Maternal considerations include an "adequate" pelvis, i.e., no evidence of contracture. This is evaluated using CT pelvimetry with minimal radiation exposure to the fetus. Generally agreed upon minimal standards are a transverse inlet diameter of 12 cm, an AP inlet diameter of 11 cm and an interspinous diameter of 10 cm. Spontaneous labor with normal progression is considered by most as a requirement, although some obstetricians will elect to induce or augment a breech. A history of a previous infant with birth trauma would make most obstetricians consider cesarean section, as will a patient's desire for permanent sterilization. Finally, experienced anesthesiology and neonatal services must be immediately available, and the patient must be able to cooperate with the delivery. Regional anesthesia sometimes improves maternal cooperation and is available if there is the need for emergent surgery, but may predispose to labor abnormalities.

As mentioned above, the conduct of a breech delivery is fundamentally different from cephalic presentation. Rarely is the breech fetus spontaneously expelled without some degree of manipulation. Therefore, the techniques of vaginal breech delivery are worthwhile reviewing, as they may be needed in an emergency. It is useful to note that the very same maneuvers are applied during cesarean section for a breech as for vaginal delivery. It is an excellent opportunity to practice one's techniques of breech extraction.

Techniques

A full description of the techniques of breech extraction is beyond the scope of this text. The resident-in-training must consult a complete text for detail.[58,59] However, the main points will be reviewed here.

In a frank breech presentation, assistance usually begins with crowning of the presenting part. The bisacromial diameter is usually in the anterior-posterior plane. Index fingers are placed at the hips and gentle downward traction is applied until the scapula are visible. At this point the feet can be delivered by flexing the knees with gentle popliteal pressure. Continue downward traction until the scapulae are delivered and an axilla is visible. Do not place fingers or hands on the fetal abdomen as the liver and spleen are easily injured. At this point an arm may be delivered by sweeping it along the thorax. The second arm can be delivered by a similar technique. The posterior and lateral maternal pelvis have the most room. If necessary, the fetus may be rotated away from the remaining arm to achieve a posterior position. A nuchal arm, or an arm tucked behind the fetal head, can often be reversed using this rotational method away from the arm. If not, the fetus may be gently pushed up into the vagina to release it, or it must be swept with risk of humeral or clavicular fracture.

Finally, the fetal head may be delivered by either Piper forceps or by the Mauriceau-

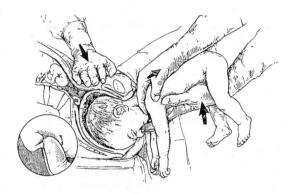

Figure 18-11. Techniques for flexion of the aftercoming fetal head. (Courtesy of Cunningham FG, et al. *Williams Obstetrics*, 20th ed. Norwalk, CT: Appleton & Lange, 1997.)

Smellie-Veit maneuver. Both techniques are designed to flex the fetal head and sequentially deliver the chin, mouth, nose, brow, and occiput. The maneuvers are aided with mild suprapubic pressure by the assistant, who supports the fetal arms (Figure 18-11).

In the event of entrapment of the aftercoming head by an incompletely dilated cervix, the cervix may be incised at 2, 6, and 10:00 positions with scissors (Duhrssen's incision). This is considered by most to be a last-ditch effort, as severe maternal hemorrhage is likely.

Version

External cephalic version is used as an attempt to convert a breech, transverse, or oblique lie into a vertex presentation, thus allowing for a vaginal delivery. The degree of success is variable and dependent on multiple factors, but reported success rates are around 70%, with a high percentage of these remaining vertex at the onset of labor.[53] Due to the decreasing incidence of spontaneous flipping of fetal poles after 36 weeks, version should be performed in the last few weeks of pregnancy. Some authors advocate use of beta mimetics for tocolysis.[54] Other factors associated with increased success are multiparity, adequate amniotic fluid volume, frank breech with an anterior spine, normal maternal and fetal weight, and a nonengaged presenting part.

External cephalic version is not without its risks. Reported complications include maternal mortality, fetal mortality, transection of the fetal spine, placental abruption, uterine rupture, fetal distress requiring emergent cesarean section, and autoimmunization from fetal-maternal hemorrhage.[52]

The technique of external version, in theory, is quite simple. In practice, it is less so. It is important that the patient be prepared for a possible emergent delivery: labor and delivery is the best place to perform the procedure. Anti-D immune globulin should be given to D-negative women before the procedure. A nonstress test before the version attempt is a useful baseline. The exact fetal position is confirmed with ultrasound and Leopold's maneuvers. Hands are placed over the fetal poles on a well-lubricated maternal abdomen. Gently but firmly, an attempt is made to exchange the fetal poles. Progress and heart tones can be frequently checked with ultrasound. After the attempt, an NST is repeated to observe for evidence of distress or contractions. If successful, some advocate frequent knee-chest position as a means of preserving vertex presentation. If unsuccessful, the option of vaginal breech delivery may be entertained.

INTRAPARTUM SURVEILLANCE

Introduction

This section is intended to review the basic principles of electronic fetal monitoring and fetal heart rate patterns. It is also intended to remind the clinician of the importance of looking at, talking to, and examining the patient. Electronic monitoring provides only a part of the overall clinical picture, despite the degree of attention that it receives.

It should be mentioned that continuous fetal heart rate monitoring has not been demonstrated to be superior to intermittent heart rate monitoring in decreasing poor neonatal outcome in low-risk populations. There appears to be an increase in the cesarean section rate in laboring patients who are continuously monitoring. Studies comparing intermittent to continuous monitoring used one-on-one patient care in the intermittently monitored group.[55]

Physical Exam

Laboring patients should be examined regularly throughout parturition. Along with interval fetal heart tones, the vital signs should be reviewed for trends in temperature, pulse, blood pressure, and respiratory rate. A quick glance at the patient can often reveal their degree of discomfort and the appropriateness of their affect. Subtle changes in her appearance can warn the observant clinician of changes in well-being. Pallor, diaphoresis, and a withdrawn affect may be a response to labor pain but may also signal the onset of a serious pathologic process (chorioamnionitis, placental abruption). Examination of the abdomen is helpful in assessing frequency, intensity, and duration of contractions. Resting uterine tone and presence or absence of pain with examination should be noted. Leopold's exam may be repeated to assess position, attitude, and engagement to the fetal head. Vaginal examinations need not be performed at regular intervals in the presence of ruptured membranes without contractions. Otherwise, interval vaginal exams should be performed during labor to track the patient's progress. It is helpful to document dilation and effacement of the cervix, station and position of the presenting part, as well as the degree of caput and molding of the fetal head if vertex. Other aspects of the physical exam should be repeated as the clinical situation requires (deep tendon reflexes in a preeclamptic on magnesium, for example).

Fetal Heart Rate Patterns

Fetal heart rate (FHR) patterns are used to assess fetal well-being. Interpretation of the overall pattern by evaluation of its components (baseline, variability, and periodic changes), can give some idea of fetal acid-base status and oxygenation. One may also identify specific FHR patterns such as sinusoidal (associated with severe, chronic anemia) and saltitory (possible fetal compromise).

It should be pointed out that a "normal" tracing with a normal baseline, normal long- and short-term variability in association with heart rate accelerations and no decelerations is virtually always reassuring. However, the converse is not true. It is difficult to accurately predict the degree of fetal acidosis and hypoxia based upon baseline changes, degree of variability, and associated decelerations. It does seem safe to say, however, that the greater the number of abnormal components of the FHR tracing, the more severe the fetal depression. For instance, a FHR with late decelerations associated with fetal tachycardia and absent short-term variability is more likely to be associated with a depressed fetus than a FHR with late decelerations alone.

The basic components of the fetal heart rate tracing include baseline, variability, and periodic changes. An average FHR baseline is between 120 and 160 beats per minute (bpm). An FHR below 120 bpm for 15 minutes or longer is termed a bradycardia. Baseline fetal heart rates between 100 and 120 bpm are generally not indicative of fetal compromise except when associated with decreased variability or late decelerations. A baseline greater than 160 bpm is also not necessarily indicative of fetal depression unless it is associated with other worrisome patterns. Persistent bradycardia may be indicative of congenital heart block seen with certain autoimmune disorders. Fetal tachycardia of 160–200 bpm is seen in such clinical situations as maternal fever, maternal drug administration, fetal compromise, and fetal arrhythmia.

Variability of the baseline is a function of the fetal autonomic nervous system. It results from a dynamic balance between sympathetic (acceleratory) and parasympathetic (deceleratory) impulses upon the myocardium. These impulses result in a heart rate that is not constant but varies from beat to beat and over time. When charted on graph paper, this variation in heart rate creates a line that is not straight but "wavy." Short-term variability refers to the variation in rate from beat to beat and can be best measured with a fetal scalp electrode. Long-term variability refers to oscillations in the baseline over the longer time period of one minute.

The average number of oscillations is three to five per minute. Long-term variability can be assessed with an external monitor or a scalp electrode.

Periodic fetal heart rate changes are upward or downward deviations of the FHR from baseline in relation to uterine contractions. An acceleration is an increase in heart rate of at least 15 bpm for at least 15 seconds. Fetal heart rate accelerations are generally very reassuring and suggest fetal well-being. They are temporally associated with certain fetal behavioral states such as wakefulness and movement. Their absence in labor, however, need not be interpreted as worrisome.

Decelerations are a slowing of the FHR below the baseline. There are three recognized forms: variable, early, and late. They are named according to their temporal relationship to uterine contractions, and each has their suspected pathophysiology. The most common form is the variable deceleration, felt to be the result of cord

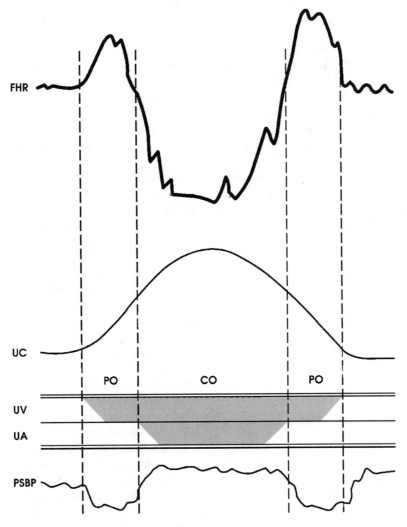

Figure 18-12. Effects of cord occlusion on fetal heart rate. UC, uterine contractions; UV, umbilical vein; UA, umbilical artery; PO, partial occlusion; CO, complete occlusion; FSBP, fetal systemic blood pressure.

occlusion (Figure 18-12). They are termed variable because they are not always associated with uterine contractions. They are often V-shaped with accelerations (shoulders) preceding and following the deceleration. Variable decelerations are typically not in and of themselves associated with fetal depression, even when frequent and severe, as normal perfusion follows between contractions. However, with prolonged deep variable decelerations (to or below 60 bpm), fetal acidemia may develop from decreased fetal perfusion and may be demonstrated as a loss of baseline variability and/or fetal tachycardia.

Early decelerations are felt to be related to fetal head compression. These decelerations are often shallow and mirror contractions in onset and duration. Early decelerations are not associated with fetal compromise.

Late decelerations are felt to be secondary to uteroplacental insufficiency. They are termed *late* because their onset lags behind the contraction and their recovery to baseline occurs after the contraction ends. Transient late decelerations are commonly seen in laboring patients and usually do not signify fetal compromise. Persistent late decelerations are felt to be more worrisome; but again only in light of associated findings. If late decelerations are accompanied by a normal baseline and with good short-term variability, they are less worrisome than if they are in the presence of fetal tachycardia and decreased or absent short-term variability. This latter situation usually is associated with some degree of fetal acidosis; the degree of which cannot be accurately determined without biochemical analysis.

External and Internal Fetal Monitors

External fetal monitors consist of an ultrasound Doppler probe to measure fetal heart rate and a tocodynamometer to measure the frequency of uterine contractions. The ultrasound probe consists of a transducer and a sensor. The transducer emits an ultrasound beam that is deflected off moving fetal heart valves, creating a

frequency change. This change in frequency is picked up by the probe's sensor. This information is fed into a microprocessor that edits out noise by searching for regular signals. Because of this, the external monitor can only give an indirect measure of fetal cardiac activity. Direct, instantaneous cardiac motion is not being recorded. This is considered to be the main disadvantage of external fetal heart rate monitoring: short-term variability cannot be clearly evaluated. Its advantages over internal monitoring are that membranes may remain intact and the fetal scalp need not be penetrated.

The tocodynamometer is a pressure gauge and transducer that creates a signal in proportion to displacement of the sensor. It gives information on frequency of contractions but unfortunately cannot be used to assess intensity, duration, or resting tone. It is dependent upon proper placement over the fundus, and its sensitivity is lessened in obesity. Its advantages are its ease of use and that membranes may remain intact.

Internal monitors consist of the fetal scalp electrode (FSE) and the intrauterine pressure catheter (IUPC). The fetal scalp electrode is a wire electrode that is attached to the fetal scalp. It senses the electric current generated by fetal cardiac depolarization. A microprocessor calculates instantaneous heart rates. Unlike the external Doppler monitor that searches for regularity out of various random noises, the FSE directly measures fetal cardiac activity and therefore is more informative of fetal cardiac status. Its major disadvantages are the need for ruptured membranes and penetration of the protective barrier of fetal skin.

The intrauterine pressure catheter is a water-filled plastic tube that is inserted into the uterine cavity beside the presenting part. The catheter is connected to a transducer that measures intrauterine pressure. The advantage of the IUPC over the tocodynamometer is that the former can accurately measure resting uterine tone, intensity and duration of contractions, as well as contraction frequency. Obviously the IUPC is clearly superior to the tocodynamometer when managing patients on oxytocin, those with labor abnormalities or those with a previous uterine scar. Its disadvantage is the need for ruptured membranes and instrumentation of the uterine cavity.

Other Methods of Fetal Surveillance

As mentioned above, interpretation of fetal heart rate tracings is an imprecise science. A normal-appearing FHR tracing with a normal baseline, good long- and short-term variability, and periodic accelerations is almost universally reassuring and correlates well with good one- and five-minute Apgar scores, normal fetal acid-base status, and favorable neonatal outcome. On the other hand, an FHR tracing with tachycardia, decreased short- and long-term variability and persistent late decelerations may or may not be associated with low Apgar scores, fetal acidosis, and poor neonatal outcome. Predicting the degree of neonatal compromise from interpretation of the FHR tracing is unreliable at best. It would be helpful, then, to employ a technique to aid in interpretation of nonreassuring FHR tracings (tachycardia, diminished variability, decelerations). Several have been evaluated including fetal scalp stimulation, vibroacoustic stimulation, and fetal scalp blood gas analysis.

Fetal scalp stimulation entails applying a strong stimulus to the fetus in the form of a pinch that changes the fetus' behavioral state and, in a healthy fetus, is associated with heart rate acceleration. The same principle applies to vibroacoustic stimulation, which is employed using a vibroacoustic stimulator to the maternal abdomen. An acceleration of the fetal heart rate in association with fetal scalp or vibroacoustic stimulation in the presence of an otherwise nonreassuring tracing is associated with a favorable fetal acid-base balance. However, the absence of a provoked acceleration does not predict fetal compromise.

A more direct form of fetal assessment is scalp blood gas analysis, performed transcervically in the presence of ruptured membranes and an adequately dilated cervix. Commercial kits are available that make sample collection rela-

tively easy. The sample is run through an analyzer that measures pH. A mixed capillary pH of 7.25 or greater is generally associated with a favorable acid-base balance. A pH between 7.20 and 7.25 is worrisome and requires a repeat analysis within 30 minutes. A pH less than 7.20 is considered critical and warrants delivery by the most expedient means.

Management of the Nonreassuring Pattern

When faced with a *nonreassuring heart rate tracing* during labor, a reasonable approach is to attempt to identify and correct the underlying cause(s). For example, late decelerations are caused by uteroplacental insufficiency. Therefore look for causes of decreased placental perfusion such as maternal supine position, maternal hypotension, uterine tachysystole or hypertonus, or maternal hypoxemia, and remedy these causes if possible. If the patient is lying supine, she should be rolled to the left or right lateral position. If she is hypotensive, a common finding after epidural placement, an IV fluid bolus can be given. If the fundus is firm between contractions or contractions are palpated one on top of another, or an IUPC demonstrates increased resting tone and tachysystole, a tocolytic agent such as terbutylene 0.25 mg IM or IV can be given. If oxytocin is in use, it should be decreased or stopped. Finally, supplemental oxygen, 8–10 L/min via face mask, may be administered to the mother in hopes of improving fetal oxygenation. Slight changes in maternal oxygenation may have significant changes in fetal status.

In the presence of severe variable decelerations, one could look for causes of umbilical cord occlusion such as a prolapsed cord or rapid descent of the presenting part. If no cord is palpated and rapid descent has not occurred, then the compression is probably intrauterine. Sometimes a change in maternal position may improve the variable decelerations. If not, amnioinfusion may be performed in hopes of replacing amniotic fluid volume, thus reducing cord compression.

The above mentioned intrauterine resuscitative measures are frequently enough to improve the FHR tracing and fetal status. If the tracing remains nonreassuring, scalp or vibroacoustic stimulation may be attempted to induce accelerations. If possible, amniotomy and placement of an FSE should be performed in the presence of decreased or absent long-term variability. If decreased short-term variability and the absence of induced accelerations are confirmed with the FSE, then biochemical assessment of fetal acid-base status by scalp blood pH, if available, is indicated. If the scalp gas is not obtainable or available, then delivery of the fetus by the most expeditious route is indicated.[56]

CONCLUSION

The intent of this introduction to normal and abnormal labor and delivery is to impress upon the resident-in-training the myriad of complications, some of them catastrophic, that can arise during parturition. Many are predictable and can be anticipated. Others strike without a moment's notice and require immediate intervention to minimize morbidity and prevent mortality. As obstetricians we are committed, to the best of our ability, to effect an optimum outcome. This requires a solid knowledge base, focused decisiveness, and above all, constant vigilance during the process of parturition.

REFERENCES

1. American College of Obstetricians and Gynecologists and American Academy of Pediatrics. *Guidelines for Perinatal Care*, 3rd ed. Washington, DC: 1992, ACOG, 72, 76.
2. Ingemarsson I, Akulkumaran S, Ingemarsson E. Admission test: a screening test for fetal distress in labor. *Obstet Gynecol.* 1986;68:800–806.
3. Whittle MJ, Wilson AI, Whitfield CR, et al. Amniotic fluid phosphatidylglycerol and the lecithin/sphingomyelin ratio in the assessment of fetal lung maturity. *Br J Obstet Gynaecol.* 1982;89:727–732.
4. Baptisti A. Chemical test for the determination of ruptured membranes. *Am J Obstet Gynecol.* 1938;35:688–690.
5. Atlay RD, Sutherst JR. Premature rupture of the fetal membranes confirmed by intra-amniotic injection of the dye (Evand's blue T-1824). *Am J Obstet Gynecol.* 1970;108:993–994.
6. Hertzberg BS, Bowie JD, Carroll BA, et al. Diagnosis of placenta previa during the third trimester: role of transperineal sonography. *AJR* 1992;159:83–87.
7. Friedman EA, ed. *Labor: Clinical Evaluation and Management*, 2nd Ed. New York: Appleton-Century-Crofts, 1978.
8. Atrash HK, Koonin LM, Lawson HW, et al. Maternal mortality in the United States, 1979–1986. *Obstet Gynecol.* 1990;76:1055–1060.
9. Rosen MG, Peisner DB. Effect of amniotic membrane rupture on length of labor. *Obstet Gynecol.* 1987;70:604–607.
10. Kilpatrick SJ, Laros RK. Characteristics of normal labor. *Obstet Gynecol.* 1989;74:85–87.
11. American College of Obstetricians and Gynecologists. Dystocia and the augmentation of labor. *ACOG Technical Bulletin 218.* Washington, DC: ACOG, 1995.
12. Borgatta L, Piening SL, Cohen WR. Association of episiotomy and delivery position with deep perineal laceration during spontaneous delivery in multiparous women. *Am J Obstet Gynecol.* 1989;160:294–297.
13. Ritgen G. Concerning his method for protection of the perineum. Monatschrift fur Geburtskunde 1855;6:21 See english translation, Wynn RM. *Am J Obstet Gynecol.* 1965;93:421–433.
14. Prendiville W, Elbourne D, Chalmers I. The effects of routine oxytocin administration in the management of the third stage of labor: an overview of the evidence from controlled trials. *Br J Obstet Gynaecol.* 1988;95:3–16.
15. Usher RM, Boyd ME, McLean FM et al. Assessment of fetal risk in postdate pregnancy. *Am J Obstet Gynecol* 1988;158:259–264.
16. Eden RD, Seifert LS, Winegar A, Spellacy WN. Perinatal characteristics of uncomplicated postdate pregnancies. *Obstet Gynecol.* 1987;69:296–299.

17. Friedman EA, Sachteleben MR. Amniotomy in the course of labor. *Obstet Gynecol.* 1963;22: 755–770.

18. Friedman EA. An objective approach to the diagnosis and management of abnormal labor. *Bull NY Acad Med.* 1972;48:842–858.

19. Hendricks CH, Quilligan EJ, Tyler AB, Tucker GJ. Pressure relationships between intervillous space and amniotic fluid in human term pregnancy. *Am J Obstet Gynecol.* 1959;77:1028–1037.

20. American College of Obstetricians and Gynecologists. Obstetric anesthesia and analgesia. *ACOG Technical Bulletin 112.* Washington, DC: ACOG, 1988.

21. O'Drischoll K, Foley M, MacDonald D. Active management of labor as an alternative to cesarean section for dystocia. *Obstet Gynecol.* 1984;63:485–490.

22. American College of Obstetricians and Gynecologists. Induction of labor. *ACOG Technical Bulletin 217.* Washington, DC: ACOG, 1995.

23. Satin AJ, Leveno KJ, Sherman ML, Brewster DS, Cunningham FG. High versus low-dose oxytocin for labor stimulation. *Obstet Gynecol.* 1992;80:111–116.

24. Acker DB, Sanhs BP, Friedman EA. Risk factors for shoulder dystocia in the average-weight infant. *Obstet Gynecol.* 1986;67:614–618.

25. Acker DB, Sanhs BP, Friedman EA. Risk factors for shoulder dystocia. *Obstet Gynecol.* 1985;66:762–768.

26. American College of Obstetricians and Gynecologists. Fetal macrosomia. *ACOG Technical Bulletin 159.* Washington, DC: ACOG, 1991.

27. American College of Obstetricians and Gynecologists. Fetal heart rate patterns: monitoring, interpretation, and management. *ACOG Technical Bulletin 207.* Washington, DC: ACOG, 1995.

28. American College of Obstetricians and Gynecologists. Obstetric forceps. *ACOG Committee Opinion No. 71.* Washington, DC: ACOG, 1989.

29. American College of Obstetricians and Gynecologists. Operative vaginal delivery. *ACOG Technical Bulletin 196.* Washington, DC: ACOG, 1994.

30. Secher NJ, Arnso P, Wallin L. Hemodynamic effects of oxytocin (Syntocinon) and methylergometrine (Methergin) on systemic and pulmonary circulations of pregnant anesthetized women. *Acta Obstet Gynecol Scand.* 1978; 57:97–103.

31. Browning DJ. Serious side effects of ergometrine and its use in routine obstetric practice. *Med J Austral.* 1974;1:957–959.

32. Hankins GDV, Berry GK, Scott TR Jr, Hood D. Maternal arterial desaturation with 15-methyl prostaglandin F2 alpha for uterine atony. *Obstet Gynecol.* 1988;72:367–370.

33. Thiery M, Delbeke L. Acute puerperal uterine inversion: two-step management with a β-mimetic and a prostaglandin. *Am J Obstet Gynecol.* 1985;153:891–892.

34. Gibbs RS, O'Dell TN, MacGregor RR, et al. Puerperal endometritis: A prospective microbiologic study. *Am J Obstet Gynecol.* 1975;121: 919–925.

35. American College of Obstetricians and Gynecologists. Antimicrobial therapy for obstetric patients. *ACOG Technical Bulletin 117.* Washington, DC: ACOG, 1988.

36. Duff P, Gibbs RS. Pelvic vein thrombophlebitis: Diagnostic and therapeutic challenge. *Obstet Gynecol Surv.* 1983;38:365–373.

37. Rosen MG, Dickinson JC, Westhoff CL. Vaginal birth after cesarean section: A meta-analysis of morbidity and mortality. *Obstet Gynecol.* 1991;77:465–470.

38. American College of Obstetricians and Gynecologists, Committee on Obstetrics, Maternal and Fetal Medicine. Guidelines for vaginal delivery after previous cesarean birth. *No. 64.* Washington, DC: ACOG, 1988.

39. American College of Obstetricians and Gynecologists, Committee on Obstetrics, Maternal and Fetal Medicine. Assessment of fetal maturity prior to repeat cesarean delivery or elective induction of labor. *No. 77.* Washington, DC: ACOG, 1990.

40. Hatcher RA, Stewart F, Trussel J, et al. *Contraceptive Technology,* 15th Ed. New York: Irvington, 1990, 391, 403, 416.

41. Husbands ME Jr, Pritchard JA, Pritchard SA. Failure of tubal sterilization accompanying cesarean section. *Am J Obstet Gynecol.* 1970;107: 966–967.

42. American College of Obstetricians and Gynecologists. Sterilization. *ACOG Technical Bulletin 222*. Washington, DC: ACOG, 1996.

43. Bohman VR, Gilstrap L, Leveno K, et al. Subcutaneous tissue: To close or not to close at cesarean section. *Am J Obstet Gynecol*. 1992; Abstract No. 481;166:407.

44. American College of Obstetricians and Gynecologists, Committee on Obstetrics, Maternal and Fetal Medicine: Obstetric forceps. *No. 59*. Washington, DC: ACOG, 1988.

45. American College of Obstetricians and Gynecologists. Operative vaginal delivery. *ACOG Technical Bulletin 196*. Washington, DC: ACOG, 1994.

46. American College of Obstetricians and Gynecologists. Management of the breech presentation. *ACOG Technical Bulletin 95*. Washington, DC: ACOG, 1986.

47. Nelson KB, Ellenberg JH. Antecedents of cerebral palsy: Multivariate analysis of risk. *N Engl J Med*. 1986;315:81–86.

48. Brenner WE, Bruce RD, Hendricks CH. The characteristics and perils of breech presentation. *Am J Obstet Gynecol*. 1974;118:700–712.

49. Gimovsky ML, Paul RH. Singleton breech presentation in labor experience in 1980. *Am J Obstet Gynecol*. 1982;143:733–739.

50. Calvert JP. Intrinsic hazard of breech presentation. *Br Med J*. 1980;281:1319–1320.

51. Westgren M, Paul RH. Delivery of the low birthweight infant by cesarean section. *Clin Obstet Gynecol*. 1985;182:752–62.

52. Hofmeyer GJ. External cephalic version: How high are the stakes? *Br J Obstet Gynaecol*. 1991;98:1–3.

53. Amon E, Sibai BM. How perinatologists manage the problem of the presenting breech. *Am J Perinatol*. 1988;5:247–250.

54. Fortunato SJ, Mercer LJ, Guzick DS. External cephalic version with tocolysis: Factors associated with success. *Obstet Gynecol*. 1988; 72:59–62.

55. American College of Obstetricians and Gynecologists. Antepartum fetal surveillance. *ACOG Technical Bulletin 188*. Washington, DC: ACOG, 1994.

56. American College of Obstetricians and Gynecologists. Fetal heart rate patterns: Monitoring, interpretation, and management. *ACOG Technical Bulletin 207*. Washington, DC: ACOG, 1995.

BIBLIOGRAPHY

Cunningham FG, MacDonald PC, Gant NF, et al. *Williams Obstetrics*, 19th Ed. Appleton & Lange, 1993.

Gabbe SG, Niebyl JR, Simpson JL. *Obstetrics: Normal and Problem Pregnancies*, 2nd Ed. Churchill Livingstone Inc. 1991.

QUESTIONS

1. A 29-year-old G3 P2002 at 36 weeks gestation presents to labor and delivery with the complaint of bleeding after intercourse. She reports no pain or contractions. Leopold's maneuvers suggest longitudinal lie with breech presentation. The most appropriate next step is to:
   a. Perform a sterile speculum exam to locate the source of bleeding
   b. Perform a digital vaginal exam to confirm breech presentation
   c. Proceed with cesarean section for breech presentation
   d. Admit to the antepartum unit for observation
   e. Verify placental location by prenatal records or ultrasound exam

2. After extraction of the fetal head by forceps, the shoulders fail to deliver with moderate downward nuchal traction. The most appropriate next step is to:
   a. Replace the head back into the pelvis and perform an emergent cesarean section (Zavanelli maneuver)
   b. Attempt to sweep the posterior arm across the fetal chest and deliver the posterior shoulder
   c. Enlist the assistance of other available personnel
   d. Manually rotate the posterior shoulder 180 degrees (Woods corkscrew maneuver)
   e. Hyperflex the maternal hips onto the abdomen (McRoberts maneuver)

3. After a prolonged induction for a macrosomic infant, your patient is noted to have excessive vaginal bleeding. The placenta was delivered intact.

The most likely etiology of her postpartum hemorrhage is
a. Uterine atony from prolonged labor
b. Cervical or vaginal lacerations due to macrosomia
c. Consumptive coagulopathy from amniotic fluid embolism
d. Retained products of conception
e. Uterine rupture from obstructed labor

4. The patient in the above question has now become pale, tachycardic, hypotensive, and lethargic. Based upon your diagnosis, what is the next most appropriate intervention?
a. Place a Foley catheter to monitor urine output
b. Employ bimanual uterine compression and massage
c. Consult anesthesia to place a Swan-Ganz catheter in order to aid in fluid resuscitation
d. Draw a blood specimen for an emergent type and cross and coagulation profile
e. Perform an emergency laparotomy and hypogastric artery ligation

5. All of the following are associated with increased neonatal morbidity and mortality at term except
a. Breech presentation
b. Prolonged second stage
c. Postterm pregnancy
d. Prolonged latent phase
e. Arrest of dilatation

6. Criteria for a vaginal breech delivery includes all of the following except

a. Fetal weight between 1600 and 3600 grams
b. Footling or frank presentation
c. Biparietal diameter less than or equal to 9.5 cm
d. Adequate maternal pelvis by CT pelvimetry
e. No evidence of intrauterine growth restriction

7. A 17-year-old G1 P0 at term presents to labor and delivery with regular, painful uterine contractions. Membranes are intact. Her vaginal exam is 5 cm dilated, +1 station, 90% effaced and vertex presenting with mild caput but no molding. Estimated fetal weight is 7 pounds. Two hours later her vaginal exam is unchanged. Of the following, the most appropriate next step in managing this patient is to
a. Proceed with cesarean section for cephalopelvic disproportion
b. Begin oxytocin augmentation of labor
c. Rupture membranes and place an intrauterine pressure catheter
d. Reexamine in 1 hour. If no change, proceed with cesarean section
e. Perform a bedside ultrasound to estimate fetal weight

8. Which of the following precludes a trial of vaginal birth after cesarean section (VBAC)?
a. Dysfunctional labor requiring oxytocin stimulation
b. Epidural analgesia
c. Previous vertical uterine scar
d. Gestational diabetes with an estimated fetal weight of 3600 grams
e. Unknown type of uterine scar

19

Anesthesia and Analgesia for the Obstetrical Patient

John R. Fisgus

INTRODUCTION

Almost every organ system of the body is effected by pregnancy. The physiologic and anatomic alterations the maternal patient undergoes and the demands of the fetus present the physician with a myriad of clinical challenges. Anesthesia personnel must also deal with the altered physiologic state of the mother when delivering care. The members of the obstetrical care team should be aware of the concerns that each member faces, and function as an integrated unit. The obstetrician should understand the physiologic and anatomic changes that occur in pregnancy which can effect anesthetic decision making, and to be able to discuss this aspect of maternal care with his or her patients.

PHYSIOLOGIC AND ANATOMIC CHANGES OF PREGNANCY THAT AFFECT ANESTHETIC CARE

Cardiovascular Changes

With increasing metabolic requirements of the developing fetus, the cardiovascular system adapts to meet those demands. As the uterus en-

larges, maternal blood volume increases by 45%.[1] This results in roughly a 1.5 liter increase in maternal intravascular volume by the third trimester. Heart rate is elevated by 15% and cardiac output increases 30%–40% by the third trimester with further elevations as labor ensues.[2,3] Cardiac output reaches its peak in the third stage of labor rising up to 80%[3] above baseline as sustained uterine contraction effectively autotransfuses the "extra" intravascular volume back into the maternal circulation. Central venous pulmonary artery pressures remain normal while maternal blood pressure declines slightly in spite of the increase in blood volume. This is probably the result of a decrease in systemic vascular resistance. The increase in heart rate, blood volume, and cardiac output can cause cardiac decompensation in patients with significant cardiopulmonary disease.

After 20 weeks gestation, if the patient is supine, the expanding uterus may compress both the aorta and the inferior vena cava, decreasing both aorto-iliac arterial flow and venous return. Aortocaval compression can produce what has been called the "supine hypotensive syndrome" where patients can develop symptoms of shock.[4] Anesthesia can inhibit the normal physiologic mechanisms which compensate for aortocaval compression, this can result in severe maternal hypotension and fetal distress. Uterine displacement is required in all patients after 20 weeks gestation when regional or general anesthesia is initiated.

The Respiratory System

The anatomic and physiologic alterations that occur in the respiratory system may significantly increase the risk of anesthetic care in the pregnant patient. Weight gain and breast enlargement along with capillary engorgement and edema which can develop throughout the respiratory tract may make mask ventilation and tracheal intubation difficult. Airway manipulation for intubation or suctioning is more likely to result in trauma, swelling, and bleeding. Use of tocolytics and trendelenberg positioning can further exacerbate swelling in the airway. As a result, there is a three-fold increase in the incidence of failed intubation in pregnancy. Examination of the airway and careful positioning of the head and neck are important prior to induction. Short handle laryngoscopes and emergency airway equipment must be immediately available in case difficulty in intubation is encountered. Edema of the larynx may require the use of smaller endotracheal tubes. Also, blind nasotracheal intubation is strongly advised against. Due to the significant risk of failed intubation in pregnancy, a failed intubation protocol should be established in each OB anesthesia department.

Many ventilatory parameters change including significant increases in minute volume (50%), tidal volume (40%), and alveolar ventilation (70%)[5] while functional residual capacity (FRC) and residual volume decrease. The increasing physiologic demands of the fetus result in a 20% increase in maternal oxygen consumption.[6] The decreased FRC and increased oxygen consumption result in rapid development of hypoxemia and hypercarbia when apnea or airway obstruction occur. Supine positioning and morbid obesity exaggerate this problem. If general anesthesia is necessary, prior to induction, the patient should be preoxygenated to prevent hypoxemia from occurring should intubation prove to be difficult.[6]

The Gastrointestinal Tract

As pregnancy progresses, the enlarging uterus alters the position of the stomach, changing the angle of the gastroesophageal junction.[3] In addition, there is a decrease in lower esophageal sphincter tone and gastric motility secondary to elevated progesterone levels. Gastrin levels are also elevated in pregnancy. These changes result in decreased gastric emptying, increased gastric acid volume, and G-E reflux of gastric contents. When labor pain ensues, parenteral administration of narcotics may further inhibit gastric emptying. These alterations of the maternal GI system have serious implications.

The patient is always considered to have a full stomach and at risk of aspiration, regardless as to when the patient actually ate last. There is an eight-fold increase in the incidence of clinical aspiration with general anesthesia in pregnancy. To minimize this risk, OB patients from the second trimester through the second week postpartum are treated with a nonparticulate antacid (e.g., sodium citrate) when they are taken to the operating room. Other therapies include H_2 antagonists to decrease HCl production, and metoclopramide (Reglan) to enhance gastric emptying and increase esophageal sphincter tone. Labor epidural anesthesia does not alter gastric emptying as parenteral narcotics do. A labor epidural may be used for emergent cesarean section, thus avoiding intubation and general anesthesia (Table 19-1).

Hematologic Effects of Pregnancy

Plasma volume increases by 45% while RBC volume increases by 35% resulting in a dilu-

Table 19-1. Anesthesia Risks in Pregnancy

1. Risk of "supine hypotensive syndrome"
2. Increased risk of failed intubation
3. Increased risk of aspiration
4. Rapid onset of hypoxemia with apnea

Source: From ref. 5.

tional anemia during pregnancy. This results in a 45% increase in maternal intravascular volume. Normally, this increase in blood volume would usually be of little significance except for patients, such as those with significant cardiopulmonary disease, that have underlying conditions in which volume increases can be detrimental. Because of the increase in maternal blood volume, blood loss as much as 1500 ccs in parturition is normally well tolerated. Unfortunately, should significant maternal hemorrhage occur, its severity may be masked by the physiologic changes of pregnancy and delay intervention.

Clotting factors I, VII, VIII, X, and XII are noted to increase significantly[3] while platelet counts remain normal or slightly decreased. The increase in coagulation factors in pregnancy produces a hypercoagulable state rendering the pregnant patient more prone to thrombotic complications (e.g., deep vein thrombosis and pulmonary embolism). At the same time, the increase in coagulation factors and intravascular volume afford protection to the parturient against the inevitable blood loss that occurs at delivery.

PAIN RELIEF IN LABOR

Labor is a painful process that has both a physiological and psychological toll on the parturient. Pain relief in labor includes both nonpharmacologic as well as pharmacologic techniques. Lamaze or psychoprophylaxis is one of the most common approaches to ''natural childbirth.'' Educating the patient about the birth process helps the parturient cope with the stress of labor and can decrease the need for medication. The Lamaze method uses special breathing techniques along with changing patient focus away from the discomfort of labor. This results in decreased maternal fear and anxiety, as well as helping the parturient feel in control of the birth process. The advantage of psychoprophylaxis is that medications that may depress the mother or the fetus are avoided. However, many parturients that begin with Lamaze or other ''natural

childbirth'' techniques require alternative methods of pain relief once labor progresses.

Systemic analgesic medications are still widely used for relief of the pain and anxiety in labor. These medications include: benzodiazepines, phenothiazines, barbiturates, and narcotics. All of these medications cross the placenta and may affect the fetus. The degree of the effect will depend on the dose, route, and timing relative to delivery.

Systemic Medications for Labor

1. Benzodiazepines
   Use: Sedation, premedication for surgery, decrease narcotic requirements, and anticonvulsant.
   Agents: Midazolam (Versed) and diazepam (Valium) are most commonly used.
   Pharmacology:
   a. Diazepam is metabolized in the liver, has a half-life of up to 36 hours, and has active metabolites with half-lives of up to 100 hours. In relatively small doses of 2.5 mg to 10 mg, beat-to-beat variability is significantly decreased,[7] FHR is increased, without changes in fetal acid-base status and minimal effect on the neonate. Larger doses may precipitate hypotonia, lethargy, and hypothermia.[8,13]
   b. Midazolam differs from diazepam in that it is water soluble, has a rapid onset of action, a short duration of action with a half-life of 1 to 2 hours. It is 4 to 5 times as potent as diazepam and produces anterograde amnesia more predictably than diazepam. Unlike diazepam, IM and IV injections are painless. Concerns with midazolam, however, include an association with lower Apgar scores even in small doses. Additionally, complaints by parturients of having no recall of the delivery if given prior to parturition.[9] As a result, the use of midazolam in labor is not recommended.

2. Phenothiazines/Hydroxyzine:
   Use: Anxiolytic, antihistamine, antiemetic, decrease narcotic requirements
   Agents: Promethazine (Phenergan), hydroxyzine (Vistaril)
   Pharmacology:
   a. Promethazine (Phenergan), is one of a group of phenothiazines that may be used in labor to decrease anxiety and decrease narcotic requirements.[10] Placental transfer is rapid and beat-to-beat variability may be decreased but it appears to lack any significant neonatal depressant effects.[11] Other phenothiazines (e.g., prochlorperazine) are not usually used due to their greater alpha adrenergic inhibition and resulting hypotension.
   b. Hydroxyzine is chemically unrelated to the phenothiazines but has similar effects. It is an anxiolytic agent that rapidly crosses the placenta yet appears to lack neonatal depressant effects.[12] Hydroxyzine is often used in labor to potentiate the effects of narcotics. The addition of hydroxyzine to meperidine during labor produces results in pain relief without adversely effecting Apgar scores.
3. Barbiturates
   Use: Sedative—hypnotic with amnestic effects,
   Agents: secobarbital (Seconal), pentobarbital (Nembutal)
   Pharmacology:
   a. Used mainly for overnight sedation. Barbiturates lack analgesic effects and in the presence of pain are antianalgesic. They can produce prolonged depressant effects on the newborn and therefore not considered appropriate for use in labor.
4. Narcotics
   Use: Analgesia
   Agents: Morphine, meperidine (Demerol), fentanyl (Sublimaze)
   Pharmacology:
   a. Narcotics are the primary systemic

agents used for pain relief in labor. The side effects of narcotics (respiratory depression, sedation, nausea/vomiting, orthostatic hypotension) limit the extent of pain relief that will be achieved. Since all narcotic agents can produce equivalent levels of pain relief with appropriate doses, the choice of narcotic should be based on the maternal and neonatal side effects, as well as the drugs duration of action.
   b. Morphine in doses of 5 to 10 mgs, has a duration of action of 4 to 6 hours. However, compared to meperidine has a more pronounced respiratory depressant effect on the neonate.[13] As a result, morphine is not routinely used in labor.
   c. Meperidine is 1/10 as potent as morphine with a duration of action of 2 to 4 hours. When doses up to 100 mg are given to parturients within one hour of delivery, neonatal depression is not seen. When delivery occurs 2 to 3 hours after giving meperidine, there is an increased incidence of neonatal depression, even with smaller doses.[14] Neonatal depression may be due to action of meperidine and its active metabolite, normeperidine.
   d. Fentanyl is a synthetic narcotic analgesic that is rapid in onset, short in duration (30 to 60 minutes), and 70 to 100 times as potent as morphine. IV administration results in a peak analgesic effect in 3 to 5 minutes.[15] Doses of 50 to 100 mcg IV (or 1 mcg/kg) produce minimal neonatal effects. Fentanyl may be a useful agent as a supplement to anesthesia for cesarean section, or even as an infusion during labor.
5. Narcotic agonist-antagonists
   Use: pain relief, reversal of side effects of spinal/epidural narcotics
   Agents: nalbuphine (Nubain), butorphanol (Stadol)
   Pharmacology:
   a. These are agents that provide pain relief while producing less maternal respira-

tory depression compared to other narcotics. Antagonist properties of these agents can be used to treat the side effects of spinal and epidural opioids such as puritis and nausea/vomiting. These agonist-antagonist agents should not be used in individuals with who are known narcotic abusers, as they may precipitate symptoms of narcotic withdrawal.

Nalbuphine and butorphanol are synthetic agonist-antagonists narcotic analgesics. Nalbuphine has a maternal half-life of approximately 2 1/2 hours, with a duration of analgesia of 3 to 4 hours. This agent is equipotent with morphine and is similar to meperidine in its effect on the neonate.[13] Butorphanol is 4 to 5 times as potent as morphine, with a half-life of about 2 1/2 hours and analgesia of about 4 hours duration. Maternal analgesia is equivalent if not superior to meperidine while it's effect on the neonate is similar.[16] However, butorphanol may produce more sedation than nalbuphine when used for pain relief.

6. Narcotic antagonists
Use: Reversal of the effects of narcotics
Agents: naloxone (Narcan), nalmefene (Revex)
Pharmacology:
These are pure opioid antagonists. They can be used to treat the side effects of spinal and epidural narcotics as well as respiratory depression. Patients who are narcotic abusers should not be given opioid antagonists

as this may precipitate symptoms of withdrawal.

a. Naloxone is used to treat both respiratory depression from narcotics and may also be used in low dose (0.1 mg to 0.2 mg) to treat side effects of spinal opioids without reversing maternal analgesia. The half-life of naloxone is relatively short (30 to 80 minutes in adults)[17] thus recurrence of respiratory depression is possible. Nalmefene is a new opioid antagonist that has a much longer half-life than naloxone. Recurrence of narcotic-induced respiratory depression would be much less likely with this agent. Use in the pregnancy, the neonate, or the treatment of spinal opioid side effects has not been evaluated yet[17] (Table 19-2).

Regional Anesthesia for Labor

Regional blocks in the obstetrical patient include: continuous epidural anesthesia, spinal anesthesia, paracervical blocks, and pudendal nerve blocks (Table 19-3). All regional blocks have a high margin of safety when properly administered and can provide excellent pain relief for labor and/or delivery without causing maternal or fetal obtundation. To provide adequate pain relief for labor, the pain pathways from T10 through L1 must be blocked to inhibit the pain of uterine contraction and cervical dilatation. At delivery, pain fibers from S2 to S4 carried by the pudendal nerve must be blocked to inhibit the pain of vaginal, vulvar, and perineal distention.

Table 19-2.   Agents with Opioid Receptor Effects

Narcotic	Classification	Potency vs. Morphine	Duration of Action
Morphine	opioid agonist	10 mg	4 to 6 hours
Meperidine	opioid agonist	100 mg (1/10 as potent)	2 to 4 hours
Fentanyl (Sublimaze)	opioid agonist	100 mcg (100× as potent)	30 to 60 min
Nalbuphine (Nubain)	opioid agonist antagonist	10 mg	2 to 4 hours
Butorphanol (Stadol)	opioid agonist antagonist	2 mg (5× as potent)	4 hours
Naloxone (Narcan)	opioid antagonist	NA	1 to 2 hours
Nalmepene (Revex)	opioid antagonist	NA	up to 10 hours

Table 19-3. Regional Blocks for Labor Pain Relief

1. Paracervical block*
2. Epidural anesthesia
3. Spinal anesthesia
4. Combined spinal-epidural anesthesia

*High-risk fetal arrhythmias.

Table 19-4. Contraindications to Regional Anesthesia for Cesarean Section

Absolute contraindications
1. Hemorrhage/hypovolemia
2. Maternal septicemia/meningitis
3. Coagulopathy/DIC
4. Skin infection in lumbar region preventing aseptic technique
5. Acute central nervous system disease
6. Patient refusal of regional anesthesia

Relative contraindications
1. Progressive neurologic disease
2. Anticoagulation?

The most commonly used local anesthetic agents for regional blockade in the obstetrical patient include lidocaine, bupivacaine, and chloroprocaine. Bupivacaine is a long-acting local anesthetic that provides more sensory than motor blockade, making it an excellent choice for the laboring patient. Epidural bupivacaine, 0.0625% to 0.25%, in combination with a narcotic (fentanyl or sufentanil) is commonly used for labor pain relief. The major concern with bupivacaine is the danger of cardiotoxicity from either an accidental intravascular injection of a large dose or from cumulative doses. At high blood levels, bupivacaine can block myocardial Na channels causing cardiac arrest[18] that may require a long period of resuscitation before enough drug metabolism occurs to allow return of myocardial function. Lidocaine and chloroprocaine inhibit motor function more than bupivacaine but also have a faster onset of action. Both of these agents may be used for epidural analgesia in the laboring patient, and are well suited for elective or urgent cesarean section. Ropivacaine is a new amide local anesthetic that is similar to bupivacaine in most respects yet it lacks the severe cardiotoxic effects with high systemic levels.[19] As a result, this new local anesthetic may eventually replace bupivacaine.

Before any regional anesthetic is performed, cardiopulmonary resuscitation equipment must always be immediately available in the labor and delivery area. Though emergencies are rare, one must be prepared to immediately treat complications of regional blockade such as local anesthetic overdose, inadvertent "high spinal" blockade, or cardiac arrest. Contraindications to regional anesthesia include patient refusal, infection at the site of injection, coagulopathy, and sepsis. Spinal and epidural anesthesia may also be contraindicated in the presence of acute CNS

disease or increased intracranial pressure. Relative contraindications include maternal infection, some cardiac lesions, and some preexisting neurologic conditions (Table 19-4). Though controversial, many anesthesiologists do not consider chorioamnionitis a contraindication for epidural anesthesia and place catheters after initiation of antimicrobial therapy.[20]

Pudendal Nerve Block

This is an easily performed block that will give the patient perineal anesthesia for delivery but not labor pain relief. Most obstetricians use the transvaginal approach. With the patient in the lithotomy position, after the area has been prepped with an antibacterial agent, the second and third fingers locate the ischial spine and the sacrospinous ligament. The needle is passed at the junction of the ischial spine and sacrospinous ligament through the mucosa until the needle passes through the ligament. After aspirating to check for accidental intravascular placement, 5 ml to 10 ml of a local anesthetic is deposited and the procedure is then repeated on the other side. This block will be useful for perineal anesthesia for forceps delivery as well as repair of vaginal lacerations that may occur during birth.

Paracervical Block

This type of block involves a submucosal injection of local anesthetics into the vaginal fornix to block the fibers of T10-L1. When used in labor, it can provide pain relief for up to an hour before needing to be repeated. Though a technically easy block to perform, this block has been associated with a number of complications during pregnancy. Uterine blood vessels are in close proximity and the danger of accidental intravascular injection exists. Rapid absorption of the local anesthetic into the uterine vasculature may decrease uterine artery blood flow. Decreased oxygen delivery to the fetus secondary to increased uterine tone[21] and/or decreased uterine artery blood flow may explain the high incidence of fetal arrhythmias that have been reported with this technique.[22] Fetal acidosis, seizures and death have also been associated with the use of this block in labor. Though excellent for D&Cs and other localized GYN procedures, the paracervical block use in labor has fallen out of favor with the availability of epidural anesthesia. Recently, a study using a superficial injection technique revisited paracervical block for labor pain relief and found minimal fetal effects but postblock fetal bradycardia was not eliminated.[23]

Epidural Anesthesia

Epidural anesthesia is one of the most effective treatments of pain related to the first and second stages of labor. When administered properly, it is a safe procedure with minimal effect on the progress of labor or the fetus. Epidural anesthesia has significant beneficial effects on the laboring parturient. This technique prevents harmful metabolic responses to the pain of labor such as hyperventilation, hypocapnia, metabolic acidosis, and lactic acid accumulation. Labor epidural anesthesia also decreases pain-induced catecholamine levels and improves intervillous blood flow.[24] In patients with preeclampsia, epidural anesthesia has a more profound effect, improving intervillous blood flow by 77%.[25] Most epidural anesthesia is placed by trained anesthesia personnel though some are still administered by obstetricians in rural areas. Due to the risks of possible respiratory embarrassment associated with regional anesthesia, individuals with expertise in airway management should be immediately available (Table 19-5).

Continuous epidural anesthesia involves the

Table 19-5. Preparations/Precautions for Regional Anesthesia in Pregnancy

1. Prophylactic fluid bolus prior to block
     500 cc for labor epidural
       1 to 2 liters for cesarean section under epidural or spinal
2. GI prophylaxis for surgery
     15–30 cc sodium citrate 15 minutes before procedure
     H_2 blocker/metaclopramide is an option if time permits
3. Left uterine displacement
     Emergency airway/resuscitative equipment immediately available

placement of an epidural catheter, with continuous infusion of local anesthetic with or without a narcotic. An initial bolus dose of bupivacaine 0.125% to 0.25% with fentanyl (2 to 7.5 mcg/cc) is administered to initiate adequate labor pain relief. A continuous infusion of bupivacaine 0.0625% to 0.125% with fentanyl (1 to 2 mcg/cc) is usually begun at a rate of 8 to 12 cc/hr. With the addition of epinephrine, the concentration of local may be decreased, helping to limit the total amount of local anesthetic infused over time. Epidural infusion concentrations of 0.0625% or less with the addition of epinephrine have also been used. Patient-controlled epidural anesthesia enables the patient to control her own epidural infusion of local anesthetic for labor. Benefits may include decreased total local anesthetic dose and the patients ability to adjust the anesthetic level. Further evaluation of this technique is needed.

Combined Spinal Epidural Analgesia

The use of combined spinal epidural analgesia for labor pain relief has recently been gaining popularity. Using intrathecal opioids such as fentanyl (25 mcgs) and sufentanyl (10 mcgs) diluted with 1 to 2 ccs of preservative-free saline, intrathecal injection provides rapid relief of first-stage labor pain lasting 90 to 120 minutes with minimal cardiovascular disturbance and no motor block.[26] The addition of small amounts of isobaric bupivacaine (1.25 to 2.5 mgs) appears to improve the quality and duration of labor analgesia with minimal motor blockade or cardiovascular impact.[27] Dural puncture headache risk does not seem to be higher with this technique than routine epidural placement when 25 gauge pencil point needles are used. Continuous spinal anesthesia (requiring placement of an intrathecal catheter) has not gained popularity in the obstetrical patient due to the risk of frequent dural puncture headaches. In the event of accidental dural puncture during epidural catheter placement, the catheter may be left intrathecal and be used for labor pain relief using small doses of a local anesthetics and/or narcotics as previously described.

Epidural and Spinal Narcotics for Labor

The addition of narcotics to local anesthetic solutions for labor epidural analgesia has proved to be beneficial, reducing the local anesthetic concentrations and minimizing local anesthetic motor blockade. Unfortunately, epidural narcotics alone have not been very successful in providing labor pain relief. In contrast, intrathecal narcotics appear to provide excellent relief from labor pain without effecting motor function. Intrathecal narcotics may be advantageous in patients with severe cardiopulmonary conditions that may be adversely effected by sympathetic blockade. Complications of epidural or intrathecal narcotics include, puritis, nausea/vomiting, hypotension, and urinary retention. Delayed respiratory depression is also a rare complication of regional use of narcotics that is easily reversed with narcotic antagonists. The risk of respiratory depression is increased, however, if parenteral narcotics are also given.

General Anesthesia for Vaginal Delivery

This technique is rarely utilized today in obstetric practice. When general anesthesia is administered, endotracheal intubation is mandatory. General anesthesia for vaginal delivery is limited to situations where uterine relaxation is required for obstetrical maneuvers such as second twin delivery, breech, shoulder dystocia, etc. After delivery, uterine relaxation may be required for conditions such as retained placenta

or uterine inversion. Volatile anesthetic agents produce uterine relaxation in a dose dependent fashion. Increasing inspired concentrations as high as 2 MAC (minimum alveolar concentration) may be required for maximal relaxation. Anesthetic overdose to the maternal patient with hypotension and hemorrhage from uterine relaxation are potential complications.

REGIONAL ANESTHESIA FOR CESAREAN SECTION

Regional blockade is the preferred anesthetic for cesarean delivery. Compared to general anesthesia, regional techniques such as epidural and spinal anesthesia have numerous advantages: decreased risk of aspiration, avoidance of depressant anesthetics, and the ability of the mother to be awake for the delivery. Cesarean delivery can also be done with only local anesthetic infiltration of the abdomen but this technique is only done in extreme circumstances.

Spinal Anesthesia for Cesarean Delivery

Spinal anesthesia has advantages and disadvantages when compared to epidural anesthesia for cesarean delivery. Spinal anesthesia can be placed quickly, is faster in onset than an epidural, and has a lower failure rate.[28] This technique tends to produce a more profound sensory block that provides the patient with less sensation during surgery. Spinal anesthetics also requires a significantly lower dose of local anesthetic which minimizes the risk of local anesthetic toxicity. The disadvantages of spinal anesthetics include limited surgical operating time, increased risk of spinal headaches, less ability to control anesthetic level, and rapid onset of sympathetic blockade that is more likely to precipitate acute hypotension. Continuous spinal catheters may be placed for anesthesia and analgesia in the obstetric patient, but their use is limited due to the high frequency of spinal headaches.

Epidural Anesthesia for Cesarean Delivery

Epidural anesthesia may be used for cesarean delivery using more concentrated local anesthetic agents than those described for labor pain relief. For patients in labor that have an epidural catheter in place, potent local anesthetics may be given to rapidly provide anesthesia if emergency cesarean section becomes necessary. Lidocaine (2%) with epinephrine (1:200,000) or chloroprocaine (3%) 15 cc to 20 cc are administered in divided doses. When lidocaine is used, the addition of 8.4% Na bicarbonate (1 cc NaHCO3 for each 10 cc's lidocaine) may significantly shorten the time of onset of surgical anesthesia.[29]

Spinal and epidural anesthesia can both be used to provide postoperative pain relief in surgical patients. Morphine given as a single dose epidurally or intrathecally can provide up to 24 hours of pain relief. Narcotics bind to mu receptors in the substantia gelatinosa in the spinal cord modulating pain perception.[30] Puritis and nausea are common side effects of spinal opioids. Puritis is treated with low-dose naloxone (0.1 mg IV), nalbuphine (2.5 mg to 5 mg IV), and/or diphenhydramine (25 mg to 50 mg IV). Respiratory depression is a rare, but serious complication, and is reversible with an opioid antagonist.

Postdural Puncture Headaches (PDPH)

When the dura is punctured either purposely for spinal anesthesia or unintentionally during epidural placement, the patient may develop a spinal headache or what is also referred to as a postdural puncture headache. The primary cause of postdural puncture headache is acute CSF loss into the epidural space resulting in a pressure differential between the spinal canal and the brain. Symptoms include the classical complaint of a positional headache that is worse when sitting or standing, and is relieved with reclining. Other symptoms include neck and shoulder pain, nausea/vomiting, depression, and

photophobia. Onset is usually 24 to 48 hours after the regional procedure was performed. Most symptoms resolve within 4 to 7 days. Conservative therapy consists of oral hydration and nonsteroidal anti-inflammatory agents. Caffeine benzoate 500 mg IV or caffeine 300 mg po has also been used to treat PDPH with some success. Unfortunately the relief of pain from caffeine is often transient. Epidural blood patch is successful in over 90% of patients with minimal risk, and is indicated in patients that do not respond to conservative treatment or those that desire rapid relief of their symptoms.[31]

GENERAL ANESTHESIA IN PREGNANCY

General anesthesia (GA) has the distinct advantage over regional anesthesia in that it can be rapidly administered, its effects are reliable, and its duration of action can be easily controlled. It is the anesthetic of choice in obstetrical patients with the following conditions: hypovolemia, sepsis, coagulopathy, dermal infections that cover the area where regional anesthetic would need to be placed, and patient refusal of regional anesthesia. GA is frequently used for the maternal patient with obstetrical hemorrhage, fetal distress (where time does not allow regional anesthetic placement), and situations where uterine relaxation is needed. GA must be approached with great caution in patients that have known or suspected difficult airways, pulmonary disease, history of malignant hyperthermia, or those at high risk for hyperkalemia from the use of succinylcholine (major burns, crush injuries, some neurologic diseases). Major complications of GA include aspiration, failure to intubate, failure to ventilate and oxygenate, and fetal depression from anesthetic agents (Table 19-6).

Nonobstetrical Surgery in the Pregnant Patient

When the maternal patient requires surgery during pregnancy for reasons other than delivery of the fetus, the short- and long-term effects of

Table 19-6. Preparations/Precautions for General Anesthesia and Cesarean Delivery

1. GI prophylaxis (sodium citrate/H_2 blockers)
2. Left uterine displacement
3. Minimize anesthesia induction time to delivery time. Prep and drape patient prior to induction of anesthesia.
4. Preoxygenation/cricoid pressure/endotracheal intubation
5. Maintain volatile inhalation agents at 0.5 MAC
6. N_2 0–50%, (avoid if fetal distress is present?)
7. Extubate patient when awake/airway reflexes returned

our anesthetic management as well as the stage of fetal development must be taken into consideration. Teratogenicity is certainly a concern in the first trimester. Fortunately, to date there is no apparent increase in congenital anomalies associated with the use of any anesthetic agents.[32] Some concern has been raised with the use of nitrous oxide during pregnancy due to its inhibitory effect on methionine synthase that could theoretically effect fetal development. The use of N_2O should be dictated by the procedure and the surgical needs. The most important factors that effect outcome of pregnancy in the surgical patient are the type and site of the surgical procedure, not the anesthetic used.

From the second trimester and on, specific precautions must be instituted for all surgical procedures.

1. All patients after 14 weeks gestation are considered to have full stomachs and are at risk for aspiration. Thus all such patients should receive a nonparticulate oral antacid or be treated with H_2 antagonists such as ranitidine or cimetidine. Metaclopramide is useful to increase gastric emptying, and may decrease postoperative nausea/vomiting.
2. Rapid sequence induction of anesthesia is indicated in the second trimester. This requires that the patient be preoxygenated and have cricoid pressure applied from the time of induction until successful endotracheal intubation has been confirmed. At the conclusion of the procedure, extubation is done only when the patient is awake, has good respiratory effort, and airway reflexes are intact.

3. Left uterine displacement is needed after the 20 week of gestation.
4. When the fetus is viable, monitoring of the FHR should be done intraoperatively to treat possible complications related to the surgery and effect delivery if fetal distress develops.

Specific Precautions for Cesarean Delivery

All patients should be prepped/draped prior to induction of anesthesia to minimize fetal exposure to inhalational anesthetic agents if cesarean delivery is anticipated. Volatile inhalational agents may produce fetal depression if used for an extended period of time at high doses. If analgesic doses (0.5 MAC or less) are utilized, neonatal depression is unlikely even if the time of anesthesia induction to delivery is prolonged.[33] Nitrous oxide is rapidly transferred across the placenta to the fetus and may produce neonatal depression. This agent depresses the neonate either as a direct anesthetic effect or as an effect of diffusion hypoxemia related to neonatal excretion of N_2O from the lungs.[34] The depressant effects of N_2O are lessened if inhaled concentrations are limited to a concentration no greater than 50% and the length of exposure is under 20 minutes. At delivery, oxygen should be administered to the neonate at birth if N_2O is used for the mother.

More important than the anesthetic time to delivery appears to be the uterine incision time to delivery interval. In situations where uterine incision to delivery time exceeded 180 seconds, an increase in fetal acidosis and depressed Apgar scores was seen.[35] After delivery, it is suggested that the concentration of volatile inhalational anesthetic be limited to 0.5 MAC in order to minimize the uterine relaxant effects of these agents that may increase blood loss.

Intravenous General Anesthetic Agents

Thiopental

Thiopental rapidly induces sleep for general anesthesia. It rapidly crosses the placenta but due to numerous factors, (rapid maternal/fetal redistribution and dilution the fetal circulation) the fetus does not lose consciousness. Doses up to 4 mg/kg do not appear to produce significant neonatal depression.

Ketamine

Ketamine is a dissociative agent that produces profound analgesia/anesthesia. In low doses (<0.25 mg/kg), it can be used for analgesia/amnesia to augment regional anesthesia without loss of maternal airway reflexes. Ketamine is indicated for induction of general anesthesia in the hypovolemic/hypotensive patient as well as severely asthmatic patients. In doses of 1 mg/kg or less, no adverse neonatal effects are seen.[36]

Propofol (Diprivan)

Propofol is a new intravenous anesthetic agent with a rapid onset and recovery. It is used for both induction of general anesthesia as well as IV sedation. Propofol is a safe alternative to thiopental for induction of anesthesia and for use in maintenance of anesthesia through delivery.[37] Benefits of propofol include rapid return of consciousness and low incidence of postoperative nausea/vomiting. In the pregnant sheep model, no significant effect was seen on uterine blood flow, fetal heart rate, or variability. Severe maternal bradycardia was noted when propofol was used with succinylcholine in this model but no adverse fetal effects were seen.[38]

ANESTHESIA MANAGEMENT CONSIDERATIONS IN THE COMPLICATED OBSTETRICAL PATIENT

Preeclampsia/Eclampsia: Anesthesia Considerations

Preeclampsia is a disorder classically defined by the presence of hypertension, edema, and proteinuria. The presence of significant intravascular volume depletion that is common in the preeclamptic, effects the anesthetic approach. With the initiation of epidural anesthesia, careful fluid preloading, left uterine displacement, and frequent monitoring of blood pressure is necessary due to the risk of hypotension. In the severe preeclamptic, there is a significant risk of pulmonary edema. Prophylactic fluid loading for regional anesthesia should be done with caution along with continuous monitoring of the patients urine output and overall volume assessment. In patients who are oliguric, a fluid challenge of 500 ccs of an isotonic crystalloid solution may be given. If there is no response to fluid challenge or if initial central venous pressures are high (>8 mm/Hg), consider pulmonary artery catheterization for fluid management.

Epidural anesthesia for labor will have multiple benefits in the preeclamptic patient: improved uterine blood flow, decreased catecholamine levels/blood pressure fluctuations with pain relief, and the ability to avoid general anesthesia in the event of fetal distress.[23,24] If cesarean section is indicated, epidural anesthesia is preferred to spinal in the severe preeclamptic due to the potential for severe hypotension that may result from rapid onset of sympathetic blockade. Spinal anesthesia may be used however with caution in the event of emergency C/S in the severe preeclamptic if the maternal risks of general anesthesia outweigh those associated with spinal anesthesia. General anesthesia in the preeclamptic for cesarean section is fraught with numerous dangers including increased airway vascularity/edema and wide fluctuations of blood pressure with induction and intubation. These complications can lead to severe morbidity and even death. Induction of general anesthesia in the severe preeclamptic should include: invasive arterial blood pressure monitoring, large bore IV access, and availability of agents to treat hypertension (labetolol, nitroprusside, nitroglycerine) or hypotension (ephedrine). If hypotension occurs, IV fluid should be given along with only small doses of vasoactive drugs, as preeclamptics are highly responsive to sympathomimetic agents.

In the event that eclampsia should occur: oxygen should be applied and the patiency of the airway should be established. If the patient is hypoxemic endotracheal intubation should be initiated, but only by individuals with expertise in airway management. An anticonvulsant such as diazepam or thiopental, is administered if the patient has persistent seizures.

Hemorrhage

With up to 20% of the maternal cardiac output perfusing the uterus in the third trimester, conditions such as placental abruption, placenta previa, and uterine rupture can lead to rapid exsanguination of the maternal patient. The increase in intravascular volume of up to 1.5 l with pregnancy is protective of the maternal blood loss that normally occurs with delivery. With maternal hemorrhage, the patient may be able to tolerate greater blood loss before becoming symptomatic. If the patient becomes acutely hypotensive, this often signifies severe hypovolemia and immediate volume resuscitation is indicated.[39] If emergency cesarean section is indicated, general anesthesia should be used if the patient is hypovolemic. A minimum of 2 large bore IV sites should be established, an arterial line is highly recommended, and blood must typed and crossed (along with blood products) as soon as possible. Type O negative blood should be immediately available for transfusion in severe hemorrhage.

Cardiac Disease

Cardiac disease complicates up to 4% of pregnancies.[40] While a comprehensive review of heart disease is beyond the scope of this manual, important concepts in regard to pregnancy and cardiac disease will be covered. Heart diseases that seriously threaten the maternal patient include pulmonary hypertension (especially Eisenmenger's syndrome), mitral stenosis, aortic stenosis, Marfan's syndrome, Tetralogy of Fallot, and coarctation of the aorta. The physiologic changes of pregnancy can precipitate cardiac decompensation in patients with significant disease. Maternal morbidity and mortality is high-

est at those points in pregnancy when maternal myocardial stress increases: in the third trimester as cardiac output and intravascular expansion peaks, during labor, delivery, and especially the immediate postpartum period. Anesthesia and obstetrical management for the pregnant patient with cardiac disease involves efforts to decrease those factors that cause sudden changes in myocardial and pulmonary status. Regional anesthesia is often appropriate for labor and delivery by decreasing pain and minimizing patient expulsive efforts, allowing for a controlled instrumental delivery. Epidural anesthesia is often indicated in patients with coronary artery disease, valvular disease and Marfan's syndrome. Patients that have Eisenmenger's syndrome and cyanotic heart lesions may not tolerate peripheral vasodilation with epidural anesthesia that can aggravate R to L shunting. These patients may benefit from intrathecal narcotics for pain management in labor. Patients with significant cardiac disease will often require invasive arterial pressure monitoring, central venous or pulmonary artery catheterization. Preoperative consultation with anesthesia, obstetrical, and cardiology physicians is important to ensure a coordinated team approach to management of these high-risk patients.

Asthma

Asthma complicates up to 7% of pregnancies. Pregnancy may improve or exacerbate the symptoms of asthma though the majority of patients symptoms are unchanged. The asthmatic patient is at increased risk of premature delivery, intrauterine fetal death, low birth weight, hemorrhage, hyperemesis, and toxemia.[41]

There are two primary objectives in treating the pregnant asthmatic patient. Optimization of the patients pulmonary status and prevention of acute episodes of bronchospasm. Analgesia for labor will help prevent anxiety and hyperventilation that can potentially exacerbate bronchospasm. Parenteral narcotics should be used with caution in the actively wheezing asthmatic as they can depress respiratory drive and precipitate bronchospasm. Regional anesthesia is preferred for labor pain relief and cesarean section. Regional anesthesia avoids the need for endotracheal intubation that can precipitate life-threatening bronchospasm with light anesthesia. Caution must be used to avoid a high thoracic regional blockade for two reasons: impairment of the accessory muscles of respiration will make breathing more difficult and cause the patient considerable anxiety. Also, a high thoracic blockade may block sympathetic outflow and leave the parasympathetic system unopposed, potentially causing bronchospasm. Epidural anesthesia may be preferred to spinal anesthesia in the asthmatic patient since the level of anesthesia is easier to control and should a high block occur, there is less motor block of the accessory muscles of respiration.

If general anesthesia is indicated, ketamine is the drug of choice for induction of anesthesia in the severely asthmatic patient. Ketamine is a bronchodilator, is not associated with histamine release, and can blunt the response to intubation that may precipitate bronchospasm. All volatile anesthetics are bronchial relaxants and excellent for maintenance of anesthesia. Beta sympathomimetics may be used to treat bronchospasm during general anesthesia and can be delivered via the endotracheal tube. If uterine atony is encountered, prostaglandin F_2 alpha is not recommended since it can precipitate bronchospasm.

Neurologic Disorders and Anesthesia

All local anesthetics are neurotoxic at concentrations far above those normally used clinically. In patients with neurologic conditions such as multiple sclerosis, there is concern that they may be more susceptible to the neurotoxic effects of local anesthetics such as those used in regional anesthesia. No clear evidence of enhanced neurotoxicity has been demonstrated.[42] If regional anesthesia is felt to be appropriate for the patient with multiple sclerosis, the smallest concentration of local anesthetic suitable is suggested. Intrathecal narcotics may be an op-

tion for the patient in labor. The risks and benefits should be discussed with the patient.

Patients with spinal cord injuries at T7 or higher are at risk for autonomic hyperreflexia. Symptoms of hyperreflexia include severe life threatening hypertension, bradycardia, ventricular arrhythmias, and sweating. Autonomic hyperreflexia is precipitated by stimulation below the level of the spinal cord lesion. Uterine contractions, genital stimulation, and bladder distention are among the maneuvers that can precipitate this phenomenon. Regional anesthesia can inhibit the reflex adrenergic response and thus is useful in preventing autonomic hyperreflexia.[43] General anesthesia can also inhibit autonomic hyperreflexia, but the use of succinylcholine for induction should be avoided as severe hyperkalemia may result.

CPR IN PREGNANCY

In the event of cardiac arrest in the pregnant patient, an organized team approach is vital to the survival of the mother and the fetus. The initiation of CPR, evaluation of the maternal and fetal condition, and the search for an etiology are vital to a successful resuscitation. What may be just as important to maternal survival is the immediate preparations for emergency cesarean delivery. There is significant evidence that pregnancy hinders adequate CPR. A suggested protocol is presented for the maternal resuscitation.

In the event of maternal cardiac arrest:

a. Begin CPR per ACLS guidelines.[44]
b. After 20 weeks gestation, left uterine displacement is vital and must be done IMMEDIATELY either manually or with a wedge (a towel, an IV bag, etc.) under the left hip.
c. If the fetus is viable, FHR should be monitored as soon as possible via external Doppler.
d. Use all standard drugs as indicated for the resuscitation. Larger than standard doses of epinephrine may be indicated as pregnancy

decreases response to alpha and beta agonists.

e. If an arrhythmia is present that requires defibrillation, the fetus is not affected. If a fetal scalp electrode is present though, it should be removed to avoid current flow through the fetus.

f. There is a significant amount of evidence that emergency cesarean section may be lifesaving to the maternal patient if the initial resuscitation is not successful. Put another way, C/S is part of the resuscitation of the mother.

Suggested Guidelines for CPR in Pregnancy[45]:

1. Fetus 25 to 27 weeks gestation: If palpable pulse or adequate FHR, continue CPR for 10 minutes. If unsuccessful, C/S.

2. Fetus 28 weeks gestation and >: If no response to initial CPR, deliver fetus via C/S within 5 minutes of arrest unless maternal cardiac function rapidly returns.

3. 25 weeks and greater: If no palpable pulse with chest compression or severe fetal bradycardia is detected during CPR, immediate C/S.

Remember the ABCDs of CPR in pregnancy: A = airway, B = breathing, C = circulation, D = delivery![45]

CONCLUSION

Labor and delivery can be an extremely painful experience for many parturients. There is no other situation in medicine where it is considered morally acceptable for pain to be left untreated. It is clear that labor pain relief can be safely provided to most parturients with the use of regional anesthesia. Anesthesiologists working together with the other members of the obstetrical care team can effectively deliver analgesia and anesthesia in almost any situation that confronts the pregnant patient. As the obstetrical care providers learn more about the challenges

and concerns that anesthesia personnel have when caring for the pregnant patient, the safer and more effective all obstetric care will be.

REFERENCES

1. Ueland K. Maternal cardiovascular hemodynamics. VII intrapartum blood volume changes. *Am J Obstet Gynecol.* 1976, 126:671–677.

2. Mashini IS, Albazzaz SJ, Fadel HE. Serial non invasive evaluation of cardiovascular hemodynamics during pregnancy. *Am J Obstet Gynecol.* 1987,156:1208–1213.

3. Cheek TG, Gutche BB. Maternal physiologic alterations during pregnancy. In: *Anesthesia for Obstetrics.* Shnider SM, Levinson G, eds. Baltimore: Williams & Wilkins, 1993, 3–18.

4. Howard BK, Goodson JH, Mengert WF. Supine hypotensive syndrome in late pregnancy. *Obstet Gynecol.* 1953, 1:371–377.

5. Camann WR, Ostheimer GW. *Understanding the Mother. Manual of Obstetric Anesthesia.* Ostheimer GW, ed. New York: Churchill and Livingstone, 1992.

6. Weinberger SE, Weiss ST, Cohen WR, Weiss W, Johnson TS. Pregnancy and the lung. *Am Rev Respir Dis.* 1980, 121:559–581.

7. Yeh SY, Paul RH, Codero L, Hon EH. A study of diazepam during labor. *Obstet Gynecol.* 1974, 43:363–373.

8. Flowers CE, Rudolph AJ, Desmond MM. Diazepam (Valium) as an adjunct in obstetric anesthesia. *Obstet Gynecol.* 1969, 34:68–81.

9. Camann W, Cohen MB, Ostheimer GW. Is midazolam desirable for sedation in parturients? *Anesthesiology.* 1983, 65:441.

10. Kerri-Szanto M. Mode of action of promethazine potentiates narcotics. *Br J Anes.* 1974, 46: 918–924.

11. Malkasian GD Jr., Smith RA, Decker DG. Comparison of hydroxyzine-meperidine and promethazine-meperidine for analgesia during labor. *Obstet Gynecol.* 1967, 30:568–575.

12. Zsigmond EK, Patterson RL. Double blind evaluation of hydroxyzine hydrochloride in obstetric anesthesia. *Anesth Analg.* 1967, 46: 275–280.

13. Levinson G, Shnider SM. Systemic medication

for labor and delivery. In: *Anesthesia for Obstetrics*. Shnider SM, Levinson G, eds. Baltimore: Williams & Wilkins, 1993, 125.

14. Shnider SM, Moya F. Effect of meperidine on the newborn infant. *Am J Obstet Gynecol*. 1964, 89:1009–1015.

15. Eisele JH Jr, Wright R, Rogge P. Newborn and maternal fentanyl levels at cesarean section. *Anesth Analg*. 1982 61:179–180.

16. Quilligan EJ, Keegan KA, Donahue MJ. Double blind comparison of intravenously injected butorphanol and meperidine in parturients. *Int J Gynaecol Obstet*. 1980, 18:363–368.

17. *Physicians Desk Reference* 50th Ed. Montvale, NJ: Medical Economics Data Production Co, 1996, 934, 1811.

18. Clarkson C, Hondegham L. Mechanism for bupivacaine depression of cardiac conduction: fast block of sodium channels during the action potential with slow recovery from block during diastole. *Anesthesiology*. 1985, 62:396–405.

19. Moller R, Covino BG. Cardiac electrophysiologic properties of bupivacaine and lidocaine compared with those of ropivacaine, a new amide local anesthetic. *Anesthesiology*. 1990, 72: 322–329.

20. Bromage PR. Neurologic complications of regional anesthesia. *Anesthesia for Obstetrics*. Shnider SM, Levinson G, eds. Baltimore: Williams & Wilkins, 1993, 445.

21. Morishima HO, Covino BG, Yeh MN, et al. Bradycardia in the fetal baboon following paracervical block anesthesia. *Am J Obstet Gynecol*. 1981, 140:775–780.

22. Cibils LA. Response of human arteries to local anesthetics. *Am J Obstet Gynecol*. 1976, 126: 202.

23. Ranta P, Jouppila P, Spalding M, et al. Paracervical block—a viable alternative for labor pain relief? *Acta Obstet Gynecol Scand*. 1995 74:122–126.

24. Jouppila R. Maternal and fetal effects of epidural analgesia during labor. *Zentralbl Gynakol*. 1985, 107:521–531.

25. Jouppila P, Jouppila R, Hollmen A, Koivula A. Lumbar epidural analgesia to improve intervillous blood flow during labor in severe pre-eclampsia. *Obstet Gynecol*. 1982, 59:158–161.

26. Norris MC, Grieco WM, Borkowski M, et al. Complications of labor analgesia: epidural versus combind spinal epidural techniques. *Anesth Analg*. 1994, 79:527–537.

27. Campbell DC, Camann WR, Datta S. The addition of Bupivacaine to intrathecal Sufentanil for labor analgesia. *Anes Analg*. 1995, 81: 305–309.

28. Glosten B, Gianas A, et al. Practical aspects of regional anesthesia for cesarean delivery: failure rates and anesthetic preparation times. Abstract presented to the Society of Obstetrical Anesthesia and Perinatologists, annual meeting 1995.

29. DiFazio CA, Carron H, Grosslight KR, et al. Comparison of pH-adjusted lidocaine solutions for epidural anesthesia. *Anesth Analg*. 1986, 65: 760–764.

30. Ostheimer GW. Intraspinal opioids in the management of Obstetric pain. *Manual of Obstetric Anesthesia*. Ostheimer GW, ed. New York: Churchill and Livingstone, 1992, 98–104.

31. Morewood GH. A rational approach to the cause, prevention, and treatment of post dural puncture headache. *Can Med Assoc J*. 1993, 149:1087–1093.

32. Duncan PG, Pope WDB, Cohen MM, et al. Fetal risk of anesthesia and surgery during pregnancy. *Anesthesiology*. 1986, 64:790–794.

33. Warren TM, Datta S, Ostheimer GW, et al. A comparison of the maternal and neonatal effects of halothane, enflurane, and isoflurane for cesarean section. *Anesth Analg*. 1983 62:516–520.

34. Mankowski E, Brock-Utne JG, Downing JW. Nitrous oxide elimination by the newborn. *Anaesthesia*. 1981, 36:1014–1016.

35. Datta S, Ostheimer GW, Weiss JB, et al. Neonatal effects of prolonged anesthetic induction for cesarean section. *Obstet Gynecol*. 1981:58: 331–335.

36. Janeczko GF, el-Etr AA, Younes S. Low dose ketamine anesthesia for obstetrical delivery. *Anesth Analg*. 1974, 53:828–831.

37. Abboud TK, Zku J et al. Intravenous propofol vs thiamylal-isoflurane for cesarean section, comparative maternal and neonatal effects. *Acta Anaesthesiol Scand*. 1995 39:205–209.

38. Alon E, Ball EH, Gillie MH, et al. Effects of propofol and thiopental on maternal and fetal cardiovascular and acid base variables in the

pregnant ewe. *Anesthesiology.* 1993 78:562–576.

39. Knuppel ZA, Hatangandi SB. Acute hypotension related to hemorrhage in the obstetric patient. *Obstet Gynecol Clin NA.* 1995:22:111–129.

40. Sullivan JM, Ramanathan KB. Management of medical problems in pregnancy: Severe cardiac disease. *N Engl J Med.* 1985, 313:304–309.

41. Schatz M. Asthma during pregnancy: interrelationships and management. *Ann Allergy.* 1992:68:123–133.

42. Bader AM, Hunt CO, Datta S, et al. Anesthesia for the pregnant patient with multiple sclerosis. *J Clin Anesth.* 1988:1:21.

43. Wanner MB, Rageth CJ, Zach GA. Pregnancy and autonomic hyperreflexia in the patients with spinal cord lesions. *Paraplegia.* 1987:25:482.

44. Emergency Cardiac Care Committee and Subcommittees, American Heart Association. Guidelines for cardiopulmonary resuscitation and emergency cardiac care. *JAMA.* 1992 268:2199–2241.

45. Fisgus JR. Cardiopulmonary resuscitation in pregnancy. *Progress in Anesthesiology.* 1995, 9:243–249.

BIBLIOGRAPHY

Chestnut DH. *Obstetric Anesthesia: Principles and Practice.* 1994, Mosby-Year Book Inc.

Datta S. *Obstetric Anesthesia Handbook*, 2nd Ed. 1995 Mosby-Year Book Inc.

Bonica JJ, McDonald JS. *Principles and Practice of Obstetric Analgesia and Anesthesia*, 2nd Ed. Baltimore: Williams & Wilkins, 1994.

Datta S. *Anesthesia for Obstetrics Management of the High Risk Pregnancy*, 2nd Ed. Mosby Yearbook Inc., 1995.

Clark SL, Cotton DB, Hankins GD, Phelan JP. *Critical Care Obstetrics*, 2nd Ed. New York: Blackwell Scientific Publications, 1991.

QUESTIONS
(choose the single best answer)

1. The pregnant patient having general anesthesia is at increased risk all of the following except:
   a. Failed intubation
   b. Cardiac arrest
   c. Aspiration
   d. Aortocaval compression
   e. Hypoxemia

2. Which statement about pregnancy is false:
   a. Patients are considered to have full stomachs after the 14th week gestation
   b. Gastrin levels are increased
   c. All patients receive H_2 blockers before surgery
   d. Gastric reflux is common in the third trimester
   e. Parenteral narcotics hinder gastric emptying

3. Which statement is true:
   a. Diazepam effects beat-to-beat variability
   b. Midazolam is equipotent with diazepam
   c. Promethazine has significant alpha adrenergic blocking effects
   d. Hydroxyzine potentiates the fetal depressant effects of narcotics
   e. Secobarbital has minimal neonatal effects

4. Meperidine:
   a. Is ten times as potent as morphine
   b. Causes neonatal depression if delivery is within one hour of administration
   c. Is antagonized by the use of hydroxyzine
   d. Has an active metabolite that may cause neonatal depression
   e. Has a duration of action of 4 to 6 hours

5. Complications of regional anesthesia include all of the following except:
   a. Postdural puncture headache
   b. Intravascular injection
   c. Local anesthetic toxicity
   d. Respiratory arrest
   e. Chorioamnionitis

6. Which regional block is associated with a high incidence of fetal arrhythmias?
   a. Pudendal nerve block
   b. Paracervical block
   c. Combined spinal epidural block
   d. Ilioinguinal-iliohypogastric nerve block
   e. Intrathecal sufentanil administration

7. General anesthesia is indicated for cesarean section if:
   a. It is an emergency
   b. If the patient has multiple sclerosis
   c. If the patient has preeclampsia
   d. If the patient is septic
   e. If the patient has placenta previa

8. Spinal anesthesia's advantages for cesarean de-

livery over epidural anesthesia includes all of the following except:

   a. It is faster in onset
   b. It tends to produce less hypotension
   c. It has a lower failure rate
   d. It requires less local anesthetic
   e. It is unlikely to cause toxicity

9. Which statement is false:

   a. Volatile anesthetic agents are not associated with congenital anomalies
   b. Nitrous oxide has no effect on the neonate if used for cesarean delivery
   c. Nitrous oxide inhibits methionine synthase
   d. Uterine incision to delivery times greater than 3 minutes are associated with neonatal acidosis and lower apgar scores
   e. Volatile inhalational agents produce uterine relaxation in a dose dependent fashion

10. CPR in the pregnant patient after 25 weeks gestation requires all of the following except:

   a. Left uterine displacement
   b. Use of electrical defibrillation if it is indicated by the maternal arrhythmia
   c. Immediate preparations for possible emergency cesarean section
   d. Monitoring of the fetal heart rate
   e. Lower doses of epinephrine due to the changes of pregnancy

20

Neonatal Resuscitation and Intensive Care

M. T. Fundzak and J. J. Moore

INTRODUCTION

Approximately six percent of all deliveries require neonatal resuscitation and stabilization in the delivery room.[1,2] In perinatal centers where high-risk obstetric patients are delivered, this number can rise significantly to as many as 35–40% of all deliveries. In an obstetric service that delivers 4000 newborns a year, this involves anywhere from 240–1600 neonates a year. Because of the large number of newborns at risk, every obstetrical facility must be able to quickly mount a resuscitation team composed of trained individuals who can assist the infant's transition from intrauterine to extrauterine life.

Purpose

At the moment of delivery, the neonate goes through a series of complex changes in the adjustment from intrauterine to extrauterine life. These changes begin with the clamping of the umbilical cord and the first breath.[3,4] They are initiated by the opening of the alveoli for oxygen and carbon dioxide exchange and the cardiac and circulatory adaptations resulting from the changes in the pulmonary vascular resistance. Expansion of the lungs decreases the pulmonary vascular resistance (PVR) and increases the pulmonary blood flow. This shift in the PVR closes the foramen ovale, completing the cardiovascular transition to extrauterine life.[4]

Neonatal resuscitation facilitates these changes when the neonate is compromised or otherwise unable to adapt to extrauterine life. The majority of neonates that require resuscitation at birth, do so as a result of difficulty in respiratory initiation. Ventilatory support is all that is required in the large majority of cases. Much less often a neonate will need cardiovascular support as well. When this occurs, it is usually secondary to prolonged intrauterine asphyxia.

Team Concept

Neonatal resuscitation is most successful with a team approach.[5,6] Individually skilled resuscitators may be ineffective if their efforts are uncoordinated. Each team member should have a designated role in the effort. A team leader is fundamental to the coordination and effectiveness of the resuscitation team. Megacode training sessions with teams formed from each hospital shift significantly improve performance.

RISK FACTORS

When factors which increase the risk of neonatal distress at birth are present prior to an impending delivery, the neonatal resuscitation team should be assembled. Risk factors are anything that increases the probability of distress in the newborn (Tables 20-1–20-3). Distress may result from an interruption in the chain that links the maternal and fetal cardiorespiratory system[7] (see Figure 20-1). Determination of risk factors is important not only to assess the need for a resuscitation team, but also to assess the need for additional procedures that may be necessary to individual cases.

RESUSCITATION TEAM

Neonatal resuscitation is best accomplished by a team. Unless the resuscitation is minimal, three members are needed. Each member should have an assigned role in the resuscitation effort.

Number One Team Member

Team member one is assigned to airway management. This person is generally the most skilled at intubation and/or bag and mask ventilation. This individual should initially dry and position the head. Endotracheal intubation and suctioning for meconium is performed by this member if indicated. Application of oxygen, continuous positive airway pressure (CPAP), positive pressure ventilation, and intubation of the infant is also performed by this member if necessary.

Table 20-1. Maternal Risk Factors

No prenatal care
Substance abuse with maternal and/or fetal distress
Toxemia/preeclampsia/pregnancy-induced hypertension
Insulin-dependent diabetes
Maternal fever > 38°C. With signs of infection, such as increased white blood cell count with a shift to the left or foul-smelling amniotic fluid
Vaginal bleeding beyond expected, such as with placental abruption, placenta previa, etc.

Table 20-2. Labor and Delivery Risk Factors

Nonvertex presentations delivering vaginally (breech, face, brow)
Emergency cesarean sections
Cord prolapse
Placenta previa and/or abruptio
Use of mid-forceps or mid-vacuum
Difficult delivery, particularly a shoulder dystocia
Use of general anesthesia
Delivery outside the labor and delivery area (on the antenatal floor or in the emergency department)

Number Two Team Member

Number two is responsible for the assessment and for the evaluation of the effectiveness of interventions performed during the neonatal resuscitation. Assessment begins prior to delivery. Information to be obtained prior to delivery includes at a minimum: (1) the gestational age; (2) the number of newborn infants; (3) the presence and degree of meconium stained fluid; (4) maternal blood loss; (5) signs of fetal distress; and (6) any anomalies.

This member should observe the birth, receive the newborn infant from the obstetrician/nurse midwife, and carry the infant to the radiant warmer. Observation during the birth should include ruling out late meconium and fetal blood loss. A quick physical exam should be done to identify anomalies relevant to resuscitation (omphalocele, gastroschisis, or scaphoid abdomen suggestive of diaphragmatic hernia).

Member two stimulates and performs the initial evaluation of the infant's status while member one is drying and positioning the head. Thereafter, with each intervention, this second

Table 20-3. Fetal/Neonatal Risk Factors

Meconium-stained fluid
Abnormal fetal heart rates (either tachycardia or bradycardia)
Late decelerations
Persistent loss of the fetal heart rate variability
Congenital anomalies
Gestational age less than or equal to 35 weeks
Small for gestational age (IUGR) or large for gestational age (LGA)
Multiple gestations

Levels at Which Fetal Distress Occurs	Condition	Fetal Signs/Symptoms
Maternal	Hypoxia	Fetal tachycardia
	Shock	Fetal hypoxia
	Drugs	Respiratory depression
Uterine circulation	Anesthesia	Decreased placental circulation
	Maternal vascular disease	Fetal hypovolemia
	Acute blood loss	
Placenta/cord		Fetal hypovolemia
	Obstruction	Fetal bradycardia
	Acute blood loss	Fetal hypoxia
Baby	Meconium	Airway obstruction
	Infection	Shock/DIC
	Congenital anomalies	Ascites
	Hemolytic disease	
Drugs/Toxins		Hypotonia, septic shock

Figure 20-1. Fetal distress. DIC = disseminated intravascular coagulation.

member performs an assessment in the following sequence: effectiveness of intervention, breath sounds, heart rate, color, and perfusion.

The effectiveness of the intervention is assessed first to preclude proceeding to further interventions if the current intervention is not being satisfactorily performed (e.g., chest compression or giving medications without adequate ventilation).

If chest compressions are necessary, member two performs these. In this case, the assessment function must be performed by an additional team member.

Number Three Team Member

Team member three documents the resuscitation as it occurs. A form for documenting the interventions and evaluations of these interventions should be completed as part of each delivery (see Figure 20-2). When extraordinary resuscitation measures are required, recording may have to be suspended to allow the team member to perform these activities.

If the resuscitation effort requires volume expansion and intravenous access, member number three is responsible for umbilical line insertion and infusion of fluids and medications. If the resuscitation becomes even more complex, extra hands beyond the three basic resuscitation members are required. The job assignments for these members are dictated by the clinical situation.

RESUSCITATION SEQUENCE

Anticipation and preparation are critical to successful neonatal resuscitation. Anticipation requires a dialogue between obstetric and neonatal teams.

Once the team is in place and the delivery is eminent, preparation also includes: gathering and checking the appropriate equipment needed for the anticipated neonate. Check for working order of the bag and mask ventilation system, laryngoscope and blade, and select the right size equipment for resuscitation (see Table 20-4). It is here that the key information indicated previously is useful. That information includes:

- How many infants are expected—how many resuscitation set-ups and resuscitators must be assembled?
- What is the gestational age of the expected baby—what size equipment should be placed at the bedside?
- Is there evidence of meconium—should plans be made for intubation or removal of meconium?
- Is there evidence of fetal blood loss—should plans be made for early volume replacement (umbilical venous catheter tray, fluids)?

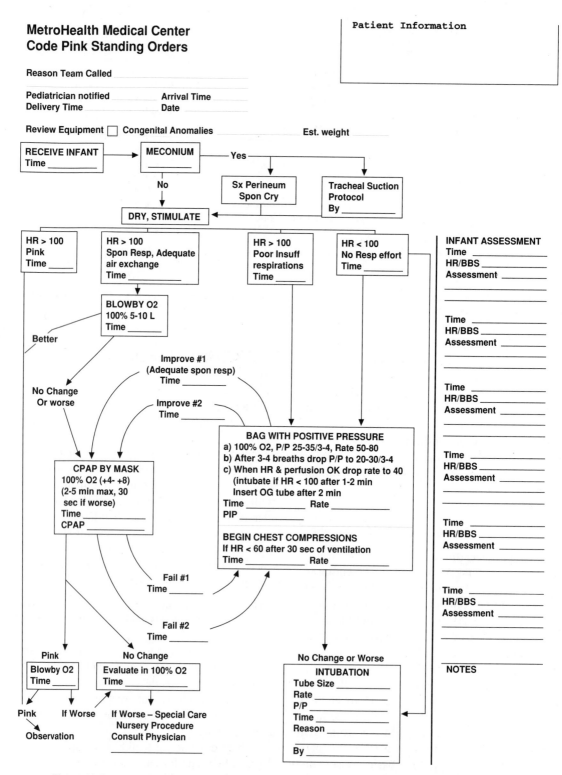

Figure 20-2. Resuscitation documentation. Sx, suctioned; HR, heart rate; BBS, bilateral breath sounds; P/P, peak inspiratory pressure/peak end expiratory pressure; CPAP, continuous positive airway pressure.

INTUBATION / PPV

Improvement after Intubation

No Change or Worse

CHECK / ADJUST OETT
Time _____
Reintubate　　YES　　NO
Tube Size _____
Pressure (20-30/3-4) Rate (50-60)

Improved

VENTILATION ADEQUATE - HR PERFUSION, WORSE OR NO CHANGE
Continue chest compressions
Time _____
Give Epi OETT 1/10,000 (0.1 mg/ml)
0.5 plus 1 cc NS

Improved

No Change or Worse

RECHECK OETT　　Time _____
Continue CPR
Insert UVC　　Time _____
Volume expander 10-20cc/kg IV
Over 1-2 min May be repeated
Every 5-10 min
Normal Saline　　Packed RBCs
Ringer's Lactate
Time _____　Dose _____
Repeat Epi per above q 3-5 min
Time _____

Improved

No Change or Worse

CONTINUE CPR
Epi per above　Time _____
NaHCO3 (0.5 mEq/ml) IV
(2mEq/kg, 1st dose) over 2 min
Time _____　Dose _____
Repeat 1 mEq/kg q 5-10 min

EVALUATE WITH OETT
PPV, O2
Stop Compressions

No Change or Worse

CONTINUE CPR
Get CXR, assess OETT, R/O Pneumo
Thorax, ABGs, Hct
Further instruction from physician

INFANT ASSESSMENT
Time _____
HR/BBS _____
Assessment _____
_____
_____

Time _____
HR/BBS _____
Assessment _____
_____
_____

Time _____
HR/BBS _____
Assessment _____
_____
_____

Time _____
HR/BBS _____
Assessment _____
_____
_____

Time _____
HR/BBS _____
Assessment _____
_____
_____

Time _____
HR/BBS _____
Assessment _____
_____
_____

NOTES

INFANT DISPOSITION

Apgars	RR	HR	Color	Tone	Activity	Total
1 min						
5 min						
10 min						
15 min						
20 min						

Team Members

_____
_____
_____

Recorder _____
Date _____ Time _____
Physician signature _____
Parental Consultation　Yes　No

DRUG TABLE	DOSE	TIME	ROUTE
1. Epi #1			
2. Epi #2			
3. Vol #1			
4. Epi #3			
5. Vol #2			
6. HCO3 #1			
7. Epi #4			
8. HCO3 #2			
9. Other			
10. Other			

Figure 20-2. (Continued) OETT, oral endotracheal tube; CPR, cardiopulmonary resuscitation; CXR, chest x-ray; ABG, arterial blood gas.

Table 20-4.   Equipment List for Delivery
                 Room Resuscitation

Ventilation bag in neonatal size (no larger than 750 ml)
Masks of various sizes, full-term and premature size
Oxygen source—preferably wall oxygen with heat and humidity
Suction apparatus
Suction catheters 6, 8, 10 Fr
Infant hat
Cord clamp
Lamps or overhead light
Warming table
Bulb syringe
Eye prophylaxis (dependent on what each institution uses, either erythromycin ointment or silver nitrate)
Vitamin K
Laryngoscope and blades, Miller size 0,1
Various endotracheal tubes, size 2.5, 3.0, 3.5, 4.0 Fr.
Stylet
Umbilical line placement tray
Umbilical catheters, size 3.5, 5.0 Fr
Umbilical tape
Adhesive tape
Benzoin
Scissors
Angiocaths/IV equipment
Heparinized saline

- Are there fetal anomalies—will special procedures be needed to protect exposed tissue (omphalocele, gastroschisis, etc.).

The information gathered from these questions allows the team to anticipate and prepare for the resuscitative needs of the neonate. This should be completed in a minimal amount of time and concurrently with the preparation of the equipment in the delivery room.

Meconium-Stained Fluid

Meconium-stained fluid (MSF) occurs in approximately 12–20% of all deliveries.[1-4] MSF is the most common risk factor requiring the presence of a neonatal resuscitation team in the delivery room.

Resuscitation of infants with MSF begins at the perineum. The obstetric team should thoroughly suction the mouth and nose and hypopharynx prior to the delivery of the abdomen to prevent aspiration of the meconium with the first breath.

When particulate/thick MSF is present, signs of fetal distress have been present during labor, or the infant is flaccid/apneic, the airway of the neonate is intubated and cleared before breathing is initiated. Drying and stimulation of the infant is delayed until this is accomplished. The neonate is placed on the radiant warmer and immediately intubated and suctioned. A meconium adapter is used with the wall suction permitting the use of the endotracheal tube as a suction catheter. The endotracheal tube is used rather than a standard suction catheter because of the wider inside diameter of the catheter for the removal of particulate matter. Repeated intubations with endotracheal suctioning are accomplished until no meconium is seen in the ET tube. Once the endotracheal tube is clear or two minutes have elapsed, the suction sequence is discontinued and drying, stimulation, and initial assessment are performed as described below.

If MSF is nonparticulate/thin, the resuscitation sequence may proceed one of two ways. If the neonate has been suctioned at the perineum and the neonate is active and crying at delivery, endotracheal intubation with suctioning is not necessary. Once the infant is crying and active, it is thought that the risk of trauma from performing the intubation is greater than the benefit of clearing the meconium.[8] If the infant is flaccid, however, the trachea is intubated and suctioned in the same manner as particulate/thick MSF (see Figure 20-3).

Immediately after Delivery

When the neonate is born, team member two receives the infant from the obstetrical team and places him/her under a radiant warmer. The neonate is positioned supine with the head in a neutral position, suctioned with a bulb syringe to removal oral and nasal secretions, and then dried and stimulated. Tactile stimulation is performed by rubbing the back along the spine. The wet linen is removed and the infant is placed on a warm, dry blanket.

Initial assessment focuses on the newborn's respiratory status. Air exchange rather than

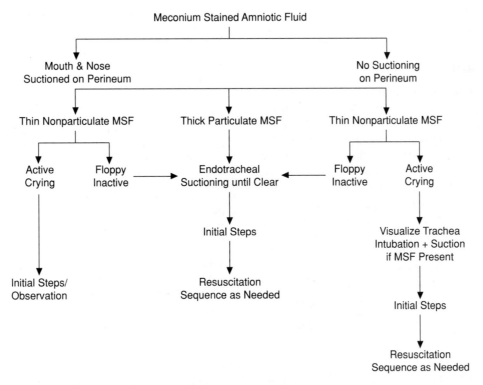

Figure 20-3. Meconium-stained fluid (MSF) decision tree.

chest wall motion must be assessed by auscultation. If air exchange is adequate, the heart rate is assessed. If the heart rate is greater than 100, the neonate's color and perfusion are evaluated. If the neonate is pink and well perfused, the infant is observed and the resuscitation effort is completed.

If after completing this initial evaluation, the neonate has adequate spontaneous respiratory effort and a heart rate greater than 100, but remains cyanotic, blowby oxygen is indicated. This is administered by free flow oxygen near the neonate's face. As the neonate's color improves, the free flow oxygen is withdrawn slowly, observing the neonate's color as the oxygen is gradually withdrawn.

Assisted Ventilation

Positive pressure ventilation (PPV) with a bag and mask is indicated whenever the new-

born has ineffective respiratory effort (gasping and/or poor air exchange), apnea, or HR < 100 following stimulation. Ventilation is initiated with 100% oxygen at a rate of 60–80 breaths per minute. Initial (3–4 breaths) inflation pressures are 25–30/4 mmHg with subsequent inflation pressures between 18–20/4 mmHg based on the newborn's chest rise and air exchange. The rate of artificial ventilation should be lowered to 40 breaths per minute when good heart rate and perfusion are established. In prematures, pressures 3–5 mmHg lower are appropriate.

PPV is continued until spontaneous respiratory effort is established with good air exchange. Once spontaneous respirations begin, the ventilation rate is titrated with the newborn's efforts. The assisted ventilation is weaned until it is eventually decreased to continuous positive airway pressure (CPAP). If at any point the newborn decompensates during the weaning process, PPV is restarted and chest rise, air exchange, heart rate, and color are reevaluated.

Endotracheal Intubation

Endotracheal intubation is indicated when the neonate requires prolonged PPV and/or has respiratory distress in conjunction with a gastrointestinal defect (diaphragmatic hernia, omphalocele, gastroschisis). Infants should be stabilized with bag and mask ventilation prior to endotracheal intubation whenever possible. Most neonates can be bagged and mask ventilated until endotracheal intubation can be performed electively.

Endotracheal intubation should be performed as a two-person procedure. The intubator requires assistance of a second person to hand the endotracheal tube, connect the bag apparatus to the tube, and to help with taping and stabilizing of the endotracheal tube. See Figures 20-4 and 20-5 for an overview of the procedure.

Once the endotracheal tube is placed and secured with tape, placement must be confirmed. It is confirmed clinically by breath sounds and chest rise, secondly by depth of insertion, and finally by a chest x-ray.

Cardiac Compressions

Cardiac compressions are rarely needed during a delivery room resuscitation. When they are needed, it is usually as a result of prolonged intrauterine asphyxia. Chest compressions are begun when the heart rate is zero at delivery or less than 60 beats per minute after ventilation has been established. Ventilation must be effective prior to the initiation of chest compressions or the effort will be fruitless. Many times the neonate is electively intubated prior to the initiation of chest compressions. Chest compressions are done at a rate of 90 compressions per minute in a 3:1 ratio with ventilation. This requires coordination between the airway manager and the person performing the chest compressions.

After 30 seconds of chest compressions, the heart rate is evaluated. If the heart rate is 80 or

1. Determine equipment required, check for working order.
   Appropriate size endotracheal tube
   Stylet
   Laryngoscope and blade
   Suction with appropriate sized catheter, 6 Fr
   Adhesive tape
   Benzoin
   Oxygen source
   Bag and mask, size appropriate
2. Insert stylet into oral endotracheal tube and secure by bending over the oral endotracheal tube adapter.
3. Insert the laryngoscope and blade into the infant's mouth.
4. Visualize the epiglottis and vocal cords.
5. Insert endotracheal tube into trachea. See Figure 20-5 for depth of insertion.
6. Hold the tube in place, remove laryngoscope and blade. Remove stylet from the oral endotracheal tube.
7. Bag the neonate, assess breath sounds over apex of lungs and over the stomach. Adjust placement as needed.
8. Tape tube into place.
9. Confirm placement with chest x-ray.

Figure 20-4.   Steps in endotracheal intubation.

greater, the chest compressions are discontinued, and PPV is continued until the neonate is stable. If after 30 seconds of chest compressions the heart rate is still less than 80, chest compressions are restarted at the same 3:1 ratio, and PPV is continued.

Medications (See Table 20-5)

Medications are used in a neonatal resuscitation when ventilation and chest compressions are not effective. The medications used in neonatal resuscitation are designed to increase the heart rate, increase fluid volume, and/or stabilize acid-base balance.[3] The medication list for neo-

Tube Size	Neonate Weight	Insertion Length (Tip to Lip)
2.5 Fr	<1 kg	6 cm
3.0 Fr	1–2 kg	7 cm–8
3.5 Fr	2–3 kg	8 cm–9
4.0 Fr	>3.5 kg	9 cm–10

Figure 20-5.   Endotracheal tube sizes.

Table 20-5. Neonatal Resuscitation Medications

Drug	Indications	Dose	Dilution	Side Effects or Precautions
Adrenalin (Epinephrine)	To restore myocardial contractility in cardiac arrest—given for flat line EKG or persistent bradycardia. Will increase BP.	0.5 cc	1:10,000 IV/ET rapidly, ET follow with NS 1 cc	Rise in BP with cerebrovascular hemorrhage from overdose. Tachyarrhythmias.
Normal saline 5% albumin or O negative blood	Shock for volume expansion Shock for volume expansion	10–20 cc/Kg 10–20 cc/Kg	IV over 5–10 minutes IV over 5–10 minutes	Transfusion reaction. Transmission of infection.
Sodium bicarbonate 4.2%	Metabolic acidosis which occurs in cardiac arrest.	2 meq/Kg	0.5 meq/cc IV (1 meq/kg/min)	High sodium levels, hyperosmolarity, intracranial hemorrhage, adequate ventilation should be established.
Narcan (Naloxone hydrochloride)	Narcotic depression	0.1 mg/Kg	0.1 mg/cc (0.1 cc/Kg) Give rapidly IV, ET, IM, SQ 0.4 mg/cc (.25 cc/Kg)	Contraindicated if mother is suspected narcotic user (will put infant into withdrawal). Observe infant for recurrent respiratory depression, as Narcan's effect may be shorter than the narcotic's effect.
Dextrose 10%	Hypoglycemia, blood sugar below 30 mg per 100 ml	2 cc/Kg IV	10% bolus, then 3–4 cc/kg/hr continuous	Hyperglycemia. Retake dextrostix in 10 minutes and at least every 30 minutes thereafter. Use infusion pump to regulate.

natal resuscitation (see Table 20-5) is short and consists of the following:

1. Epinephrine: Epinephrine is indicated when the heart rate is zero or less than 60 with effective ventilation. It has a rapid onset of action and is easily administered through the endotracheal tube or intravenously.

2. Volume Expanders: Volume expanders are indicated in the neonate when there is an acute blood loss or there are signs and symptoms of hypovolemia. The latter may be present in asphyxia. The neonate may be pale, have weak to absent pulses with poor perfusion and severe peripheral vasoconstriction. Fluids are administered via the umbilical vein through an umbilical catheter. The fluid administered can be normal saline, lactated ringers, 5% albumin, or whole blood. Blood products are generally reserved for those instances when acute blood loss has occurred (cord accident, placental abruption).

3. Narcan: Narcan (Naloxone) is indicated for a neonate when the mother has received a narcotic analgesia within 4 hours of delivery and the neonate shows signs of respiratory depression after birth. Narcan, however, is not indicated for neonates born to narcotically addicted mothers. Narcan given to these neonates may elicit withdrawal symptoms and seizures.

4. Sodium Bicarbonate: Sodium bicarbonate is indicated during the neonatal resuscitation if the effort is prolonged (longer than 10–15 minutes) or there is documentation of a metabolic acidosis. In order for the drug to be effective, the neonates must be properly ventilated. Without effective ventilation, the sodium bicarbonate will be converted to CO_2, increasing respiratory acidosis. Sodium bicarbonate is administered IV via the umbilical vein or peripheral IV, and may be given every 10 minutes as necessary. Sodium bicarbonate should be administered slowly because of its osmolarity. A rapid infusion has been shown to contribute to intraventricular hemorrhage, particularly in premature neonates.[3]

STABILIZATION

The stabilization period begins once the neonatal resuscitation is completed. During this time period, it is important to maintain a neutral thermal environment for the neonate. This may require additional heat sources such as warming pads and extra blankets.

Depending on the status of the neonate, stabilization may take place in the delivery room or in a nursery setting. If facilities for a special care nursery or neonatal intensive care nursery are available, unstable neonates are transferred for further treatment.

A newborn is considered stable after the resuscitation if: (1) the temperature is normal and stable; (2) glucose level is within normal limits; (3) blood gases are monitored and acceptable; (4) hematocrit is stable and not dropping; and (5) chest x-ray is completed and read.

CONCLUSION

The transition to extrauterine life for the neonates is usually uneventful, but a coordinated, skilled neonatal resuscitation team must be available to support those neonates who need assistance with this transition.

REFERENCES

1. Neonatal resuscitation. *JAMA.* 1992;268:2276–2281.

2. Schuman, AJ. Neonatal resuscitation: What you need to know. *Contemp Pediatr.* 1991;6:92–114.

3. Bloom RS, Cropley C, eds. *Textbook of Neonatal Resuscitation.* AHA/AAP Neonatal Resuscitation Program Steering Committee.

4. Fanaroff AA, Martin RJ, eds. Delivery room resuscitation of the newborn. In: *Neonatal Perinatal Medicine Diseases of the Fetus and Infant,* vol. 1. St. Louis: Mosby Year Book, Inc., 1992, 301–324.

5. Moore JJ, Andrews L, Henderson C, Zuspan KJ, and Hertz RH. Neonatal resuscitation in community hospitals: A regional-based, team oriented training program coordinated by the terti-

ary center. *Am J Obstet Gynecol.* 1989; 161: 849–855.

6. Bailey C, Kattwinkel J. Establishing a neonatal resuscitation team in community hospitals. *J Perinat.* 1990;X:294–300.

7. Aucott S, Moore JJ. Neonatal Resuscitation. *Manual of Obstetrics and Gynecology,* Iams J, Zuspan F, eds. St. Louis: CV Mosby, 1990;231–244.

8. Cunningham AS. When to suction the meconium stained newborn? *Contemp Pediatr.* 1993;1:91–109.

9. *Guidelines for Perinatal Care.* Third Ed. American Academy of Pediatrics/American College of Obstetricians and Gynecologists, 1992. Developed through the cooperative efforts of the AAP Committee on Fetus and Newborn and the ACOG Committee on Obstetrics: Maternal and Fetal Medicine.

QUESTIONS

1. Bag and mask ventilation with positive pressure should be done:
   a. With all newborn infants
   b. With apnea, gasping newborn infants
   c. With abdominal defects
   d. None of the above

2. Endotracheal intubation for meconium suction is:
   a. Done for all meconium stained infants
   b. Best done by a person skilled in endotracheal intubation
   c. Done when the newborn is flaccid and not breathing
   d. B and C

3. Neonatal resuscitation is best performed:
   a. By one individually skilled person
   b. When a team approach is used
   c. By anyone in the delivery room

4. Chest compressions in neonates are:
   a. Done whenever the heart rate is less than 60
   b. Require effective ventilation prior to the initiation of
   c. Performed in a 3:1 ratio with ventilations
   d. All of the above

5. Neonatal resuscitation requires medications for:
   a. All deliveries
   b. A heart rate of zero at delivery
   c. Respiratory depression

21

Perinatal Pathology

Josephine Wyatt-Ashmead

PREGNANCY LOSS

The loss of a baby in utero or ex utero is an abnormal event. Finding the cause of the loss depends on combined information obtained from the parents, their health care providers, and perinatal pathologist. Unless the etiology of the pregnancy loss is searched for in each instance, a cause will not be found.

Knowing the reason(s) for the parent's loss helps them focus on the cause and not blame themselves or others. After a time of grieving which varies with each couple, understanding and identifying the cause ought to help the parents plan future pregnancies.

The following chapter is prepared to help others to look for the cause or causes of pregnancy loss and console the parents.

EXAMINATION OF THE PRODUCTS OF CONCEPTION TO FIND THE CAUSE OF PREGNANCY LOSS

The products of conception (POC) (embryonic and extraembryonic tissues) must be examined. Consent for the pathologic examination of the baby (embryo-fetus-neonate) and the extraem-

bryonic tissues (gestational sac-placenta) must be obtained from the parents or parent's guardian. After the parents have had an opportunity to be with their baby, the POC must get to the perinatal pathologist.

The perinatal pathologist needs the baby, the extraembryonic tissues (gestational sac-placenta), and clinical history to determine the cause of pregnancy loss. Without all the pieces, the puzzle cannot be completed (see flowsheet in Figure 21-1).

Embryonic Tissues

Determination of sex is critical to the parents. In immature babies, the external genitalia may be easily confused. The large clitoris is often mistaken for a penis. If the sex is in doubt, then one should wait for pathologic confirmation by external and internal examination. If, after external and internal examination, the genitalia are still ambiguous, then one should wait for cytogenetics studies before telling the parents the sex of their baby.

For example, one set of parents pressed the resident to tell them the sex of their baby who had died in utero. They were told by the resident that the baby was a boy. They named the baby after the father and chiseled the name in a gran-

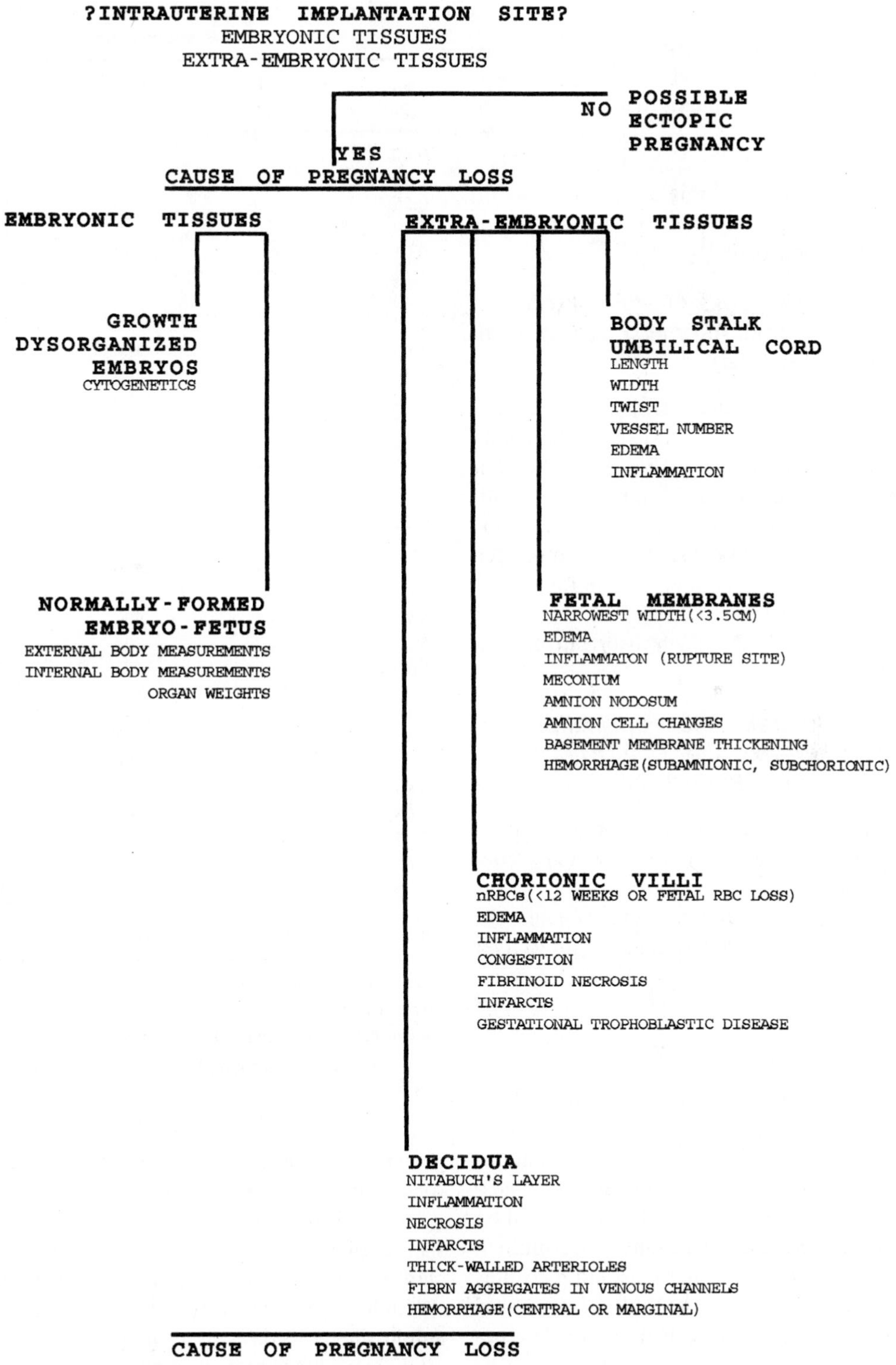

?INTRAUTERINE IMPLANTATION SITE?
EMBRYONIC TISSUES
EXTRA-EMBRYONIC TISSUES

NO **POSSIBLE
ECTOPIC
PREGNANCY**

YES
CAUSE OF PREGNANCY LOSS

EMBRYONIC TISSUES   **EXTRA-EMBRYONIC TISSUES**

**GROWTH
DYSORGANIZED
EMBRYOS**
CYTOGENETICS

**BODY STALK
UMBILICAL CORD**
LENGTH
WIDTH
TWIST
VESSEL NUMBER
EDEMA
INFLAMMATION

FETAL MEMBRANES
NARROWEST WIDTH (<3.5CM)
EDEMA
INFLAMMATON (RUPTURE SITE)
MECONIUM
AMNION NODOSUM
AMNION CELL CHANGES
BASEMENT MEMBRANE THICKENING
HEMORRHAGE (SUBAMNIONIC, SUBCHORIONIC)

**NORMALLY-FORMED
EMBRYO-FETUS**
EXTERNAL BODY MEASUREMENTS
INTERNAL BODY MEASUREMENTS
ORGAN WEIGHTS

CHORIONIC VILLI
nRBCs (<12 WEEKS OR FETAL RBC LOSS)
EDEMA
INFLAMMATION
CONGESTION
FIBRINOID NECROSIS
INFARCTS
GESTATIONAL TROPHOBLASTIC DISEASE

DECIDUA
NITABUCH'S LAYER
INFLAMMATION
NECROSIS
INFARCTS
THICK-WALLED ARTERIOLES
FIBRN AGGREGATES IN VENOUS CHANNELS
HEMORRHAGE (CENTRAL OR MARGINAL)

CAUSE OF PREGNANCY LOSS

Figure 21-1. Products of conception flowsheet. nRBC, nucleated red blood cells.

ite tombstone. A month later, when the parents were going over the autopsy findings, the parents were distressed to find out their baby was actually a girl. They thought that if the resident was mistaken about the sex, then the resident might have mixed babies up altogether. They thought that their baby might be still alive or, at least, might not have all the malformations attributed to their baby.[1-7]

Embryo (<8 Weeks After Fertilization and <10 Weeks After First Day of Last Menstrual Period)

The embryo must successfully reach certain milestones which can be seen using a dissecting scope or magnifying glass. For example, four limb buds can be seen at 28 days after fertilization, finger rays can be seen by 41 days, toe rays can be seen by 44 days, elbows can be seen by 50 days, etc. If the embryo fails to form completely or the embryo fails to form normally, then the embryo is a growth-disorganized embryo.

Fetus (>8 Weeks After Fertilization and >10 Weeks After First Day of Last Menstrual Period)

Although the fetus has all the organ systems formed, the fetus and the organ systems continue to grow at a certain rate (see Table 21-1). Normally, the head circumference equals the crown-rump length and the brain weight to liver weight ratio equals 3:1.

Extraembryonic Tissues

The gestational sac-placenta is a diary of the pregnancy. Pathologic examination of the gestational sac-placenta may show changes that impact the baby as well as the mother. Every gestational sac and placenta should be examined by a perinatal pathologist. If resources are limited, then, at least, the gestational sacs and placentas of complicated pregnancies (Table 21-2) should be examined by a perinatal pathologist. If a perinatal pathologist is not available in your institution, then the complicated gestational sac or

Table 21-1.   Foot Length, Crown-Rump Length, Body Weight, and Gestational Age

Foot Length[a]	Crown-Rump Length[a]	Body Weight[b]	Gestational Age[c]
0.42	2.7	1	8
0.46	3.1	2	9
0.55	4.0	4	10
0.69	5.0	7	11
0.91	6.1	14	12
1.14	7.4	25	13
1.40	8.7	45	14
1.68	10.1	70	15
1.99	11.6	100	16
2.30	13.0	140	17
2.68	14.2	190	18
3.07	15.3	240	19
3.33	16.4	300	20
3.52	17.5	360	21
3.95	18.6	430	22
4.22	19.7	501	23
4.52	20.8	600	24
4.77	21.8	700	25
5.02	22.8	800	26
5.27	23.8	900	27
5.52	24.7	1001	28
5.70	25.8	1175	29
5.92	26.5	1350	30
6.12	27.4	1501	31
6.30	28.3	1675	32
6.50	29.3	1825	33
6.82	30.2	2001	34
7.05	31.1	2160	35
7.35	32.1	2340	36
7.65	33.1	2501	37
7.85	34.1	2775	38
8.10	35.2	3001	39
8.25	36.2	3250	40

[a] Mean lengths in centimeters.
[b] Mean weight in grams.
[c] Gestational age (last menstrual period) in weeks.

Source: Adapted from Streeter QL, Contributions to Embryology 11:143, 1920.

placenta can be sent to a perinatal pathologist for a complete examination.[8-16]

In our institution, we sign out the placentas within 24 hours of receiving them. Our health care providers find the placental information invaluable in making treatment decisions. For example, in these days of short postpartum hospital stays for mother and baby, knowing whether or not the placenta shows an intrauter-

Table 21-2. Indications for Sending the Placenta
to Pathology

Death of baby and/or mother
Multiple gestation
Fetal stress
Growth retardation [symmetric/asymmetric] of baby
Malformations/deformations of baby
Oligohydramnios
Hydramnios
Fetal hydrops
Umbilical cord accidents [tangles/knots/hematoma]
Prematurity
Postmaturity
Infection [ascending/hematogenous]
Maternal vaginal bleeding
Maternal drug use and abuse
Maternal diabetes mellitus
Maternal hypertension
No prenatal care

If in doubt, send it to pathology.

---

ine infection helps in effectively caring for that
mother and baby who may not show evidence
of sepsis for several hours.

Body Stalk/Umbilical Cord

The gastrointestinal tract normally herniates
into the body stalk, but returns to the abdomen
by 10 weeks after fertilization.

The umbilical cord length increases up from
32 centimeters at 20 weeks gestation (LMP) to
60 centimeters at 40 weeks gestation (LMP).
The length increases slowly after 35 weeks gestation (LMP), after the relative volume of amniotic fluid is decreased. At birth, the minimal,
safe, functional length for a normal delivery is
32 centimeters.

The umbilical cord may become narrowed,
especially in case of asymmetric growth retardation with brain sparing and postterm gestations. When the amount of Wharton's jelly decreases, the danger of umbilical cord vessel
compression (vein > arteries) increases.

Most umbilical cords (9 out of 10) have a
left twist.

The umbilical cord normally has three blood
vessels. The vein takes oxygenated blood to the
baby and the two arteries take deoxygenated
blood to the placenta. If an umbilical cord has

only a single artery (incidence 1.5:1000 singleton deliveries), then the baby may have associated anomalies of the genitourinary system (usually ipsilateral) and cardiovascular system.

Normally, the umbilical cord is inserted
slightly eccentrically on the fetal plate of the
placenta. At times, the blastocyst may implant
upside down to form a potentially dangerous
velamentous insertion. At delivery, the unprotected vessels in the membranes may rupture
with massive loss of the baby's blood.

Membranes (Amnion and Chorion)

Normally, the amnion (ectoderm) is composed of flat or short columnar cells overlying
a thin basement membrane and a layer of loose
fibrous tissue. The chorion (mesoderm) is
formed by denser fibrous tissues in which tissue
macrophages exist. Between the amnion and the
chorion is a potential space.

If there is an irritant (meconium, infection) in
the amniotic fluid, then the amnion cells often
become columnarized and necrotic. With certain
irritants like friction, the amnion cells may even
exhibit squamous metaplasia. With irritants and
other stresses like maternal diabetes mellitus, the
amnionic basement membrane may become thick
and glassy. In intrauterine infections, maternal inflammatory cells may infiltrate the amnion.

Edema fluid may collect between the amnion
and chorion. If blood collects between the amnion and chorion, the blood is from the baby and
is often due to avulsion of a vein or artery near
the umbilical cord insertion onto the fetal plate.
The subamnionic hemorrhages can be large
enough to cause hypovolemic shock to the baby.

The chorionic macrophages may ingest meconium in cases of fetal stress or hemosiderin
in cases of placental abruption. In ascending or
hematogenous infections, the chorion may become infiltrated by maternal inflammatory cells.

Chorionic Villi

The chorionic villi are units for exchange of
oxygen and wastes between the baby and the
mother. The exchange is between the baby's
blood in the capillaries of the villi and the moth-

er's blood in the intervillous space. The baby's blood and mother's blood do not normally mix. As the pregnancy advances, the villi branch to increase the surface area for exchange.

In hypoxic-ischemic conditions, the chorionic villi become fibrotic. Fibrotic stroma consumes less oxygen. The villi sprout syncytial knots and form many, small villi which increases the surface area for exchange. The villi may also have increased numbers of capillaries. The capillaries of the villi may become damaged and leak fibrin to form nodules of "fibrinoid necrosis" or rupture to form intravillous hemorrhages. Groups of villi may become infarcted. First, because there is no maternal blood flow to the area, the villi become crowded together and congested in an attempt to extract what little oxygen is available. Later, the trophoblasts and stroma become necrotic and maternal neutrophils pour into the edge of the infarct. Finally, the infarct stains pale pink and ghost-like. Infarcts of varying ages suggest pregnancy-induced hypertension. Infarcts of the same age suggest trauma and abruption.

The chorionic villi may become edematous and crowd out the maternal blood in the intervillous space. This occurs most often in acute ascending amniotic fluid infections in which the infectious organisms and the maternal neutrophils release prostaglandins which cause the villous capillaries to leak. Villous edema may also occur in fetal hydrops from heart failure of the baby, Rhesus incompatibility, and hematogenous intrauterine infection. In the latter two conditions, the baby's red blood cells are destroyed. Extramedullary hematopoiesis is flagrant in the baby's liver which slows down the production of alpha-fetoprotein.

In hematogenous intrauterine infections, the chorionic villi may also develop thick-walled stem vessels, fibrotic stroma, rounded contours, and acute or chronic villitis with matting. At times, viral inclusions in the nuclei and cytoplasm may be recognized. In *Listeria monocytogenes* infections, the villi show subtrophoblastic abscesses.

In maternal diabetes mellitus, the villi vary in maturation from microscopic field to microscopic field. The villi have thick and glassy basement membranes. The stem vessels are thick-walled and hyalinized with intimal proliferation.

The intervillous space may contain hematomas. Subchorionic hematomas (Breus's mole) may break fetal stem vessels in which case fetal blood mixes with maternal blood. Intervillous hematomas in the body of the placenta (Kline's hemorrhage) may show defects on ultrasound examination. Fibrin deposition can also occur in the intervillous space. Intervillous fibrin deposition seems to occur with poor venous outflow of the placenta. In mothers with sickle cell trait or disease, sickled maternal red blood cells may aggregate in the hypoxic environment of the intervillous space. In malaria, the affected maternal red blood cells may also aggregate in the intervillous space. If marked, these intervillous accumulations can keep oxygenated maternal blood from entering the placenta.

Decidua

Grossly, if the decidua is not delivered intact, then there may be fragments of placenta still attached to the mother's uterine wall (placenta accreta) from which the mother may bleed to death.

If there is a hematoma indenting the placenta, then this indicates an abruption. In abruptions at the center of the placenta, the blood may not communicate with the vagina. The silent, central hematomas may push the baby's blood out of the placenta and into the baby. The baby's heart may become overloaded with too much blood too fast and the baby may die quickly. The mother may not bleed too much, but she may develop disseminated intravascular coagulopathy and labor. In abruptions at the margin of the placenta, the mother may bleed to death out into her vagina. The baby may die from lack of oxygen, because the placenta is separated from the uterus and its oxygen supply by clot. In recent abruptions, the placenta may not be indented, but may seem to float on top of a massive clot in the uterus.

The marginal decidua which is the margin of the placental blood supply may show infarction, necrosis, fibrin deposition, and hemorrhage. The hemorrhage may be recent or remote with he- mosiderin-laden macrophages. A placental bed biopsy of the decidua may show hypertensive or diabetic vessel changes.

The decidua may also show infection. A few lymphocytes are normally seen in the decidua, if the mother labored; but acute and chronic in- flammation including plasma cells may be seen in true infections. Rarely, inclusions and orga- nisms may also be seen.

In remote fetal distress, meconium-laden macrophages may be seen in the decidua.

No Embryonic or Extraembryonic Tissues—Rule Out Ectopic Pregnancy

If no embryonic or extraembryonic tissues are found and the decidua exhibits Arias Stella reaction, then an ectopic pregnancy must be ruled out[21] (see below).

Timing of Fetal Stress and Fetal Death (Meconium Passage, Maceration, Growth Retardation)

Little stress is needed to cause a term baby to pass meconium into the amniotic fluid space; but great and often prolonged stress is needed to cause a preterm baby to pass meconium into the amniotic fluid space. Once meconium is in the amnionic fluid space, the amnion cells lining the space become columnarized and necrotic with loss. If the stress subsides, the baby may swallow the meconium-stained amniotic fluid with clearing of the amniotic fluid. The meco- nium (fine, red-yellow granules) is taken up by macrophages (minimum of 3 hours) in the pla- cental membranes. With more time from the in- sult to birth, the meconium-stuffed macrophages travel into the maternal decidua and into the mother's circulation. If the stress continues, the baby may aspirate the meconium-stained amni- otic fluid deep into the lungs. At birth, although no meconium is seen below the vocal cords, the baby may already have massive meconium as- piration.

If a baby dies and is retained in utero, the baby can still be thoroughly examined for anomalies. The degree of maceration can, along with placental examination, give a crude time of death. If the epidermis is slipping off and the underlying dermis is red, then the baby has been dead for <2 days. If the denuded dermis is pink- tan, then the baby has been dead for <7 days. The baby will become gray-tan and dry, the longer the baby is retained in utero. After sev- eral weeks, the baby will become mummified or paper like (papyraceous) and may even fuse to the placental membranes. The degree of mac- eration may be accelerated by edema of the baby, intrauterine infection, and maternal fever.

Even if a grossly malformed baby is mark- edly macerated, tissue for cytogenetic studies can be taken from the placenta which is still receiving blood supply from the mother. The amnion is stripped from the fetal plate to avoid vaginal flora contamination. Then, pieces of the underlying chorion and villi are submitted for culture (Figure 21-2).

CAUSES OF ABNORMAL PREGNANCIES

Ectopic Pregnancy

An ectopic pregnancy is a pregnancy which implants outside the uterine cavity. The most common site for an ectopic pregnancy is in the fallopian tube. The most common cause of an ectopic pregnancy is chronic salpingitis. In chronic salpingitis, the inflamed plicae fuse to form a baffle of the lumen. Sperm may be able to negotiate the baffle to fertilize the egg, but the fertilized egg is too big to make it through the baffle and implant in the uterine cavity.

Once the pregnancy has implanted in the fal- lopian tube, the syncytiotrophoblasts invade vessels in the wall of the fallopian tube. Bleed- ing occurs. The blood and the products of con- ception distend and may rupture the tube. The mother may bleed to death.

The clinical diagnosis of ectopic pregnancy is confirmed by examining the contents of the

SUBAMNIONIC CULTURE OF PLACENTA

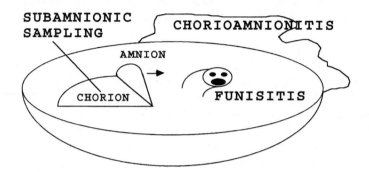

NOTE: SWAB OR TISSUE MAY BE SUBMITTED TO CULTURE FOR ORGANISMS.   TISSUE MAY BE TAKEN FOR CYTOGENETIC STUDIES, TOO.   IN THIS TECHNIQUE, THE CONTAMINATION OF THE PLACENTA BY VAGINAL FLORA IS ELIMINATED.

Figure 21-2.   Chorionic culture technique.

uterine cavity for embryonic and extraembryonic tissues. If no definitive evidence of an implantation site is found and the human chorionic gonadotropin levels remain elevated, then the patient has an ectopic pregnancy.

Treatments of an ectopic pregnancy include Methotrexate, removal of the tube and products of conception, and removal of the products of conception without the tube. The latter salvage procedure may be complicated by rupture, because not all of the invading trophoblasts are removed, and by recurrence of an ectopic pregnancy, because the cause of the ectopic is still present.

Intrauterine Infection

Intrauterine infections may ascend from the mother's vagina or may invade from the mother's blood. Some infectious organisms like *Listeria monocytogenes* may reach the baby by both routes. In our perinatal autopsy population, intrauterine infections account for 30% of the deaths.

Acute Ascending Amniotic Fluid Infection (AFI)

The AFI is the major cause of preterm labor which is resistant to tocolytic agents and pre-

term delivery. The baby may not be infected, but may be delivered too immature to survive *ex utero*.

Small numbers of organisms from the vagina probably infiltrate the placental membranes throughout pregnancy. The bacteriostatic amnionic fluid usually fend these organisms off. However, if the organisms are too great in numbers or are too virulent, then an infection takes hold. A subamnionic culture of the placenta (Figure 21-2) along with cultures of the baby (stomach contents, swabs of ear canals, blood, cerebro-spinal fluid) may identify the infectious organism.

An AFI causes morbidity-mortality of the baby by causing preterm birth, sepsis (Figure 21-3), and hypoxic-ischemic damage due to villous edema (Figure 21-4).

WEAKENING OF PLACENTAL MEMBRANES. The placental membranes become weak due to the effects of the infectious organisms and of the maternal neutrophilic response to the AFI. The weakening of the membranes results in the preterm rupture of the placenta membranes, sudden loss of amniotic fluid, and preterm labor.

PRETERM LABOR.   The AFI, through the infectious organisms and the maternal neutrophil

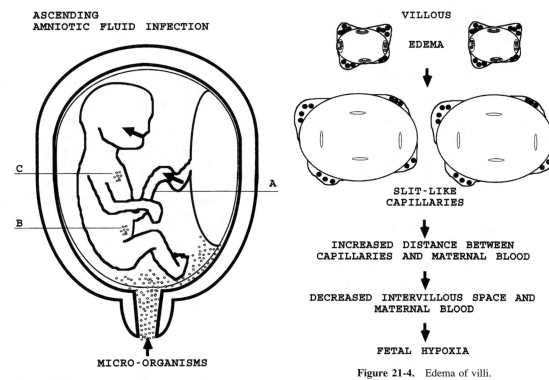

**ASCENDING
AMNIOTIC FLUID INFECTION**

C

B

A

MICRO-ORGANISMS

Figure 21-3. Acute ascending amniotic fluid infection (A = fetal blood percolating through infected vessels of fetal plate; B = ingestion of infected amniotic fluid; C = aspiration of infected amniotic fluid).

VILLOUS

EDEMA

**SLIT-LIKE
CAPILLARIES**

**INCREASED DISTANCE BETWEEN
CAPILLARIES AND MATERNAL BLOOD**

**DECREASED INTERVILLOUS SPACE AND
MATERNAL BLOOD**

FETAL HYPOXIA

Figure 21-4. Edema of villi.

response, releases prostaglandins that cause preterm labor (contractions and cervical dilatation).

SEPSIS OF BABY [FETUS AND NEWBORN]. The baby may become infected by several routes (Figure 21-3).

The baby's blood precolates through the infected membranes of the placenta.

The baby swallows the infected amniotic fluid.

If stressed, the baby may aspirate the infected amniotic fluid.

VILLOUS EDEMA WITH CROWDING OUT OF OXYGENATED MATERIAL BLOOD. The prostaglandins released during the AFI can also cause the villous capillaries to leak. The villi become edematous (Figure 21-4). In edematous villi, the distance between the capillaries and the surface is increased. In addition, the edematous villi crowd out the oxygenated maternal blood from

the intervillous spaces. Consequently, the baby develops hypoxic-ischemic damage.

Hematogenous Infection (Toxoplasmosis, Rubella, Cytomegalovirus, Herpes, Syphilis, Tuberculosis, etc.)

In hematogenous infections, the infectious organism come from the maternal circulation. The villi often show acute and/or chronic villitis. Sometimes the organism or viral inclusions are seen which identify the offending organism. For example, Cytomegalovirus induces the formation of large cells with "owl-like" intranuclear inclusions and cytoplasmic inclusions. A subamnionic culture may help identify the infectious organism (Figure 21-2). The placenta provides a barrier to these hematogenous infections. If, however, the baby becomes infected, the baby often becomes growth retarded with a small head, but a large liver and spleen. Often, the baby's red blood cells are attacked and destroyed. Nucleated red blood cells can be seen in the vessels of the villi which may become edematous.

Malformations of Baby (Fetus and Neonate)

Chromosomal Anomalies (See Genetics Chapter)

When a symmetrically growth retarded baby has multiple, symmetric malformations, chromosomal anomalies should be suspected. The following chromosome anomaly syndromes are particularly common causes of pregnancy loss.[20-21]

TURNER SYNDROME (45, X).   Occurrence is often sporadic and is not related to advanced maternal age. The missing X is usually paternal. Some are mosaic.

The incidence is 1:5000 liveborns, but many die in utero.

Externally (Figure 21-5), the small for gestational age baby girl has a wide chest with widely spaced breast buds and anomalies of her lymphatic system. The dorsum of her hands and feet are often swollen (lymphedema). Cystic hygromas may be present along both sides of her posterior neck. The cystic hygromas are probably due to failure of the thoracic ducts to drain into the jugular veins. The cystic hygromas may act as a sink for protein and fluid. The baby may become intravascular volume depleted and hydropic and die. If the cystic hygromas resolve (drain into jugular vein or rupture), then a web

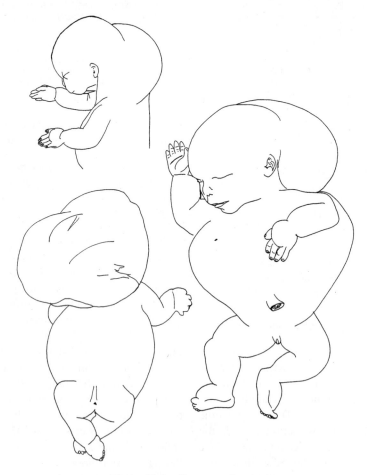

Figure 21-5.   Turner syndrome.

neck will develop. Cystic hygromas and web neck may occur in babies with other chromosomal anomalies including Trisomy 21 and Tetraploidy.

Internally, the baby girl may have a hypoplastic aortic arch or other anomalies of the aorta and the aortic valve and dysplastic ovaries. In mosaic 45, X/46, XY, tumors may develop in the dysplastic gonads.

If the baby girl is liveborn, she may only have lymphedema of the dorsum of her hands and feet which resolves quickly. If the lymphedema is not recognized, she may be lost to follow up until she returns as a teenager with short height and late menarche.

In Turner-like syndrome or Noonan syndrome, the babies (girls or boys) may have a normal karyotype and a hypoplastic pulmonary artery instead of a hypoplastic aortic arch. Noonan syndrome may be autosomal dominant.

TRISOMY 21 (47, XY, +21 OR 47, XX, +21). Occurrence is related to advanced maternal age, because about 92% are due to nondisjunction (70% maternal meiosis I) and about 5% are due to translocation.

The incidence is 1:650 livebirths. Affected boys slightly outnumber the affected girls.

Externally (Figure 21-6), the symmetrically growth retarded baby has a small, round head

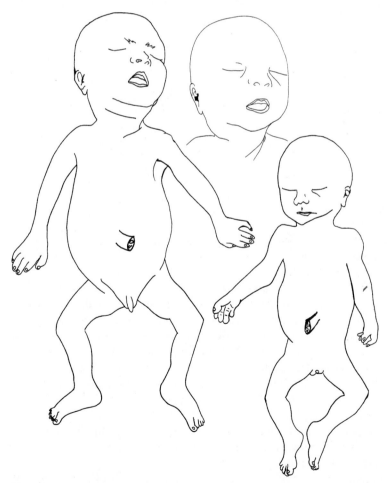

(a)

Figure 21-6A.   Trisomy 21.

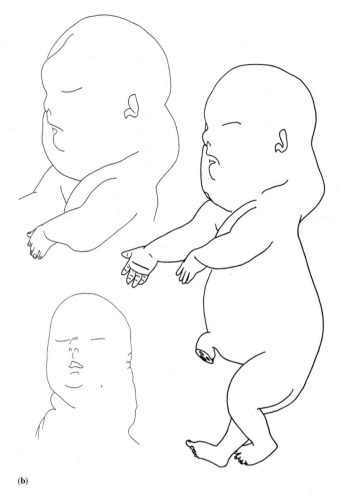

(b)

Figure 21-6B. Trisomy 21. Baby with edema and thick skin folds at back of neck may be confused with a Turner syndrome baby.

with flat occiput. The eyes slant upward and have epicanthal folds. The face is often flat. The tongue often protrudes through the open mouth. Their ears are low-set and square-shaped with a prominent antihelix. The neck is short and may have skin folds (web neck). The posterior hairline is often low. The hands have transverse palmar (simian) creases, because the baby cannot oppose his/her thumbs. Both hands also have short, broad fingers and in-curving fifth finger. There is often a deep cleft between toes 1 and 2 and fusion of toes 2 and 3, bilaterally.

Internally, the brain is round with short frontal lobes and flat occipital lobes. The baby may have major cardiac malformations with the most common and lethal being a common atrioventricular valve. They may have gastrointestinal anomalies including aganglionosis and duodenal atresia with hydramnios and meconium staining of placental membranes.

If liveborn, cardiac malformations and acute leukemia may be life limiting.

If they survive infancy, mental retardation may be severe. In adulthood, they may develop Alzheimer's dementia.

TRISOMY 18 (47, XY, +18 OR 47, XX, +18). Occurrence is related to advanced maternal age,

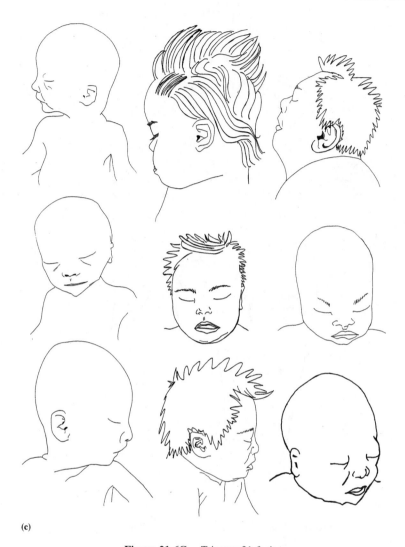

(c)

Figure 21-6C. Trisomy 21 facies.

because about 80% are due to nondisjunction (double primary nondisjunction in 10–15%) and about 10% are due to translocation.

Incidence is 1:7000 livebirths. There is a female predominance (Male:Female = 1:3).

Externally (Figure 21-7), the symmetrically growth retarded baby has a small, but elongate head with prominent occiput. The eyes, mouth, palate (V-shaped), and chin are small. The ear canals are low-set. The dysplastic auricles are backwardly and downwardly rotated. The neck may be short and narrow. The clenched fists (fixed) have fingers two overlapping the other fingers, but these hand anomalies are also seen in Pena-Shokeir syndrome and dominant distal arthrogryposis. The rocker-bottom feet of the Trisomy 18 babies have short, #1 toes.

Internally, the elongate, small brain, especially motor tracts and brain stem nuclei, showed delay in development. They may have cardiac malformations (ventricular septal defect) and gastrointestinal malformations (esophageal

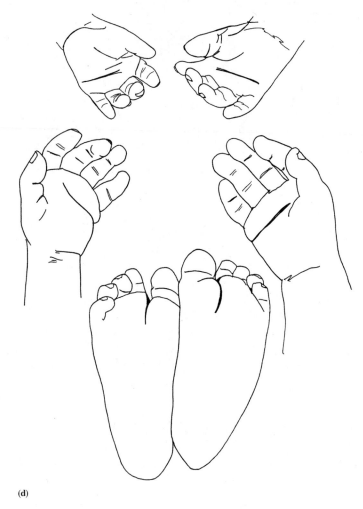

(d)

Figure 21-6D.   Trisomy 21 hand and foot anomalies.

atresia and tracheo-esophageal fistula and ectopic pancreatic tissue and Meckel's diverticulum). They may also have diaphragmatic eventration or defect and renal dysplasia.

If liveborn, the hypotonic baby has difficulty feeding. Even with supportive care, most die within the first few months of life. Girls tend to live longer than boys. A few (10%) live past infancy.

TRISOMY 13 (47, XY, +12 OR 47, XX, +13). Occurrence is related to advanced maternal age, because about 75% are due to nondisjunction and about 20% are due to translocation.

Incidence is 1:12,000 livebirths for nondisjunction and is 1:24,000 livebirths for translocation. There is a slight female predominance.

Externally (Figure 21-8), the symmetrically growth retarded baby often has a small head and facies indicating alobar holoprosencephaly (cyclopia, ethmocephaly, premaxillary agenesis, cebocephaly) or other form of arhinencephaly. The scalp over the parietal-occipital region may show defects of the skin. The hands are clenched with overlapping fingers. There may be postaxial polydactyly of hands and/or feet. The feet have prominent heels and may be rockerbottom.

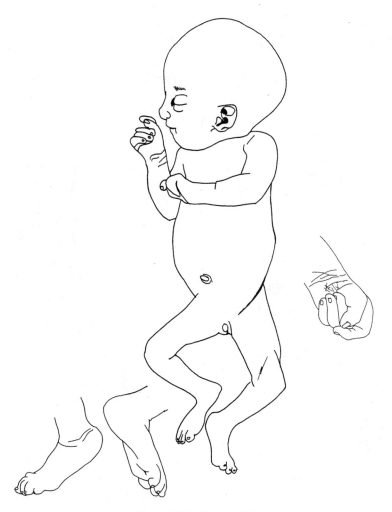

Figure 21-7.   Trisomy 18.

Internally, the small brain may exhibit alobar holoprosencephaly or other form of arhinencephaly. However, one should remember that not all Trisomy 13 babies have arhinencephaly and not all arhinencephaly babies have Trisomy 13. The eyes are small and are narrow-set and even fused. The frontal cranial vault bones may be fused. Cardiac (septal defects), diaphragmatic (eventration), gastrointestinal, and renal anomalies may be found.

If liveborn, the baby, who often does not have a functional nose, may not be able to breath and may die soon after birth. Even with supportive care, these babies often die in infancy.

TRIPLOIDY (69, XXX; 69, XXY; OR 69, XYY). About 65% are due to dispermy. About 25% are due to fertilization of a haploid ovum by a diploid sperm due to abnormal first meiotic division in the father. About 10% are due to a diploid egg due to error in first meiotic division in the mother.

Incidence is 1:2500 livebirths, but most die in utero.

Externally, the growth retarded baby (Figure 21-9) has a large posterior fontanelle (small parietal and occipital cranial vault bones). Some have neural tube defects. Some have facies of arhinencephaly. The eyes and chin are small. The ears are low-set and dysplastic. One side of

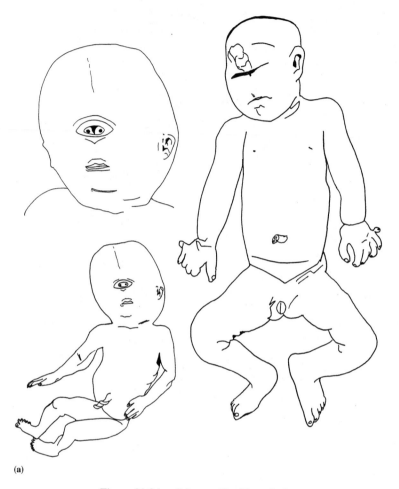

(a)

Figure 21-8A.   Trisomy 13 with cyclopia.

the body may be smaller than the other side. The fingers 3 and 4 are fused. The toes 2 and 3 are less often fused. There may be an omphalocele with hydramnios. In 69, XXY triploids, the external genitalia are hypoplastic; but, in 69, XXX triploids the external genitalia are unremarkable. The bulky, heavy placenta has edematous villi and sometimes partial hydatidiform molar change with pregnancy-induced hypertension.

Internally, the brain may show arhinencephaly. The baby may have septal defects of the heart. Renal dysplasia is not uncommon. The adrenal glands may be hypoplastic. In girls, the ovaries are hypoplastic. In boys, the Leydig cells are hypoplastic.

Most of the 69, XXX triploids are stillborn.

If liveborn, most die within the first day or two. Mosaics, who can be detected with fibroblastic culture of the baby or placenta, often live a normal life span.

Gestational Trophoblastic Disease

All products of conception, whether from spontaneous or elective abortions, should be thoroughly examined for gestational trophoblastic disease in which the hydatidiform mole is the most common. In the complete hydatidiform mole, all the villi have edema, avascularity, cistern formation, and nonpolar trophoblastic proliferation. In the partial hydatidiform mole, only one population of villi show these changes. Villi of the complete or partial hydatidiform moles

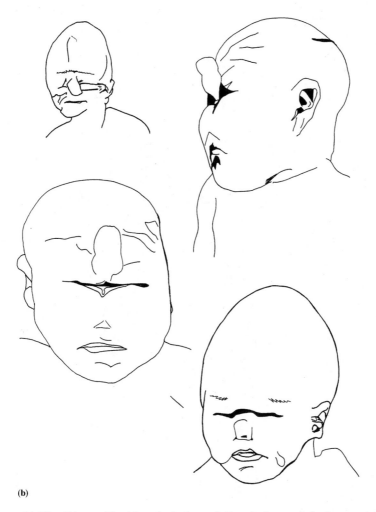

(b)

Figure 21-8B. Trisomy 13 with cyclopia (upper left) and ethmocephaly (bottom right).

must not be confused with degenerating chorionic villi. In choriocarcinoma, sheets of atypical, trophoblasts are seen without villi. In the hydatidiform moles and the choriocarcinoma, the syncytiotrophoblasts seek out and invade vessels to cause massive maternal bleeding.

Central Nervous System Anomalies

NEURAL TUBE DEFECTS [NTDs]. Embryologically, the lateral edges of the neural plate (ectoderm) curl and fuse by a process termed neurulation. The edges fuse in the middle at 22 days from fertilization and then fuse anteriorly and posteriorly. The anterior neuropore fuses completely at 24 days. The posterior neuropore fuses completely at 26 days. If the neural tube fails to fuse, then the various components of the central nervous system remain unfused and open to the amniotic fluid. In addition, the neural crest, mesoderm (cranial vault and dorsal spine and muscle), and skin may fail to fuse.

The remaining caudal spinal cord is formed by canalization. The distal spinal cord resorbs as the tail is resorbed, but the filum terminale continues to have central and peripheral nervous system components and an ependymal cell-lined space.

Later, if there is increased intraventricular

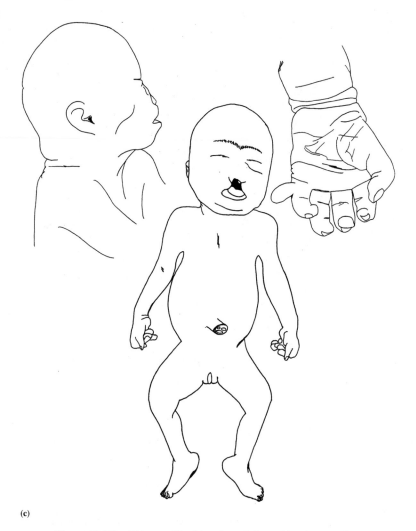

(c)

Figure 21-8C.   Trisomy 13 with cebocephaly and hand anomalies.

pressure, the neural tube may rupture to form skin-covered neural tube defects.

Occurrence of NTDs is increased in people of Scottish, Welsh, Irish, and English ancestry (genetic predisposition) and in malnourished (vitamin B6 deficiency) people.

Incidence is 1:1000 livebirths in most of the United States. If a population has a Scottish, Welsh, Irish, and/or English ancestry and malnutrition, the incidence may be up to 9:1000 livebirths. There is a male:female ratio of 1:2.

If the entire neural plate fails to fuse, then craniorachischisis (splaying of entire brain and

spinal cord) occurs (Figure 21-10). Only the caudal spinal cord will develop properly.

If the anterior neuropore fails to fuse, then anencephaly occurs. With earlier failure, anencephaly, holoacrania type (all cranial vault bones absent), with rostral rachischisis occurs (Figure 21-11). With later failure, anencephaly, meroacrania type (occipital cranial vault bone present), with intact posterior fossa structures occurs (Figure 21-12). In both types of anencephaly, the eyes, which begin to form at 16 days, project above the skull base which is also malformed and convex. These anencephalic ba-

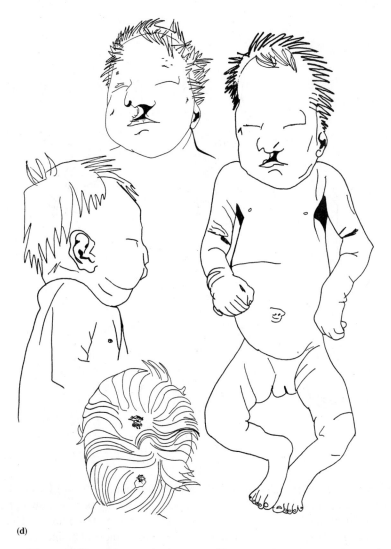

(d)

Figure 21-8D. Trisomy 13 with premaxillary agenesis and scalp defects.

bies have "frog facies." In both types of an-encephaly, a cerebrovascular mass, unprotected by cranial vault bones, is exposed directly to the amniotic fluid at body temperature. In both types, the anterior pituitary, if searched for, is present; but the hypothalamus is not formed properly. With the absent hypothalamic-pituitary connection, the anencephalic baby often has small adrenal glands and a large thymus. With brain absence, the blood shunts to the arms which become overgrown.

The "brain-absent," anencephalic babies can provide an excellent source of organs (kidneys, liver, pancreas, heart) for transplantation to chil-dren and adults. For example, the kidneys can be transplanted in block to a recipient. Within a year, the fetal kidneys grow to adult size. Since the kidneys are fetal, immunosuppressive ther-apy is not needed.

If the posterior neuropore fails to fuse, then a neural tube defect will developed at the dorsal lumbosacral region. The spectrum can range from an open myelomeningocele (Figure 21-13) to a sacral dimple. Even with the open myelo-

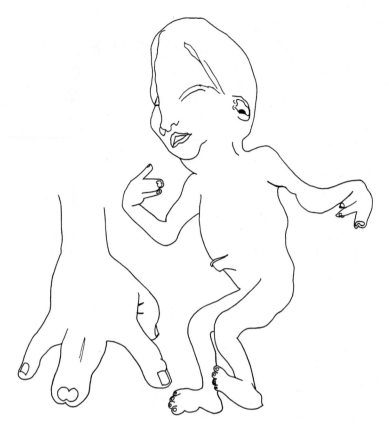

Figure 21-9.   Triploidy.

meningocele, there may be reflex activity of the legs, since the spinal cord distal to the myelomeningocele is formed by canalization and not by neurulation. Posterior NTDs are often not isolated and may be associated with Arnold-Chiari malformation (small posterior fossa, elongate and kinked brainstem with beaked colliculi, herniation of brainstem and cerebellar vermis through foramen magnum, compression and obstruction of fourth ventricle and foramen Magendie with proximal hydrocephalus), cerebral aqueductal stenosis, and hydrocephalus.

Later, the neural tube may rupture. The defects are often covered by skin which may become eroded. The defects include encephaloceles which are in the midline of the skull. In oriental people (especially from southeast Asia), frontal meningoceles and encephaloceles are more common. These may be surgically cor-

rected without significant loss of brain tissue. In caucasian people, occipital encephaloceles (Figure 21-14) are more common. These are usually lethal, since they also include the cerebellum and brain stem which becomes kinked and transected. Iniencephaly clausus is a rare, skin-covered, often lethal neural tube defect of the posterior fossa and rostral spinal cord. In this NTD, the head is retroflexed onto the spine to form a craniorachitic space. The space is too small for the brain stem, cerebellum, and rostral spinal cord. These structures become compressed and attenuated. These babies have fusion of the foregut with the brain stem and rostral spinal cord ventrally. Because the foregut does not migrate down relative to the baby's body, the diaphragm cannot close on the left. Because of diaphragmatic hernia and brain stem damage, these baby's have lung hypoplasia as well.

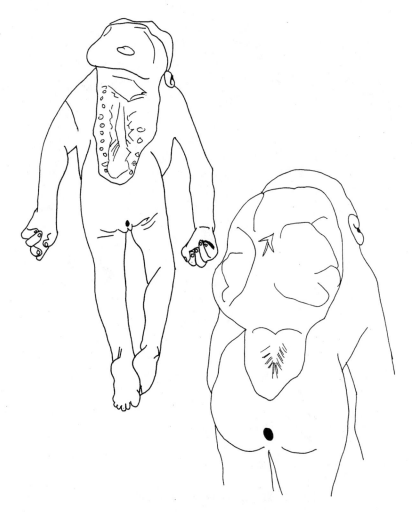

Figure 21-10.   Craniorachischisis.

Many of the NTDs are associated with hydramnios. When the NTD is open, the cerebrovascular mass brimming with capillaries is exposed to the amniotic fluid. Alpha-fetoprotein leaks out of these capillaries and carries fluid with it. In addition, if the brain stem is involved in the NTD, the baby cannot swallow and hydramnios may develop.

Many of the babies with NTDs affecting the posterior fossa structures have lung hypoplasia.

The recurrence of NTDs in subsequent pregnancies is often stated to be 5%, but these figures often included Meckle-Gruber syndrome babies. Meckel-Gruber syndrome includes a NTD (usually encephalocele), polydactyly, and polycystic kidneys and is autosomal dominant.[23-28]

ARHINENCEPHALY. This group of central nervous system anomalies range from absent olfactory tracts and cribriform plate to alobar holoprosencephaly in which the prosencephalon fails to divide into two telencephalic hemispheres. Alobar holoprosencephaly may be isolated, but often accompanies Trisomy 13 and other chromosome anomalies. Due to a defect in the notocord, alobar holoprosencephaly is of-

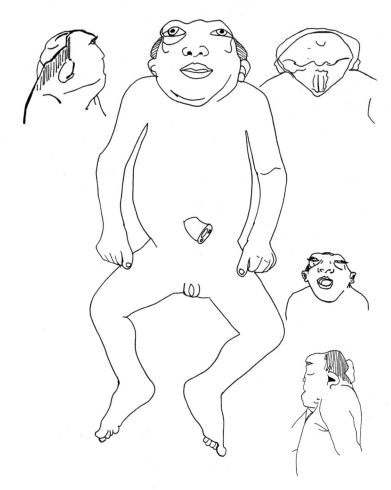

Figure 21-11. Anencephaly, holoacrania type.

ten associated with peculiar facies (cyclopia, ethmocephaly, cebocephaly, and premaxillary agenesis) (Figure 21-8). In these peculiar facies, the nose is usually nonfunctional. Since newborns are obligate nose breathers, these babies often die at birth, unless they are intubated.

Heart Anomalies

The heart forms by canalization of angioblastic cords and subsequent fusion of the two hollow, endothelial tubes. The heart folds onto itself and develops three dilatations. Septae partition the heart into four chambers. The last portion of the heart to form is the membranous septum which fuses the ventricular septum and the spiral septum dividing the great vessels in the seventh week after fertilization. Thus, a membranous ventricular septal defect is one of the most common heart defects, since the window of opportunity is open longer. The membranous ventricular septal defect may be very small and clinically insignificant or very large with maldivision and malrotation of the great vessels. If a ventricular septal defect is large, the left anterior descending artery will not be visible on external examination of the heart. If malrotation of the great vessels is present, the great vessels will be of unequal diameter on external examination of the heart.[1-7]

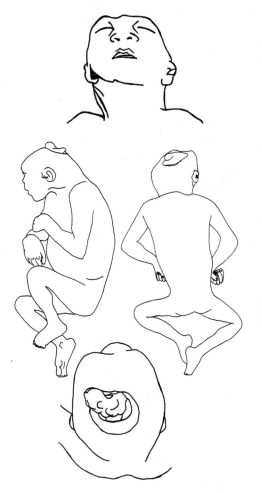

Figure 21-12. Anencephaly, meroacrania type.

RIGHT HEART ANOMALIES. Because, in utero, most of the oxygenated blood from the placenta is shunted through the ductus arteriosus to the systemic circulation, obstruction to the outflow of the right heart may lead to congestive failure, fetal hydrops, and death.

If ductus arteriosus closes suddenly, the blood suddenly stops flowing through the ductus arteriosus and backs up in the right heart chambers and the viscera. A near-term baby can die in hydrops fetalis in less than 3 days.

If the pulmonary artery and/or valve are stenotic or the right ventricular outflow tract is baffled by an Ebstein anomaly of the tricuspid valve. Ebstein's anomaly consists of a low-slung tricuspid valve with atrialization of the right ventricle and with baffling of outflow of the right ventricle. The right side of the heart may become massively distended with blood. The heart may fill the entire chest cavity to the point that the lungs are wafer thin and unable to support the baby ex utero.

LEFT HEART ANOMALIES. Because, in utero, most of the oxygenated blood from the placenta is shunted through the ductus arteriosus to the systemic circulation, obstruction to the flow to and from the left heart is rarely life limiting. However, once the baby with left heart anomalies (left hypoplastic heart, atresia of mitral valve and/or aortic valve) is born, the baby's life will be limited. Some of these left heart anomalies are ductal dependent. In other words, the anomalies become symptomatic only when the ductus arteriosus closes after birth.

DUCTUS ARTERIOSUS. The ductus arteriosus closes when the oxygen tension is elevated and/or indomethacin is increased. At first the ductus closes by contraction of the smooth muscle in its wall. Only much later (up to 1 year), does the lumen of the ductus arteriosus become completely obliterated by fibrous tissue. Thus, potentially, the ductus arteriosus may open anytime during infancy.

In utero, if the ductus arteriosus closes prematurely, then the right heart fails and little oxygenated blood flows to the systemic circulation. The baby may die quickly in utero.

Ex utero, if the ductus arteriosus fails to close, then the heart is put under added stress (more work and less oxygenated blood to the myocardium). This is a common problem in premature babies with immature lungs. At times, the ductus arteriosus closes with indomethacin administration; but, sometimes, the ductus arteriosus must be surgically ligated. Complications of surgical ligation of the ductus arteriosus include ligation of the left pulmonary artery and damage of the left recurrent laryngeal nerve.

Lung Anomalies

Embryologically, in the fourth week, the lung bud divides from the ventral foregut. The bud

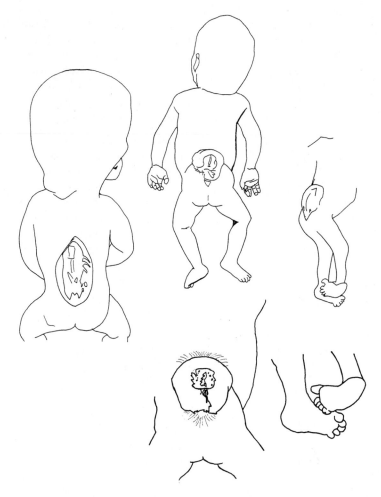

Figure 21-13. Myelomeningocele.

then divides by twos to form the airways and the lung spaces. The surrounding mesoderm is induced to form the intervening lung parenchyma. Surfactant is produced by 23–24 weeks gestation (late canalicular phase). After birth, the lungs continue to develop until the adult number of alveoli are obtained.[1-7]

CYSTIC ADENOMATOID MALFORMATIONS PERINATAL PATHOLOGY. Cystic adenomatoid malformations are hamartomatous malformations. If these malformations communicate with the airways, they can secrete protein-rich fluid into the amniotic fluid space. Hydramnios may

result. In addition, these space-occupying lesions may cause lung hypoplasia.

LUNG HYPOPLASIA. Lung hypoplasia may occur when the amount of room in which the lungs are growing is decreased by internal or external forces or when the baby is not neurologically intact.

Internally, the chest cavity may be filled by a mass (diaphragmatic defect with herniation of abdominal organs into the chest cavity, enlarged heart, cystic adenomatoid malformation, tumor, etc.) or fluid (hydrops fetalis, immune or nonimmune).

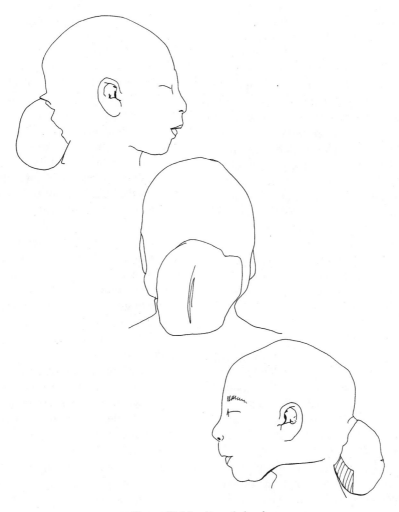

Figure 21-14.   Encephalocele.

The rib cage may be abnormally small in many of the osteochondrodysplasia syndromes. Again, the lungs may be markedly hypoplastic.

Externally, if there is too little amniotic fluid around the baby (oligohydramnios due to genitourinary tract anomalies and amniotic fluid leak), the chest may be compressed by the uterus. In addition, the chest may be compressed by a malformed uterus (bicornuate uterus, or uterus with large leiomyomas).

Finally, lung hypoplasia may occur in babies who are not neurologically intact. Babies practice breathing in utero. This activity helps the lungs to grow properly. If they cannot practice breathing in utero, then their lungs may be hy-poplastic (anencephaly, Arnold-Chiari malformation associated with myelomeningocele, occipital encephalocele, iniencephaly, severe Dandy-Walker malformation, leptomeningeal cysts of posterior fossae, tumors of the posterior fossa, etc.).

Diaphragmatic Defects

Embryologically, by the sixth week, the diaphragm develops between the thoracic and abdominal cavities. The left side of the diaphragm is the last to close. Thus, the left side is the most vulnerable to teratogens. Again, the window of opportunity is open longer. When the gastrointestinal tract returns from the body stalk in the tenth week and the diaphragm is still open, then the gastrointestinal tract herniates up into the chest cavity (usually left). The midline structures are often pushed into the right chest. The lungs become hypoplastic (left smaller than right). At birth, the baby develops respiratory distress. On bagging, the gastrointestinal tract may balloon up with further compromise of respiration. In addition, the markedly hypoplastic, left lung may blow apart. If suspected (bowel sounds in chest cavity), pushing the chest tube into the less hypoplastic, right lung may give more time until surgical correction can be done. Even after surgery, the left lung may act as a vascular shunt which can overwork the heart which is undersupplied with oxygen from the less, hypoplastic, right lung. In addition, the ductus arteriosus may remain patent in these hypoxic conditions further compromising the baby.[1-7]

Gastrointestinal Anomalies

FOREGUT ANOMALIES. If, in fourth week, the lung bud fails to separate completely from the foregut, then a tracheoesophageal fistula develops. The esophagus is often atretic and ends in a blind pouch. After birth and upon feeding, the baby spits up and may aspirate. Surgical correction is needed.

Several anomalies (pyloric hypertrophy, duodenal atresia often seen in Down syndrome, and annular pancreas) may lead to upper gastrointestinal obstruction, hydramnios, meconium reflux, and meconium histiocytosis.

MIDGUT ANOMALIES. The most common, life-threatening anomaly of the midgut is stenosis-atresia of the distal ileum which the end-artery zone for the midgut. Proximal distention, perforation, and meconium peritonitis may result.

In cystic fibrosis, the bowel may become obstructed by a inspissated, meconium plug. Meconium peritonitis may result.

Malrotations may also occur. With malrotations, volvulus and torsions may result.

HINDGUT ANOMALIES. Aganglionosis (Hirschsprung's disease) of the distal colon may cause obstruction. This is more common in Down syndrome babies.

Urinary Tract Anomalies

RENAL AGENESIS. The definitive ureteral buds form the ureters and renal pelvices and branch by twos to form the collecting system of the kidneys. The ureteral buds induce the surrounding mesenchyme to form the renal parenchyma including the glomeruli. By term, most of the nephrogenic zone (glomerular forming tissue just beneath the capsule) is gone.

If the ureteral buds are ablated and do not form, then the renal system will not form. This may be isolated or associated with abnormalities or loss of the lower part of the body distal to the umbilical cord. The lower limb buds may fuse to form a single limb with the knee posterior and a few digits at the end (merman or sirenomelia) (Figure 21-15). In sirenomelia, the aorta continues into the single lower limb. A midline branch of the distal aorta curves into the umbilical cord giving rise to a "true" single umbilical cord artery.

When the kidneys fail to form, urine production is zero. In the late second and early third trimester, because urine is the major component of amniotic fluid, oligohydramnios results. Oligohydramnios with uterine constraint defects results (Figure 21-16). Before birth, the baby may die from umbilical cord compression; and after birth, the baby often dies from lung hypoplasia.

The kidneys initially form in the pelvis. The kidneys rotate medially and migrate rostrally relative to the baby's body. As they migrate up, they received consecutive blood supply from the iliacs and varying levels of the aorta. If migration is interrupted, an aberrant vessel may cross one of the ureters to cause obstruction to urine flow and hydronephrosis of the ipsilateral kidney. Since this is usually unilateral, oligohydramnios does not result. At birth, the hydronephrotic kidney may rupture. The abnormal kidney may be removed soon after birth.

If the kidneys fail to form or fail to migrate up, the adrenal glands remain pancake-shaped with their lower poles near the usual site of the lower pole of the kidney. In fact, the adrenals have been mistaken for kidneys in babies with renal agenesis on ultrasound. In renal agenesis,

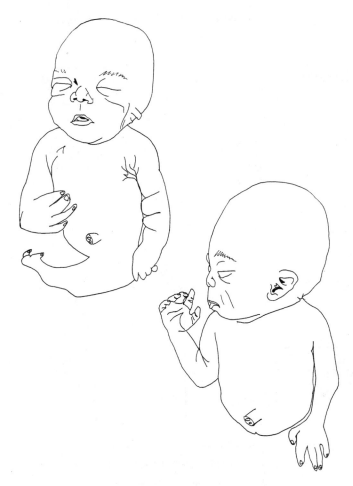

Figure 21-15. Sirenomelia.

oligohydramnios hampers visual resolution of baby from uterus on ultrasound examination. Often, amnioinfusion is necessary to improve ultrasound visualization of the baby.

In boys, the urethra is long and more vulnerable to anomalies. Posterior urethral valves or duplications and baffling of the urethra may cause bladder outlet obstruction. The urine distends the bladder which may fill the abdominal cavity. The massively distended bladder may push the diaphragm up and compress the developing lungs. The distended bladder may keep the testes from descending. The distended bladder may rupture and the urine is absorbed with the development of a ''prune belly.'' The ureters

and renal pelvices become distended, too. The increased pressure of the backed up urine may damage the developing kidneys which become multicystic and dysplastic. Depending on the time that the kidneys become damaged, they may be small or large. If recognized before irrevocable renal damage has been done, a stent may be placed through the abdominal wall between the bladder and the amniotic cavity to bypass the bladder outlet obstruction.

Musculoskeletal Anomalies

Floppy babies at birth may be due to central nervous system depression, but spinal muscular atrophy and other myopathies should be ex-

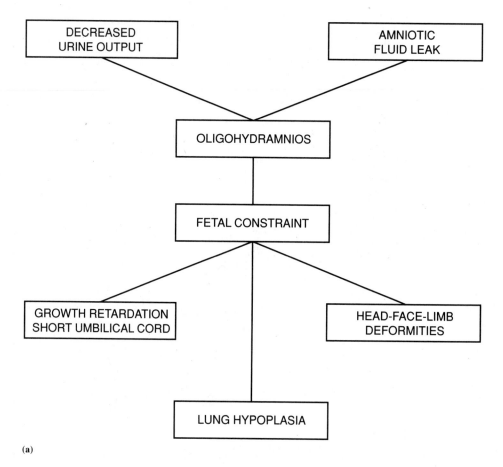

Figure 21-16A.   Oligohydramnios—uterine constraint.

plored. A percutaneous needle biopsy of the affected muscle can help determine the cause.

Skeletal dysplasia are rare. The lethal ones have narrow chests with lung hypoplasia. The most common one we see at our institution is osteogenesis imperfecta (Figure 21-17). In osteogenesis imperfecta, there is collagen defect. The soft tissues are also easily torn. The bones are not well ossified and are the consistency of butter. Because the cranial vault bones are not well ossified either, the unprotected baby's brain is pulped during delivery.[1-7,20-21]

Deformations of Baby

Oligohydramnios/Uterine Constraint Sequence (Potter Syndrome)

Amniotic fluid buoys the baby in order for the baby to develop symmetrically. At first, the amniotic fluid is formed by the placental membranes, umbilical cord, lung secretions, and urine. Later, urine forms the major component of the amniotic fluid. If urine production is zero (bilateral renal atresia, bladder outlet obstruction due to posterior urethral valves or baffled ure-

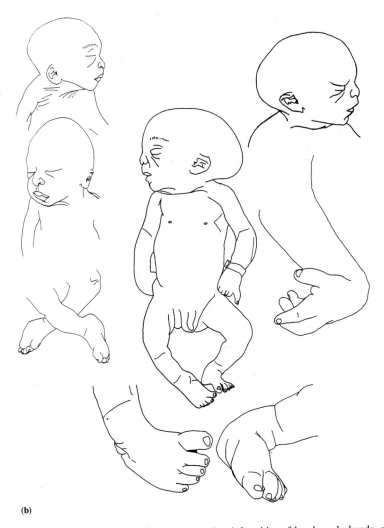

(b)

Figure 21-16B. Oligohydramnios—uterine constraint deformities of head, neck, hands, and feet.

thra), then there will not be enough amniotic fluid to buoy the baby from the muscular uterus. The baby develops secondary deformities due to uterine constraint (Figure 21-16). The baby may be caught in breech position. The breech-positioned head has the muscular uterus contracting over it like a stocking over a robber's head. The face develops epicanthal folds, beaked nose, and small chin. The auricles are pulled down and back. The occiput becomes quite prominent. The head may be deviated to one side with torticollis of the neck. The hands may become deviated outwardly. The feet may become deviated

inwardly and upwardly. The chest may be compressed with lung hypoplasia. At birth, the lung hypoplasia is the most life-limiting deformity.

Amniotic Band Syndrome (Early Amniotic Rupture Syndrome)

The amnion alone may rupture after an amniocentesis in which the needle has been wiggled and acted as a knife. In addition, the amnion has been known to rupture after other traumas like a maternal riding accident and falls downstairs during a maternal seizure.

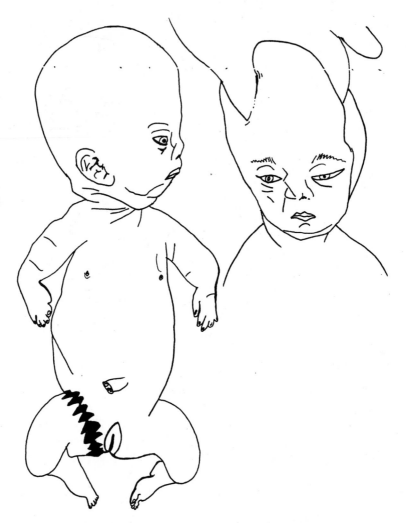

Figure 21-17.   Osteogenesis imperfecta.

If only the amnion ruptures (Figure 21-18), the amnion collapses around the umbilical cord insertion site on the placenta. The vascular chorion quickly sops up all the amniotic fluid. The baby is compressed by the muscular uterine walls and may die immediately due to umbilical cord compression. If the baby survives, the baby may develop asymmetric fusion deformities and contractures. The chorion soon thickens and stops absorbing the amniotic fluid. The baby continues to form urine and the amniotic fluid reaccumulates. Then, amnionic bands and chorionic strands develop. The baby must navigate between and around these. The umbilical cord may become entangled and compressed with death of the baby. The baby may swallow or touch the amnionic bands (ectoderm) and chorionic strands (mesoderm). The portion of the baby that touches these amnionic bands and chorionic strands become disrupted and/or amputated. Depending on how early the amnion rupture occurs, the more severe the deformations. The deformities may be horrible and are always asymmetric.

AMNIOTIC BAND SYNDROME
(Amniotic Band Syndrome, Early Amnion Rupture)

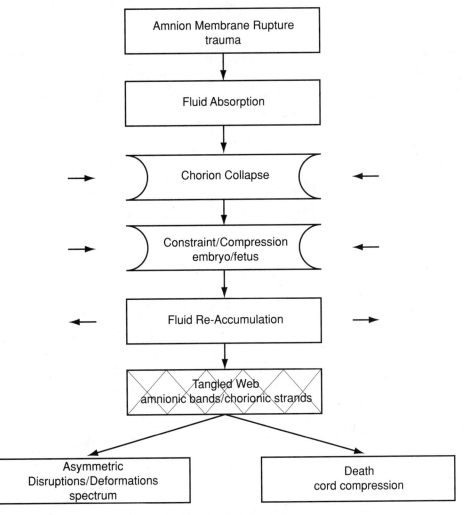

Figure 21-18. Amnionic band syndrome.

Umbilical Cord Accidents (Figure 21-19)

Long Umbilical Cords (>100 centimeters) and Tangles

The umbilical cord length is determined by the size and activity of the baby. The longest, human umbilical cord recorded was 3 meters. Boys have longer umbilical cords. The longer the umbilical cord, the more vulnerable the umbilical cord to become tangled. An active baby may entangle his neck in the umbilical cord (nuchal cord incidence = 211:1000 singleton deliveries) and limbs in the umbilical cord (body cord incidence = 25:1000 singleton deliveries). The nuchal cords are associated with low Apgar scores at 1 and 5 minutes and death than the

Umbilical Cord Length and Vulnerability

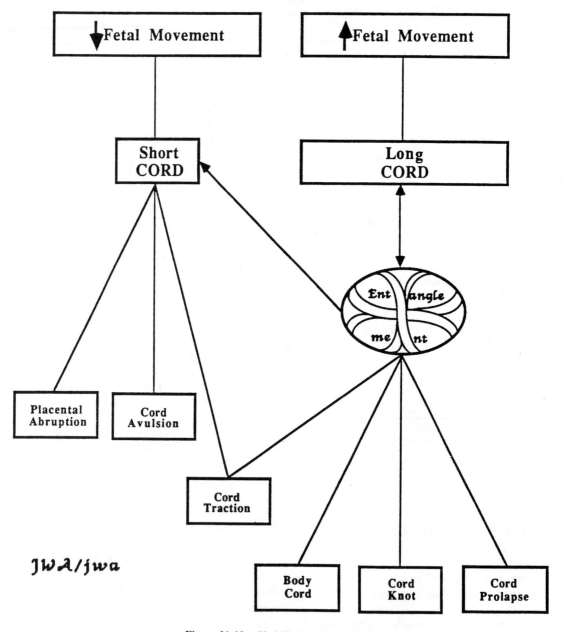

Figure 21-19. Umbilical cord accidents.

body cords are. In those babies that died, the nuchal cord was usually tight with compression of the vessels of the umbilical cord and the neck vessels. The dural sinuses of these babies were markedly engorged and their brains were markedly congested and edematous. A few babies may tie the umbilical cord into true, "lover's" knots (true cord knot incidence = 7:1000). Most of the umbilical cord knots are loosely tied and only become tightly tied at the time of delivery. These knots tied at the time of delivery do not usually damage the baby.

Short Umbilical Cords (<32 centimeters)

If the baby cannot move due to oligohydramnios or brain abnormality or neuromuscular abnormality, the umbilical cord stays short. In addition, if the active baby's umbilical cord becomes markedly tangled, then the functional length is short. The functional umbilical cord length must be at least 32 centimeters long at term for the baby's nose to be delivered before the placenta separates. With a short umbilical cord, the placenta may abrupt or the umbilical cord may be avulsed at its placenta insertion site with massive subamnionic hemorrhage of fetal blood. The baby may suffer hypoxic-ischemic damage or bleed to death before the baby can be born.

Short umbilical cords (<40 centimeters) seem to predict along with low Apgar scores and other neonatal abnormalities, subsequent low IQ scores, and neurologic abnormalities.

Umbilical Cord Prolapse and Compression

When there is rupture of the membrane, the umbilical cord, especially long ones, may prolapse (incidence up to 3:1000 singleton deliveries) and become compressed.

When there is a decreased amount of amniotic fluid (preterm rupture of placental membranes, oligohydramnios, early amnion rupture), the baby's body may compress the umbilical cord.

Decreased amounts of Wharton's jelly with narrowing and flattening of the umbilical cord

makes the umbilical cord more vulnerable to significant compression. Wharton's jelly is decreased in chronic hypoxic-ischemic placental damage with asymmetric fetal growth retardation. In post-term babies, the Wharton's jelly becomes decreased as well.

Whenever the umbilical cord is compressed, the relatively thin-walled vein, which takes the oxygenated blood from the placenta to the baby, is the first to collapse. The heart continues to pump fetal blood out of the baby and into the placenta. If umbilical cord compression continues, the two arteries are finally collapsed. If the baby dies, the baby is often pale and bloodless at the time of autopsy.

Physical Trauma

Mother and Baby

Acute trauma to the mother (motor vehicles accidents even at rather low speeds of ≤25 miles per hour, falls, blunt trauma from an enraged spouse) may cause placental abruption.

If the center of the placenta abrupts, no maternal blood may escape into the vaginal (concealed abruption). However, the maternal blood squeezes the fetal blood suddenly out of the placenta and into the baby. The baby's heart is overloaded and fails. Fetal blood backs up in the thoracic organs. The vessels burst due to overdistention of vessels with hypoxic-ischemic damage of their walls. The thoracic organs exhibit a "leopard-spot" appearance due to multiple recent hemorrhages of varying sizes. Often, labor will intervene within 24–32 hours of the abruption. With the clot of maternal blood sequestered behind the placenta, the mother may develop disseminated intravascular coagulopathy.

The edge of the placenta or the whole placenta may separate from the uterine wall with maternal bleeding into the vagina, fetal hypoxic-ischemic damage, and precipitous delivery. If only a portion of the placenta abrupts the abrupted portion becomes infarcted.

In abruption, blood may be found in the amniotic fluid and hemosiderin-laden macrophages may be found in the decidua and placental membranes.

In abruption, the mother's blood is spilled, and the baby's blood is rarely spilled. The maternal blood usually dissects along a decidual plane between the placenta and the uterus. Sometimes, the mother's blood ruptures under the fetal plate at the margin. The fetal stem vessels under the fetal plate of the placenta may rupture causing fetal blood loss and subchorionic hemorrhages. Sometimes, abruption, along with other entities, may cause hypoxic-ischemic damage to villi with intravillous hemorrhage. These villi turn into blood filled sacs which may rupture to cause fetal-maternal blood mixing. Thus, transfusion of fetal blood into the mother is rare in fetal abruption.

Baby

In precipitous breech deliveries, the sharp lower edge of the occipital bone, which is not firmly fused to the spine or skull, may be rammed into and transect the caudal brain stem and rostral spinal cord. With such an injury at birth, the baby cannot breathe on his/her own and is flaccid. Unless heroic efforts are taken, the baby dies. Only by examining the structures of the posterior fossa in situ may this injury be confirmed.

During manipulations of the head during delivery, the first cervical vertebra may telescope into the foramen magnum. The vertebral arteries may be distorted with ischemic damage to the brainstem.

Rarely, the tentorium cerebelli and veins may be torn during a heavily manipulated delivery. Subarachnoid hemorrhage with stiff neck may result. Transforaminal herniation and/or arterial spasm may result.[1-6]

Multiple Gestations

All multiple gestations (dizygotic or monozygotic) may be complicated by premature labor (increased volume of baby, placenta, and amniotic fluid with stretching of the uterus and preterm labor) and/or acute ascending amniotic fluid infection (increased surface area of membranes exposed to vaginal flora) and preterm labor. Because the markedly enlarged uterus lies over the aorta, the aorta may be compressed with decreased utero-placental blood supply and pregnancy induced hypertension.

Dizygotic twins have dichorionic-diamnionic placentas which may be fused (Figure 21-20).

Monozygotic twins may have dichorionic-diamnionic placentas due to division before implantation, monochorionic-diamnionic placenta (Figure 21-20) due to division soon after implantation, and monochorionic-monoamnionic placenta due to division later after implantation. All monochorionic twins are monozygotic, but not all monozygotic twins have monochorionic placentas. If division occurs after the primitive streak has developed, conjoined twins of varying types and, possibly, some teratomas occur.

With a monochorionic-diamnionic twin placenta, the twins often share chorion (mesoderm) and, thus, vessels. The deep vascular anastomoses are the most life-threatening, because a twin-twin transfusion may result. In a deep vascular anastomosis (Figure 21-21), an artery from the donor twin supplies 1+ cotyledons which drain through a vein to the recipient twin. Both twins are at risk for death. The donor may die due to overwork of his heart. The recipient may die due to volume overload of his heart. There may also be superficial vascular anastomoses. These superficial anastomoses are usually insignificant, because these anastomoses are usually vein-vein or artery-artery and under equal pressures. Rarely, one twin may be delivered and the second twin may die of loss of blood through a vein-vein, superficial anastomosis. Since vessels are shared, if one twin becomes infected; then, the other is infected. If one twin dies, the other may develop disseminated intravascular coagulopathy with possible thrombosis of internal carotid arteries and hydranencephaly/porencephaly. The dead twin may become a fetus papyraceus or be totally resorbed.

FUSED TWIN PLACENTAS
T-SECTION OF DIVIDING MEMBRANES

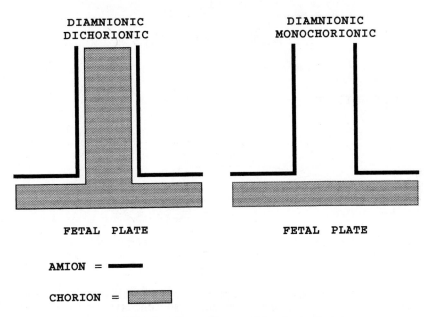

Figure 21-20. Dividing membranes of fused twin placentas.

With monochorionic-monoamnionic twin placenta, the twins share a common amnionic space which is filled with twice as much amniotic fluid. The umbilical cords of these twins may become entangled and both babies may die (50% mortality rate).

Monozygotic twins may develop anastomoses of umbilical cord vessels in which deoxygenated arterial blood is shunted from the donor twin backwards through the umbilical artery to the recipient twin. What little oxygen available in this arterial blood is directed toward the lower body. The upper body resorbs often leaving a craniopagus parasiticus or acardiac monster (Figure 21-22).

Curiously, there seems to be a spectrum from monozygotic, separate twins → conjoined twins → teratomas (Figure 21-23). Teratomas usually occur in the midline. They can involve the pineal gland, palate, thyroid gland, and gonads; but the most common site is the sacrococcygeal area.[30]

Hypoxic-Ischemic Damage (Maternal Drugs (Tobacco, Cocaine), Hypertension, Diabetes Mellitus, Sickle Cell Disease or Trait) with Infarcts, Hemorrhage, and Abruption

With chronic hypoxic-ischemic damage, the baby will shunt blood preferentially from the splanchnic circulation and to the brain and heart. While the brain continues to grow appropriately for gestational age in size and weight, the gastrointestinal tract (especially the end artery boundary zone of the distal ileum, appendix, and cecum) develops submucosal fibrosis and even ischemic necrosis, stenosis/atresia, and rupture with meconium peritonitis. With meconium in the peritoneal cavity, the vessels may spasm and cause further ischemic damage. The meconium, a toxic substance, may also cause a marked fibrotic reaction with adhesions.

With acute hypoxic-ischemic damage, the ba-

DETECTING
DEEP VASCULAR ANASTOMOSIS
IN
MONOCHORIONIC-DIAMNIONIC
TWIN PLACENTAS

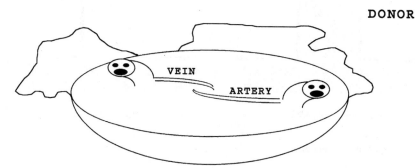

THE DIVIDING MEMBRANES ARE EXAMINED. AFTER THE
PLACENTA IS DETERMINED TO BE MONOCHORIONIC, THE
PLACENTA MUST BE CHECKED FOR DEEP VASCULAR
ANASTOMOSES. THE AMNION IS STRIPPED BACK. THE
VESSELS ON THE FETAL PLATE ARE EXAMINED FOR AN
ARTERY THAT TRAVELS TOWARD THE OTHER TWIN AND IS
DRAINED BY A VEIN THAT TRAVELS TOWARD THE OTHER
TWIN. THE ARTERY IS INJECTED WITH A SYRINGE OF
CONTRASTING FLUID. WHEN THE INJECTED FLUID FLOWS
FROM THE VEIN OF THE RECIPIENT'S UMBILICAL CORD
STUMP, THE SYRINGE INJECTED VOLUME IS MEASURED.
THUS, THE DEEP VASCULAR ANASTOMOSIS CAN BE
QUANTITATED.

Figure 21-21.   Deep vascular anastomosis in twin-twin transfusion syndrome.

by's brain may swell so rapidly that even the open fontanelles will not circumvent transforaminal herniation and death.[1-16]

MATERNAL DEATH

Placental Abruption and Uterine Rupture

Placental abruption may lead to massive maternal blood loss and death.

If a mother is allowed to labor less than a year after a vertical C-section (especially associated with an acute ascending amniotic fluid infection), the uterus may rupture spilling the baby and/or placenta into the mother's abdominal cavity. If part or all of the baby and/or placenta remain in the uterine cavity, the uterus cannot contract. Massive bleeding continues. The mother may die.

Embolization

One of the most common causes of death in pregnant women is massive thromboembolization to the lungs. Pregnancy is a hypercoagulable state. If the mother becomes dehydrated, in-

Amniotic fluid embolism may lead to maternal death. In violent labor in the older mother, amniotic fluid which contains a surfactant-like material and fetal cellular debris can gain entry into the mother's circulation. The amniotic fluid may become foamy when it is mixed in the right heart chamber. At autopsy, foamy fluid may be found in the right heart and squamous debris, vernix, and fetal hair may be found in vessels of the mother's lung.

Infection

Since pregnancy is an immunocompromised state, infection may also cause death. For example, a mother, who was first exposed to chickenpox during the pregnancy, died along with her baby at our institution.

Brain Lesions

During pregnancy, because of increased circulatory volume, vascular lesions (arteriovenous malformations and aneurysms) may enlarge and rupture.

In pregnancy-induced hypertension, acute hemorrhages may occur (especially in basal ganglia and pons).

In addition, during pregnancy, brain tumors (especially meningiomas) may enlarge due to hormonal changes and increased circulatory volume.

All the above lesions may cause increased intracranial pressure, transforaminal herniation of the brain (cerebellar tonsils), and death.

Accidents/Trauma

In preparation for a C-section, the mother's esophagus may be intubated erroneously.

The mother may be directly traumatized with lethal penetrating wound or indirectly traumatized (shearing forces) with resultant placental abruption.

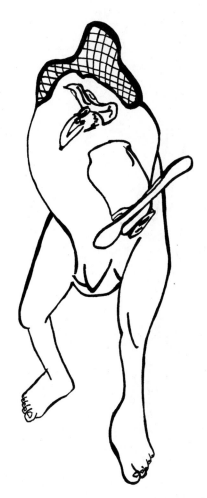

Figure 21-22.   Craniopagus parasiticus with craniorachischisis.

fected, and immobilized, then she is vulnerable to massive thromboembolization to the lungs.

For example, a pregnant woman with asthma became dehydrated and immobilized and threw a massive thromboembolus to her lungs. During transfer to our institution, she developed brain edema, trantenstorial and transforaminal herniation, and brain death.

For another example, a pregnant woman with an intrauterine infection (hematogenous) developed leptomeningitis with thrombosis of the artery of Adamkiewicz and infarction of her distal thoracic spinal cord. She became paralyzed. While immobilized, she threw thromboemboli to her lungs.

(a)

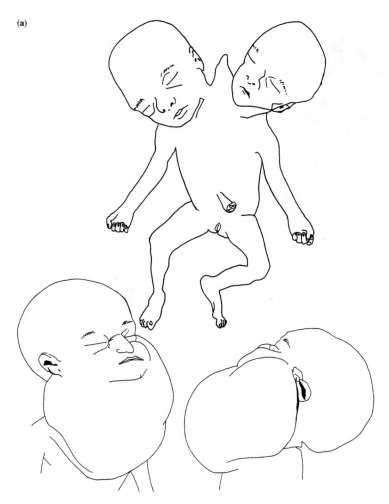

Figure 21-23A.   Spectrum of twins-to-teratomas.

COMMUNICATING WITH PARENTS AND THE NEED FOR A PATHOLOGIC EXAMINATION OF THE BABY AND PLACENTA (Figure 21-24)

Parents who have lost a baby suddenly in utero have not had time to prepare for the loss. Many parents have bonded early on to their baby in utero and the sudden death of their baby is like the loss of a loved one in a motor vehicle accident, except they didn't have a chance to know their baby. They only know their hopes and expectations for that baby. In other words, the loss of a baby in utero seems to be a more

intangible loss and more difficult to work through. Any tangible, concrete evidence that their baby existed will help the parents work through their loss. We refer to the fetus as a baby and not a specimen. We ask if they have named the baby and then we refer to their baby by that name. We try to provide the parents with time to be with their baby, baptism and blessing by representatives of every religion, foot and hand prints, blanket, hat, lock of hair, photographs, certificate, and cremation or burial services. Each set of parents is different and one must listen and ask open-ended questions to figure out what they need and want.

Parents want to know, as soon as possible, the cause of death of their baby and will often

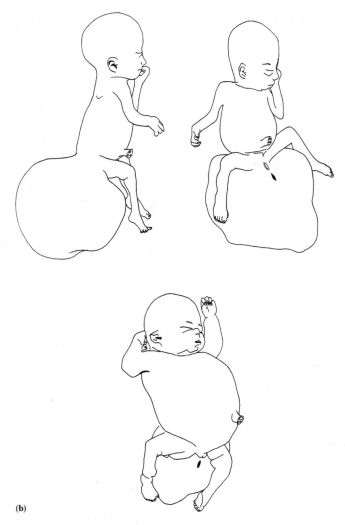

(b)

Figure 21-23B. Spectrum of twins-to-teratomas (Continued): sacrococcygeal teratomas arise from the coccyx. The lower one is dumbell shaped with an intraabdominal component.

agree to a postmortem examination of their baby. It is best for the health care provider who knows the family best to ask for the postmortem examination, but this is not always possible. At our institution, the perinatal pathologist or a specialized representative of the pathology department (mortality specialist) usually ask the family for the examination. At that time, one can find out what the family is concerned about and address that concern during the postmortem examination. Sometimes, one finds that the family wants others to learn from their baby to help other babies. One should try to obtain permis-

sion for a full, postmortem examination in all deaths. The families deserve a complete, prompt, accurate postmortem examination.

Sharing accurate information as soon as possible circumvents the parents blaming each other or their health care providers for the death of their baby. If one gives incorrect information, like wrong sex of the baby, to the parents, then the family may never trust any information.

In our institution and others, the family often meets with their primary health care provider and/or perinatal pathologist to go over the postmortem examination findings. Copies (2) of the

PREGNANCY LOSS FLOW SUMMARY

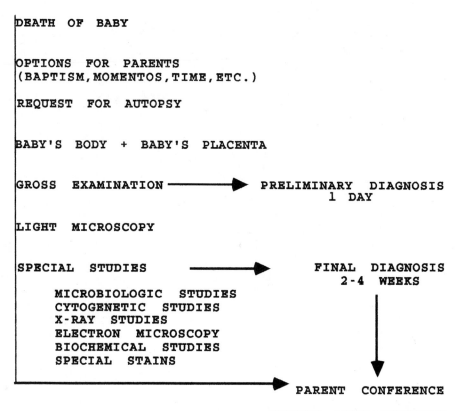

DEATH OF BABY

OPTIONS FOR PARENTS
(BAPTISM,MOMENTOS,TIME,ETC.)

REQUEST FOR AUTOPSY

BABY'S BODY + BABY'S PLACENTA

GROSS EXAMINATION ⟶ PRELIMINARY DIAGNOSIS
                                    1 DAY

LIGHT MICROSCOPY

SPECIAL STUDIES ⟶ FINAL DIAGNOSIS
                                2-4 WEEKS
    MICROBIOLOGIC STUDIES
    CYTOGENETIC STUDIES
    X-RAY STUDIES
    ELECTRON MICROSCOPY
    BIOCHEMICAL STUDIES
    SPECIAL STAINS

                                PARENT CONFERENCE

                        HEALTH CARE PROVIDER
                    HIGH-RISK OBSTETRICIAN
                                PATHOLOGIST
                        GENETIC COUNSELOR
                                GENETICIST
                            SOCIAL WORKER
                            PSYCHIATRIST

Figure 21-24.   Pregnancy loss summary.

postmortem findings may be given to the parents to review, to keep, and take with them, if they move.

The full, perinatal, postmortem examination, which includes the placenta, is invaluable to the family in understanding the loss of that baby and in understanding the impact on future children.

However, the postmortem examination is also invaluable in many other ways. In most of the postmortem examinations, unexpected entities which could have contributed to morbidity-mortality are found. The postmortem examination findings can be compiled to uncover epidemiologic trends of disease processes. The findings can confirm new diagnostic tests (ultrasound, triple screens, chorionic villous sampling) and treatments (surfactant for immature lungs, ECMO). The postmortem examination can uncover treatment misadventures. For example, four premature babies with pneumothoraces requiring chest tube placement and mechanical suction died. At postmortem examination, Pseudomonas empyemas and sepsis were found. The tubing of the suction machine was cultured and found to be contaminated with the same Pseudomonas species. The tubing was sterilized and changed after that and no further deaths occurred.

In every perinatal death, the baby and placenta must be examined in order to find the cause of death.

REFERENCES

1. Barson AJ. *Laboratory Investigation of Fetal Disease*, Bristol, UK: John Wright & Sons Ltd., 1991.
2. Dimmick JE, Kalousek DK, eds. *Developmental Pathology of the Embryo and Fetus*. Philadelphia: JB Lippincott, 1992.
3. England MA. *Color Atlas of Life Before Birth*. Chicago: Year Book Medical Publishers, Inc., 1983.
4. Keeling JW, ed. *Fetal and Neonatal Pathology*, Second Ed. New York: Springer-Verlag, 1993.
5. Moore KL and Persaud TVN. *The Developing Human*, Fifth Ed. Philadelphia: WB Saunders, 1993.
6. Wigglesworth JS. *Perinatal Pathology*, Second Ed. Philadelphia: WB Saunders, 1996.
7. Wigglesworth JS and Singer DB, eds. *Fetal and Perinatal Pathology*, Boston: Blackwell Scientific Publications, 1991.
8. Altshuler G. Role of the placenta in perinatal pathology (revisited). *Ped Path Lab Med*. 1996; 16:207–233.
9. Beebe LA, Cowan LD, Altshuler G. The epidemiology of placental features: associations with gestational age and neonatal outcome. *Obstet Gynec*. 1996;87:771–778.
10. Benirschke K, Kaufmann P. *Pathology of the Human Placenta*, Third Ed. New York: Springer-Verlag, 1995.
11. College of American Pathologists Conference XIX on the Examination of the Placenta. *Arch Path Lab Med*. 1991;115:660–721.
12. Kassberg M. Placental pathology. The neglected defense. *OBG Man J*. 1995;35–41.
13. Kassberg M. Deciding when to save the placenta. *OBG Man J*. 1995;43–45.
14. Perrin EVDK, ed. *Pathology of the Placenta*. New York: Churchill Livingstone, 1984.
15. Roberts DK. Medical-legal aspects of placental examination. *Obstet Gynec Surv*. 1993;48:777–778.
16. Salafia C, Vintzileos AM. Why all placentas should be examined by a pathologist in 1990. *Am J Obstet Gynec*. 1990;163:1282–1293.
17. Genest DR. Estimating the time of death in stillborn fetuses: I. histologic evaluation of fetal organs; an autopsy study of 150 stillborns. *Obstet Gynec*. 1992;80:575–584.
18. Genest DR. Estimating the time of death in stillborn fetuses. II histologic evaluation of the placenta; a study of 71 stillborns. *Obstet Gynec*. 1992;80:585–592.
19. Genest DR. Estimating the time of death in stillborn fetuses: III. external fetal examination; a study of 86 stillborns. *Obstet Gynec*. 1992;80: 593–600.
20. Goodman RM and Gorlin RJ. *The Malformed Infant and Child*. New York: Oxford University Press, 1983.
21. Jones KL. *Smith's Recognizable Patterns of Human Malformation*, Fifth Ed. Philadelphia: WB Saunders, 1996.
22. Kurman RJ, ed. *Blaustein's Pathology of the Female Genital Tract*, Fourth Ed. New York: Springer-Verlag, 1994.
23. Duckett S, ed. *Pediatric Neuropathology*, Baltimore: Williams and Wilkins, 1995.
24. Larroche JC. *Developmental Pathology of the Neonate*. New York: Excerpta Medica, 1977.
25. Lemire RJ, Beckwith JB, Warkany J. *Anencephaly*. New York: Raven Press, 1978.
26. Lemire RJ, Loeser JD, Leech RW, Alvord EC. *Normal and Abnormal Development of the Human Nervous System*. New York: Harper and Row, 1975.
27. Volpe JJ. *Neurology of the Newborn*, Third Ed. Philadelphia: WB Saunders, 1995.
28. Wyatt-Ashmead J. Postmortem perinatal brain removal: the value of the posterior approach method. *Ped Path*. 1993;13:875–880.
29. Naeye RL. Umbilical cord length: clinical significance. *J Ped*. 1985;107:278–281.

30. Baldwin VJ. *Pathology of Multiple Pregnancy.* New York: Springer-Verlag, 1994.

31. Cartlidge PHT, Dawson AT, Stewart JH, Vujanic GM. Value and quality of perinatal and infant postmortem examinations: cohort analysis of 400 consecutive deaths. *Brit Med J.* 1995; 310:155–158.

32. Chiswick M. Perinatal and infant postmortem examination. *Brit Med J.* 1995;310:141–142.

33. Dahms B. The autopsy in pediatrics. *Am J Diseases Childhood.* 1986;1140:335.

34. Rahman HA, Khong TY. Perinatal and infant postmortem examination. Survey of women's reactions to perinatal necropsy. *Brit Med J.* 1995;310:870–871.

35. Valdes-Dapena M. The postautopsy conference with families. *Arch Path Lab Med.* 1984;108: 497–498.

QUESTIONS

1. The minimal, functional, umbilical cord length for a safe vaginal delivery is — centimeters.

2. In an acute ascending amniotic fluid infection the baby may die from
   a. preterm delivery due to lung immaturity
   b. infection
   c. hypoxic-ischemic damage from villous edema
   d. all of the above

3. If an abnormally formed baby is markedly macerated, cultures for cytogenetic studies can still be taken from the _____.

4. If the dividing membranes of a fused twin placenta are monochorionic-diamnionic, then
   a. the twins are monozygotic (identical)
   b. the vessels of the fetal plate must be checked for anastomoses
   c. the twins are dizygotic (fraternal)
   d. none of the above

5. A long umbilical cord is associated with
   a. prolapse
   b. entanglements
   c. fetal activity
   d. none of the above

6. Determining the sex of the baby is not important to the parents.
   True/False

Part VI

LEGAL AND STATISTICS

22

Medico-Legal Aspects of Maternal Fetal Medicine

William D. Bonezzi

INTRODUCTION

The term *malpractice* in *Stedman's Medical Dictionary* is defined as follows: Mistreatment of a disease or injury through ignorance, carelessness, or criminal intent.[1] This chapter will focus on ignorance and carelessness, and defer the criminal intent aspect. Hopefully, at the conclusion, some light will be focused on what can be done to prevent it.

The term *malpractice*, or medical negligence, falls into the legal classification of a civil wrong as opposed to a criminal act. As such, there is a different burden of proof which must be produced in a courtroom, and that proof, for the party suing, must be a *probability* instead of a certainty. Probability occurs when the facts presented are likely to produce a result 50.1% of the time compared to 49.9%. In other words, the balance of proof falls ever so slightly in favor of something happening as not.

It is important to keep in mind that malpractice, or medical negligence, is not only the commission of an act, but may also involve the omission of an act, i.e., the failure to do something which should have been done. How does one go about proving that something was done wrong, or not done at all? Very simply, a phy-

sician retained by a party, known as the expert witness, will testify that the term standard of care requires that a certain act be carried out or omitted, and the failure to do so constitutes a departure from acceptable medical practice.

As one can see, each *answered* question brings with it a new set of questions. The easiest and probably the best way to provide an answer to this dilemma is to direct you, the reader, to common sense. In theory, law and medicine have their own guidelines, their own terms and principles. These guidelines ultimately cross paths in a courtroom and, when that happens, all the theory and pretense initially relied upon in defending a position come crashing to the ground. Theory is then replaced with reality. There is nothing so deafening as the silence that exists in the courtroom when the defendant physician, when asked a question by the plaintiff's attorney, realizes at that moment the error that was committed, and sits in silence, unable to answer the question for fear of the answer.

One doesn't wish to be told why something occurred, for common sense, at times, provides the answer. It is more important to learn how to stay out of a courtroom than to be told what happens when one gets there. Sometimes the most important lessons learned are the easiest to follow. The easiest one is communication.

COMMUNICATION

The act of communication is something that may need to be refined. We all possess the power to transfer information from one person to another. What needs to be taught is the vehicle used. The spoken word is effective during social engagements, but not when addressing the progress of a patient. The reasons why tests were or were not ordered, or why a nurse's assessment of your patient may not be accurate, are very important. In those circumstances, and to a physician who has been placed in a compromising situation, the chart becomes both a shield and a sword on one's behalf when a decision is being made by a patient's attorney "to sue or not to sue."

It would be easy to suggest that each action or comment regarding a patient be charted. Unfortunately, that is not always realistic given where and when a decision to do something is made. However, let common sense be your guide when charting your patient's progress or memorizing phone calls, when a chart is not available. The high-risk obstetrical patient cries out for mandatory charting in a sequential fashion, including all phone calls, complaints, or questions. In those circumstances where the initial confinement was at an institution other than your own, be circumspect albeit decisive regarding the reason(s) for the transfer of the patient to your institution. Ensure that a complete, concise, and accurate assessment has been made and charted by the referring physicians. Review the notes of the transport team to ensure the accuracy of the condition of the patient, and note any discrepancy. Do not chart the etiology of the reason for the transport of a newborn based upon conjecture and speculation—you must have all the facts and lab data. The easiest hypothesis which can be drawn involving a newborn with APGARS of 1 and 2 at 1 and 5 minutes is to conclude that the infant suffered from an intrauterine hypoxic event, and now has

hypoxic ischemic encephalopathy. If this is charted without proof, the person charting will become the plaintiff's expert years down the road when the lawsuit is filed, and may look somewhat foolish when attempting to justify the remarks, assuming the initial assessment is inaccurate.

A good rule-of-thumb to follow is to document everything when dealing with a patient whose problems are many and the outcome for survival unlikely, or morbidity high. In that situation, a well-documented course of care may dispel the notion of suing the physician for a bad outcome. Bad outcomes do not justify a lawsuit, but certainly trigger the possibility of one. When a decision is made that is completely justifiable, chart the reason(s). It is very difficult to explain to a jury why one acted, or failed to act, in a certain fashion when there is no supporting data in the chart reflecting the physician's thought process. A jury deals in common sense, and common sense suggests that a chart will provide a written chronology of the events as they occurred. Years later, when faced with the need for reasons why something was or was not done, and being questioned about same in a courtroom, the only thing which can be relied upon is the chart. A memory is a poor substitute.

A lawsuit in many instances is driven by emotion and the need of a loved one or patient to justify death or serious injury. Explain matters to the patient and/or family, and then record the important aspects of the conversation in the chart. Please remember that what separates the physician from the patient is a profession. The physician and the patient are both human beings striving to obtain answers. Give the patient answers and, lest she forget, chart it.

THE EXPERT WITNESS

Nothing sounds so profound as the information dispensed by an individual who has been asked to deliver an answer to what seems to be an extremely complex problem. Just ask the person providing the answer. At times, that individual is the plaintiff/patient's expert witness.

Just what is an expert? This individual, who has been asked to provide the key that will unlock wherein the alleged medical malpractice lies, is usually a physician who practices in the same specialty as the physician who has been sued. What is it that allows an expert physician who has never seen the patient to provide an answer which, for a period of time, remained elusive to the treating physician? In a word, the chart.

The expert physician is usually a board-certified physician, who can also be boarded in a subspecialty such as maternal fetal medicine. Prior to providing an expert report and/or testimony, the expert will request that the medical records of both the mother and infant be sent to one for review. In conjunction with the chart, the expert will also ask for and review all monitor tracings. Inasmuch as the outcome of a particular situation is known to the expert, it is easier for one to map out a plan or strategy which should have been followed by the defendant treating physician, as opposed to what was done. If the expert's strategy is not followed in the chart, the expert will opine that the expert's plan defines the minimal standard of care, and the failure of the defendant treating physician to adhere to the expert's plan creates a departure from same, thereby establishing negligence.

Long ago I inquired what constituted the "standard of care." I was told that it was "whatever the expert said it was from the witness stand in the courtroom." After that remark, I became acutely aware, first of all, of the need to correlate the written record with the available, current medical literature. Second, the importance and significance of the contents of a patient's chart are elemental and, hopefully, not lost on the reader. Lack of information in the record allows an expert to hypothesize what could have been, instead of what was!

The expert not only establishes the standard of care, but also provides a correlation to proximate cause. In other words, did the departure from the standard of care cause the injury? To arrive at an opinion on the element of proximate cause, the expert will review the chart(s), coupled with the expert's knowledge, experience, training, and review of the literature. Sometimes the only item which separates acceptable care from unacceptable care is the lack of documentation in either the office records of the treating physician, or the confinement records. This lack of charting allows speculation and conjecture to replace fact. Unfortunately, a defensible position which is not memorialized winds up sounding like an excuse.

A patient's expert will review the progress notes of the patient, correlate the complaints of the patient with those found in the record, and then determine whether or not the patient should have been referred to a consultant, i.e., an expert in the field. In many instances the lack of an appropriately timed consult, coupled with the knowledge a plaintiff's expert has regarding the outcome of a given situation, spell problems for the treating physician. This situation can be countered with a well-documented record as to the purpose of current treatment. This type of charting not only confounds the expert's position but, more importantly, advances the treating physician's reasons for not recommending a consult. A well-documented chart also provides the basis and support for the conclusions reached by the expert who has been retained to defend the treating physician. What exists for the patient's expert also exists for the treating physician's expert.

CAUSES OF LAWSUITS

The preceding information highlights an area of special concern that can ultimately establish the cornerstone of a lawsuit, i.e., charting or the lack thereof. As explained previously, the lack of written information allows speculation to replace fact. In any instance where either death or injury occurs, the family or patient will question the physician in an attempt to determine *why*. Further, the questions will start to take on the appearance of blame.

Treating the patients and/or family with respect instead of indifference during this question and answer period is one of the techniques which can either stop inquiries at inception, or prevent inquiries from escalating. It is extremely important to talk with the patient or family. When an unforeseen event occurs, human nature attempts to find a scapegoat, especially when a physician chooses to avoid answering questions or returning calls from the family. It is very difficult to blame someone for a bad outcome when all information has been shared, and the physician treats the patient or family with kindness, when kindness is due.

The reasons for lawsuits are many, some avoidable, some not. It is the lawsuit that can be avoided which is within the control of the physician, and control it one must! Certain causes of lawsuits occur more commonly than others, and these will be discussed hereafter, with suggestions on how to avoid them.

Emotional Problems

After the unexpected death of a loved one, family members turn to the physician who last saw the patient for answers. This is not an easy time for anyone but, most importantly, it is not a time for abrupt behavior on the part of the physician. Answer questions carefully in language which is understandable to the grieving family, and not in medical jargon. It is important to maintain control of the situation and provide guidance, if not answers. If a question arises relative to filing a suit, those who have assisted the family and dealt with them in a compassionate manner will not (as a rule) be sued. Physicians who fail to develop a rapport with the family, who exhibit an unwillingness to provide counsel, and who overall demonstrate a lack of concern, will be sued. As indicated earlier, the family may seek someone to blame for the bad outcome, and the physician not liked will wear the cloak of the villain and be sued.

Expectations

It is easy to overlook the fact that in certain situations, the patient is looking for a miracle. As a result, she does not hear what you are saying, but only what she wants to hear. Be concise but complete in your explanation(s). Lack of thoroughness is usually the foundation for a lawsuit based upon "lack of informed consent." This term is one of art, but basically means that she is mentally competent to understand the risks and benefits of the proposed procedure and, after weighing both, is competent to elect to proceed or not. The key to informed consent is to ensure that all risks (most likely to occur) have been explained to the patient. Without this explanation, true informed consent cannot be obtained and the expectations of the patient are inappropriate. Request that other family members, if possible, be present when information is provided. Chart the exchange of information and, if you question the patient's understanding, have the patient sign your charted conversation.

Charting

An entire chapter in a book could be devoted to this topic, for it can become the lynch pin for the patient's lawsuit, or the strength of its defense. Good medical record keeping with proper explanations can win the same lawsuit in which incomplete record keeping could lose it. A cavalier approach to charting will spell trouble years later if a suit is filed.

The clinical record documents the patient's history and physical findings. An accurate, clear, well-organized record reflects and facilitates sound clinical thinking. It leads to good communication among the many professionals who participate in caring for a patient. Most importantly, this record serves to document the patient's problems and health care for medicolegal purposes.[2] For this reason, placing a diagram in the chart that adequately describes a finding is an extremely helpful aid, not only in caring for the patient, but also in retracing steps which were taken in the past.

In the State of Ohio, an action for medical negligence must be filed within one (1) year from the date of injury, two (2) years from date of death, or within one (1) year after a minor reaches the age of eighteen (18). If a lawsuit is commenced, it may be years from the event before the physician is called upon to provide testimony. If the chart is incomplete from the standpoint of (a) progress notes, (b) orders, (c) summaries, (d) consultation requests, and/or (e) admission note, the physician must rely upon memory to provide information. At best, this is difficult. There is a maxim which states: If it wasn't written, it didn't happen. Remember this! Further, the chart may be the only means of communication between caregivers. If this is not believed, it will be driven home in a courtroom by the plaintiffs' attorney and the lesson will never be forgotten! Read the chart, including the nurses' notes. If a discrepancy exists regarding the patient's condition as described by a nurse versus your own assessment, note it in the chart. Do not allow it to go uncorrected; otherwise, the physician may end up at cross purposes with a nurse who has charted one thing, and the physician who believes something else.

Becoming an Expert Witness

In the tertiary care setting, many an infant will be transferred to your institution from a community hospital. When this occurs, be careful to obtain all necessary information regarding the infant from the attending or, if possible, from the original record. Do not hypothesize as to the cause of the problem without sufficient data. It is easy for an assigned resident to hastily and, perhaps, arbitrarily assign a cause to the problem, because the etiology of the problem "most likely" is "X." I have seen numerous situations occur involving this type of conjecture, only to find that sufficient information was not available to the physicians who formed the opinions. Then, years later, these same physicians couldn't support what they charted.

In the case involving an infant who has suffered from what appears to be a hypoxic episode in utero, who subsequently develops a severe neurological disorder, the parents will often attempt to find someone to blame for the problem. Once they confer with an attorney who specializes in medical negligence, the attorney will obtain the medical record of both the mother and infant, as well as the medical record(s) from

both the "delivery" and "transfer" institutions. If a physician writes that the infant, upon transfer, suffers from hypoxic ischemic encephalopathy, that practitioner, years later, will become either the parents' expert witness, or will become the foundation for the opinions held by the retained expert. Either way, the physician is placed in a compromised position, unless all data necessary to form such a diagnosis was available to him or her at the time of the transfer.

Be careful in criticizing another physician in the course of conversations with a patient or family members. In times of disappointment or grief, your statements will be remembered and may come back to haunt you. Do not hypothesize, but be as truthful and forthright as possible. The patient may take your "critical" comments as gospel and, unwittingly, you will have provided the basis for a lawsuit against the previous physician, hospital, or nurse.

Informed Consent

A fundamental premise of Anglo-American law is that no one can touch or treat a competent adult without the adult's informed consent.[3]

The issue of informed consent is one of importance, but easily and readily understood. What is the physician's responsibility to the patient? It is one where the physician has an obligation to provide significant information, so that the patient can intelligently decide what to do, based on the material presented. This information must be concise and direct enough to influence the patient's choice, whether it be to accept treatment or not, or to determine which method to invoke if there is more than one available to manage a condition. All positive and negative factors should be provided to the patient relative to the proposed treatment.

The positive factors include all information which will benefit the patient; the negative factors are those which would be detrimental, i.e., the risks involved. A patient is not in a position to choose among treatment options until all appropriate information has been communicated. Once this is done, chart it and have the patient sign your progress note. There will be no dispute later as to what was said or what was understood if this is done.

All consents for surgery should include the immediate reason for the surgery, plus anticipated problems and procedures. If a nurse is the individual who obtains the signed consent, it is still the responsibility of the physician to ensure that the patient understands what he or she has signed. Nurses cannot, as a general rule, provide the data necessary to ensure informed consent, only the physician can. It is the absolute obligation of the physician to obtain informed consent.

In summary, informed consent must include disclosure of the nature and purpose of the proposed treatment and/or surgical procedure, the risks and consequences,[3] including the possibility of death. Many physicians choose not to mention this simply because the likelihood is so small as to be nonexistent. *Mention it!* A physician cannot and should not minimize any known danger.

SPECIAL/UNIQUE PROBLEMS

In the past, obstetricians were at risk for being sued as a result of recognized or unrecognized complications associated with labor and delivery. In many instances, a lawsuit was filed on behalf of the neurologically impaired infant. The fetal monitor tracings which provided valuable information to the physicians and nurses prior to delivery wound up becoming a sword against the physician/nurse as a result of those findings. With the advent of technology and a better understanding of what the fetal monitor tracings provide but, more importantly, what they don't provide, suits against the obstetrician started to diminish slightly.

Currently, a fertile source of potential lawsuits involves the referral, or lack thereof, to consultants, especially with the patient who is pregnant and discovers a mass in her breast. The relationship of breast cancer to pregnancy is problematic. Diagnosed breast cancer occurs in between 1:10,000 and 1:3000 pregnancies, mak-

ing this malignancy almost as common as that of the uterine cervix.[3] A thorough breast examination is important at the first obstetrical visit, and a thorough charting of the findings or lack thereof is mandatory. During pregnancy, an increasing firmness, nodularity and hypertrophy occurs, obscuring subtle mass lesions. As a result, many abnormalities are missed, as well as the opportunities to diagnose same. The importance of thorough charting cannot be stressed enough, especially when it involves the patient who complains of a mass in the breast, nipple retraction, or other abnormality ultimately associated with a finding of breast cancer.

Normally the specific management for a breast abnormality is usually beyond the expertise of the obstetrician, and an appropriate consult should be obtained. Since each trimester has its own problems and its own unique management needs when a breast abnormality appears, allow the physician with knowledge in the appropriate field to guide you in your decision-making.

A vast majority of these cases can be defended on the basis of proximate cause, but this is not likely when there is no information in the physician's records to contradict the patient's claims and/or information other than the memory of the defendant physician.

Listen to the patient's complaints, chart the exact area (by diagram) where the patient claims to have found the abnormality, and chart whether you concur in the finding, or not. On the next office visit, specifically inquire whether or not the problem complained of at the previous month's visit still exists and, if it does, investigate it. Your chart, together with appropriate questioning, will lead to appropriate conclusions appreciated by all parties, especially a jury, if a lawsuit is filed.

This chapter has set forth the basic tenet that thorough charting is mandatory. One must keep in mind that a medical negligence suit takes the patient's compliants from the physician's office or hospital to the courtroom. As an example, when a "mother of two, who has just delivered a third child, is diagnosed with breast cancer shortly after delivery, and the mass is located in the same location where she testified (by video, since she has died by the time of the trial) she found it in the 1st trimester, but her doctor told her not to worry,'' a jury will believe the mother and not the physician, in the absence of any written material to the contrary.[4,5]

MEDICAL MALPRACTICE

All of the previously supplied information can and at times becomes the basis for a lawsuit. For the uninitiated, the following provides a road map for the establishment of a medical malpractice lawsuit.

There are four specific elements a plaintiff must establish to pursue a medical malpractice lawsuit. The absence of any one will defeat the case. These are:

1. Duty (standard of care)
2. Breach of duty
3. Proximate cause (relationship to injury)
4. Damages

At the conclusion of this chapter, the reader will find definitions of these terms drawn from *Black's Law Dictionary*.[6]

For purposes of this chapter, the *duty* addressed is the standard of care that a practicing OB/GYN must follow. (Remember, this duty is what the patient's expert says it is from the witness stand.)

A *breach of duty* occurs when the physician either (a) fails to do something which he/she should have done, i.e., an act of omission; or, (b) does something he/she should not have done, i.e., an act of commission.

The most important element (to me) is *proximate cause*, i.e., did the alleged breach of duty (standard of care) proximately cause or contribute to the injury? An example would be the physician who fails to order a timely biopsy of a mass detected in the breast after palpation. The patient is then diagnosed four (4) months later with breast cancer, with >4 positive nodes and distal metastasis. In this example, the physician breached a duty in not obtaining a biopsy; however, the end result may very well have been the

same, with earlier intervention not having altered the outcome. In this case, there would be a failure on the part of the patient/plaintiff to proximally connect the breach of duty (failure to order a breast biopsy) to the alleged injury (4-month delay in the diagnosis/treatment of breast cancer) and claim for damages. Unless the injury was caused by someone's act or failure to act (breach of duty) and this failure caused the injury (proximate cause), the patient cannot sustain her burden of proof and claim for damages.

Duty
(standard of care)
↓
Breach of Duty
(negligence)
↓
Proximate Cause
(relationship of breach
of duty to injury)
↓
Damages

THE IMPACT ON THE PERINATOLOGIST

In today's environment, problems now encountered were not recognized 20 years ago. Medical technology and advancements have raised as many questions as they have answered. In large part, physicians utilize statistics generated by various studies published on an ongoing basis. These statistics are part and parcel of a physician's knowledge in his field of expertise. Unfortunately, yesterday's statistics may be significantly different from today's. As a result, opinions and/or guidelines published by various organizations, for our purposes the American College of Obstetricians and Gynecologists, provide a continuing and current source of information for the practicing physician.

For example, in 1989, the Committee on Professional Standards of the American College of Obstetricians & Gynecologists published a ''standard of care'' to be followed by obstetricians regarding genetic counseling and prenatal diagnosis.[7] This publication provided guidelines for when genetic counseling should be recommended and what to look for in screening for genetic diseases. The failure to adhere to such published guidelines will have a deleterious impact on the perinatologist, since the very organization to which the practitioner most likely belongs has published such guidelines. These guidelines theoretically provide pertinent data which can be crucial in defining the standard of care for genetic screening. Guidelines such as the aforementioned keep a physician current in his/her specialty. The practitioner must be mindful of current literature, not only in publications of a general nature, but especially those in his/her field of expertise.

An extremely good publication to review for some of the more current problematical issues is *Legal and Ethical Issues in Perinatology* by George J. Annas and Sherman Elias.[7] Problems involving genetic screening, forced cesarean sections, abortion, fetal research, consent, and the human genome initiative are highlighted.

CONCLUSION

It is very difficult to set forth all problems that may lead to a lawsuit, and what to do about them. My purpose in writing this chapter was to provide an insight into the origins of a lawsuit and trial, and how to avoid them. In your efforts to avoid being sued, benefits occur both for you and your patients. The patient is provided quality care, and you as a physician are able to conduct your practice without interruption due to a lawsuit and trial.

If you end up in a courtroom, remember that in the absence of written material, a jury is more apt to believe the statements of a patient for it is the patient who is claiming to be wronged, and our society likes to correct wrongs. That

same jury, however, will listen intently to the testimony, and, when it sees (a) a thoroughly charted record authored by a physician who has provided good medical care, and (b) a physician with a caring demeanor, the jury will listen to you.

REFERENCES

1. Stedman TL. *Stedman's Medical Dictionary*, 24th Ed. Baltimore: Williams & Wilkins, 1982, 830.
2. Bates B. *A Guide to Physical Examination and History Taking*, 5th Ed. Philadelphia: Lippincott, 1991, 651.
3. Shiffman MA, Brook J, Haig PV, eds. *Attorney's Guide to Oncology Cases*. New York: John Wiley & Sons, Inc., 1994.
4. Petrek JA. Breast disease and pregnancy. In: *Breast Diseases*, 2nd Ed., Harris JR, Hellman S, Henderson IC, Kinne DW, Lippincott, 1991.
5. Creasy RK, Resnik R, eds. *Maternal Fetal Medicine: Principles and Practice*, 3rd Ed. Philadelphia: W. B. Saunders, 1994.
6. Black HC. *Black's Law Dictionary*, 4th Ed. St. Paul, MN: West Publishing Co., 1968.
7. Annas GJ, Elias S. *Obstetrics: Normal and Problem Pregnancies*, Chapter 42: Legal and Ethical Issues in Perinatology, 1333–1350.

QUESTIONS

1. What is a physician's first-line defense when a patient has instituted a lawsuit?
2. What four elements must a plaintiff satisfy to successfully pursue a lawsuit?
3. What is a breach of the standard of care?
4. What is proximate cause?
5. What should be done to ensure informed consent has been obtained when a physician is confronted by a patient who does not seem to grasp the risks to possible consequences of a particular course of treatment or procedure?

23

Statistics

Saeid B. Amini

INTRODUCTION

Statistics is the science of collecting, summarizing, presenting, and interpreting data, and of using it for risk factor assessments, testing hypotheses and model building. Statistical methods have assumed an increasingly central role in medical investigation and decision making.

Many physicians reading an article, assume the stated statistics are correct and do not scrutinize them. Also, many readers uncertain of their understanding of statistics tend to skim over statistical discussions in articles. Despite this, it is important to have a sufficient knowledge of basic statistics so that one is able to evaluate the validity of the conclusions drawn. Thus, this short chapter provides some discussion of elementary statistics which hopefully the readers will find useful. The discussion includes topics in study designs, descriptive and epidemiological measures, and testing the hypothesis. For a more comprehensive discussion of the topics, the reader is referred to references at the end of the chapter.

THE USE OF STATISTICS IN MEDICAL RESEARCH

In general medical studies are either descriptive or inferential. A descriptive study tends to report findings of a study through descriptive statistics such as sample mean and variance and epidemiological measures such as rates and proportions. These studies have no underlying hypothesis and are used to describe a study population and sometimes for generating hypotheses for subsequent studies. However, most of the studies in medical and behavioral sciences are inferential and conducted in order to test hypotheses which are derived from some underlying theories. Having stated a specific hypothesis, one collects data from either the whole population of study or from a representative sample drawn from that population. The collected information should enable the researcher to make a decision concerning the hypothesis. The decision may then lead to retaining, revising, or rejecting the hypothesis and the theory which was its source. To reach an objective decision as to whether a particular hypothesis is confirmed by a set of data, one must have an objective procedure for either rejecting or accepting that hypothesis. Objectivity is emphasized because one important aspect of the scientific method is that one should arrive at conclusions by methods that are public and which may be repeated by other investigators. The quality and reliability of final results are generally dependent on the many factors including proper choice of hypothesis, study design, study population, study sample, sample size, data, statistical power, statistical analyses methods, and interpretation.

The procedure usually followed involves several steps. In the following we list these steps in order of performance.

1. State the null hypothesis (H_0) and its alternative (H_1).
2. Decide on the study population (i.e., whole population or sample).
3. Decide on the study design (i.e., case control, cohort, randomized, prospective, etc.).
4. Decide on the sampling techniques (e.g., random, stratified, cluster, etc.).
5. Decide on the types of data to collect, and types of statistics to report.
6. Decide on the significance level (α), statistical power and sample size (N).
7. Decide on the test statistics appropriate for testing the null hypothesis (H_0).
8. Select the most powerful test available.
9. Use the most appropriate sampling distribution and rejection region for test statistics under the null hypothesis (i.e., normal, t, χ^2, Gamma distributions).
10. Be aware of multiple comparison problems.
11. Be aware of very small and very large samples. If the null hypothesis was not rejected (accepted) make sure there was enough power associated with the acceptance. Also, remember that with a sample large enough any tiny differences can be found statistically significant regardless of clinical significance.
12. Interpret the results properly.

A basic understanding of each of these steps is essential to understanding the role of statistics in medical studies.

LITERATURE ANALYSIS

There are, of course, different reasons for reading the medical literature. Some articles are of interest because the physician wants only to maintain an awareness of advances in a field. In these instances, the reader may decide to skim the article with little consideration of how the study was designed and carried out. The reader may be able to depend on experts in the field who write review articles providing a relatively superficial level of information. On other occasions, however, the reader wants to know whether the conclusions of the study are valid, perhaps so they can be used to determine patient care or to plan a research project. In these cases, the reader will read and evaluate the article with a critical eye in order to detect poorly done studies with unwarranted conclusions.

To assist these kind of readers, several checklists are provided by various authors.[1] In general, one can evaluate the paper as it is structured starting from abstract to conclusion. From a statistical point of view one needs to check the 12 steps just provided. Obviously for doing so one needs to have enough knowledge of the issues involved including statistical design, formulation of statistical hypothesis, sample size requirement, statistical power and use of proper statistical methods. Improper use of some or all of these will greatly affect the result of the study.

THE NULL AND ALTERNATIVE HYPOTHESIS

The first step in the decision-making procedure is to state the null hypothesis (H_0). The null hypothesis is a hypothesis of ''no effect'' and is usually formulated for the express purpose of being rejected. If it is rejected, the alternative hypothesis (H_1 or H_a) is supported. Once the null hypothesis is set up, we then evaluate the probability that we could have obtained the test statistics (or data that were more extreme) if the null hypothesis were true. This probability is usually called the P value; the smaller it is the more untenable the null hypothesis. The method is called *testing* because of the aspect of deciding whether or not we can *reject* the null hypothesis in favor of an alternative which can be either one sided or two sided. Examples of the null and various alternative hypotheses for a mean birth weight (*BW*) for a given population are given below:

Hypothesis	Testing
The null:	
H_0: $\mu_{BW} = 2,500$ g	Mean population of *BW* for a group of neonates is equal 2,500 g
One-sided alternatives:	
H_A: $\mu_{BW} > 2,500$ g	Mean population of *BW* is more than 2,500 g
H_A: $\mu_{BW} < 2,500$ g	Mean population of *BW* is less than 2,500 g
Two-sided alternatives:	
H_0: $\mu_{BW} \neq 2,500$ g	Mean population *BW* for a group of neonates is equal 2,500 g

Note that we always test a null against one alternative which should be stated before the study.[1-4]

How do we evaluate the probability of obtaining our data if the null hypothesis is true? For most problems we calculate a quantity called *test statistic*—a value which we can compare with a known distribution (e.g., standardized normal, t, chi-square) of what we expect when the null hypothesis is true. In many cases the hypothesized value is zero (e.g., differences in two population means, regression coefficients, etc.), so that the test statistic becomes the ratio of the observed quantity of interest to its standard error. The idea that the magnitude of the quantity of interest is evaluated as a multiple of its standard error is common in the main

method of stastistical analysis. The general formula for test statistics is:

test statistic

$$= \frac{\text{sample statistics} - \text{hypothesized value}}{\text{standard error of the sample statistics}}. \quad (1)$$

For example, for testing the population mean (i.e., H_0: $\mu = \mu_0$, where μ_0 is known), with a large sample (e.g., $n > 30$), the appropriate test is either

$$Z = \frac{(X - \mu_0)}{(\sigma/\sqrt{n})} \text{ or } t = \frac{(X - \mu_0)}{(s/\sqrt{n})}$$

dependent on whether the population variance (σ^2) is known or not. In other words, when σ^2 is known the appropriate test statistic is Z and it follows standardized normal distribution while when σ^2 is not known the appropriate test statistic is t which follows a t distribution with appropriate degrees of freedom.

CHOOSING A STUDY DESIGN

Study design is probably the most important aspect of the statistical contribution to medical research. It is for this reason that for many years statisticians have been urging medical researchers to consult them at the planning stage of their study, rather than at the analysis stage. The data from a good study can be analyzed in many ways, but no amount of sophisticated analysis can compensate for problems with the design of a bad study. To familiarize you with various designs, we note that medical research can be crudely divided into observational and experimental studies which can be either prospective or retrospective which is conducted at one time point (cross-sectional) or over time (longitudinal). In the following we will further discuss these studies.[3,5]

In observational studies researchers collect information about one or more groups of subjects, but do nothing to influence the outcomes. Observational studies can be prospective, where subjects are recruited and data are collected about subsequent events, or retrospective, where information is collected about past events. Examples include case-control studies, cohort studies and all surveys and most epidemiological studies. Experimental studies on the other hand are those in which the researcher offers and controls the intervention. Examples include clinical trials and many animal and laboratory studies. In general stronger inferences can be made from experimental studies than from observational studies. Experimental studies are usually carried out to make comparisons between groups with at least one control group.

Prospective or Retrospective Study

In prospective studies data are collected forward in time from the start of the study, and in retrospective studies, data may be acquired from existing sources, such as patients' charts, or by interview. In general, experimental studies are prospective, but observational studies may be prospective or retrospective.

Longitudinal or Cross-Sectional

Longitudinal studies are those which investigate changes over time, possibly in relation to an intervention. Observations are taken on more than one occasion, although they may not all be used in the analysis. Clinical trials are longitudinal because we are interested in the effect of treatment on outcome at a later time. Cross-sectional studies are those in which individuals are observed only once. Most surveys are cross-sectional. Observational studies may be longitudinal or cross-sectional, but experiments are usually longitudinal. There is also the so called pseudo-longitudinal study in which each subject is seen only once but the data are used to describe changes over time. A neonatal birthweight chart is an example of this type of study.

Case Control and Cohort Studies

Case control and cohort studies are the two main types of observational studies which are used to investigate causal effects. In a retrospective case control study a number of subjects with the disease of interest are identified (cases) along with some disease-free subjects (controls). The past history of these groups in relation to the exposure(s) of interest is then compared. In contrast, in a prospective cohort study a group of subjects is identified and followed prospectively, perhaps for many years, and their subsequent medical history recorded. The cohort may be subdivided at the outset into groups with different characteristics, or the study may be used to investigate which subjects go on to develop a particular disease. (There is also the historical cohort study, in which a past cohort is identified.)

The main advantages of the case control approach are practical: it is relatively simple, and thus quick and cheap. The case control design is also valuable when the condition of interest is very rare. The disadvantages of this design are possibility biases that can occur when comparing cases and controls. There are as many as 35 different biases that can occur in a case control study.[6]

The prospective cohort study (follow-up or longitudinal study) is the method of choice for an observational study. The essence of the cohort study is to identify a group of subjects of interest and then follow them for a period of time. Because of the need to observe unaffected individuals until a fair proportion develop the outcome of interest, cohort studies can take a long time and may thus be very expensive. They are usually not suitable for studying rare outcomes as it would be necessary to follow a very large number of subjects to get an adequate number of events. In cohort studies, there is usually one particular event of interest, such as delivering preterm birth or occurrence (or recurrence) of one or several diseases. The main purpose of this type of study is to use the information collected for each cohort to try to identify those subjects most at risk of developing the outcome of interest (e.g., premature births). Because the study is prospective the nature and quality of the data recording can be carefully controlled.

The Cross-Sectional Study

In a cohort study subjects with different characteristics are identified and followed to see what happens. By contrast, in a cross-sectional study all the information is collected at the same time because subjects are only contacted once. Many cross-sectional studies are descriptive, and these are often called surveys. Some cross-sectional studies are, however, carried out to investigate associations between a disease and possible risk factors, so that this design is an alternative to the case control and cohort approaches. The cross-sectional study does not suffer from many of the difficulties that affect these other designs, such as recall bias and loss to follow-up. It is relatively cheap and easy to carry out. Needless to say, there are different special problems associated with cross-sectional studies.

Change Over Time Studies

Change over time studies are appropriate when two or more independent sets of cross-sectional data are used to make inferences about changes over time. For example, ultrasound measurements of the fetus obtained in two periods (e.g., 20 and 30 weeks) can be used to estimate average fetal growth during this period. There are many other types of studies such as matched-pair design, cross-over design, single- and double-blind design that are mainly used in clinical trials.[7]

Sample Selections

The most common method of sampling is the random sampling. Random means that every observation has an equal chance of being selected to the sample. A sample will represent the population from which it is drawn if it meets the following requirements: (1) The sample must be large enough; and (2) the sample must be selected randomly. For convenience, however, selection from the population is sometimes carried out systematically rather than randomly, by taking individuals at regular intervals with the starting point being chosen at random. For ex-

ample, to select 1 in 10, sample of the population, the starting point is chosen randomly from numbers 1 to 10, and then every 10th person on the list is taken. There are many situations in which a simple random sample is not appropriate and a more complex sampling scheme is necessary. The most common complex sampling methods used are stratified, multistage and cluster sampling. These may be used alone or in combination. In general the aim is to apply these schemes in such a way as to give every individual an equal chance of being selected, that is, to use them with an equal probability selection method.[8] Also, it is important to select a sample not just to be a fair representative of the current population but also be representative of some future class of patients to whom the findings may be applied.

Stratified Sampling

Stratified sampling is used when the population consists of distinct subgroups, or strata, which differ with respect to the feature under study and which are themselves of interest. A simple random sample is taken from each stratum to ensure that they are all adequately represented.

Multistage Sampling

Multistage sampling is carried out in stages using the hierarchical structure of a population. For example, a two-stage sample might consist of first taking a random sample of hospitals with a maternal fetal diagnostic center and then taking a random sample of mothers from each selected center. The centers would be called first-stage units and the mothers second-stage units.

Cluster Sampling

Cluster sampling is a multistage sampling that includes all the secondary units of the primary unit. This method is preferred if some benefit is being offered to the participants which would be ethically or logistically inappropriate to offer only to some members of the unit. For example, in sampling maternal fetal diagnostic centers to estimate the prevalence rate of PKU, it would be preferable to examine all mothers in the selected centers rather than just a sample of them. The disadvantage of these types of sampling is that the overall estimate is less precise than that based on a simple random sample of the same total size.

There are many other sampling techniques such as double sampling, network sampling, capture-recapture sampling, line-intercept sampling, spatial sampling, and adaptive sampling that may be more relevant and practical to some projects. For a further reading, see Thompson.[8]

DESCRIPTIVE STATISTICS

Populations and Samples

Almost all statistical analysis is based on the principle that one collects data on a sample of individuals or objects and uses the information to make inferences about all such individuals. The set of all subjects (or whatever is being investigated) is called the *population* of interest (target population). In short, the collection of all items of interest in a study is called population and a portion of the population selected to represent the whole population is called sample.[1-4] The way the sample is selected is clearly very important, and is discussed later.

In practice we take samples because it is rarely possible to study the whole population. For example, one might be able to study all fetuses diagnosed as having cystic fibrosis in one country on a particular date, but it is still only a sample of all people with cystic fibrosis, restricted by time and geography, and undiagnosed cases are excluded. In practice, fortunately, we do not need to study the whole population since a carefully chosen sample can yield reliable answers. We cannot usually count or identify all the members of the population, but the sample allows us to draw inferences about the population, both collectively and individually. The relation between sample and population is subject to uncertainty, and probability theory has been used to indicate this uncertainty. The idea of a theoretical probability distribution is important in this context.

Types of Data and Descriptive Statistics

Since most statistical methods are specific to a certain type of data, it is important to know what types of data or variables will be collected (Table 23-1). In medical studies many different types of data are collected which in general can be classified as qualitative (or categorical) or quantitative (or numerical). A qualitative variable is nonnumerical, for instance, hospital of birth, ethnic group, or type of drug. A particularly common sort is a binary variable, where the response is one of two alternatives. For example, sex of a fetus is either male or female, a patient delivers prematurely or not. A quantitative variable is numerical and can either be discrete or continuous. The values of a discrete variable are usually whole numbers, such as the number of patients having amniocentesis in a given month. A continuous variable, as the name implies, is a measurement on a continuous scale. Examples are height, weight, abdominal circumference, and gestational age. Also, in some situations the data is naturally ordered (e.g., births in trimesters), or continuous variables grouped in order (e.g., age groups of 10–19, 20–29, etc.) or continuous variables ranked from 1 to N.

Once the data is collected appropriate descriptive statistics should be calculated. A table presentation is perhaps the simplest means of summarizing all types of data. All elementary statistics or biostatistics text books show how to summarize the data (e.g., see[2,4]). In short, nominal and ordinal data are presented by proportions and/or by relative and cumulative frequencies.[4] These frequencies can be presented in graphical form as bar charts, stacked bar charts, histograms, frequency polygons, scatter plots, box plots and line charts.[2,4]

For numerical data, a set of summary measures can be provided. The most frequently used measure is the measure of central tendency which includes mean (average), median (50th percentile), and mode (values occur most frequently). Obviously a data set can have more than one mode (e.g., bimodal or higher). Other

Table 23-1. Measurement Scales and their Presentations

Type of Measurement	Character of Variables	Example	Presentation (how to report)	Value of Measurement
Categorical				
1. Nominal Names only	Unordered categorical	Race, gender, delivery hospital, blood type	Rate, proportion counts, relative risk odds ratio, histograms frequency tables, charts	Low
2. Ordinal Ranks or Likert scale	Ordered categories with intervals that are not quantifiable	Degree of pain, severity of illness, apgar scores	All the above + median, mode, range	Moderate
Continuous				
3. Interval Differences are meaningful	Measures defined in terms of fixed and equal units. Items can be ordered.	Body temperature (e.g., 80° is not twice as warm as 30°)	All the above + mean, variance, SD CV, correlation	High
4. Ratio Like interval, but with inherent point (there is a fixed zero)	Measures defined in terms of fixed and equal units. Items can be ordered.	Neonatal length, femoral length, gestational age, birth weight	All the above + regression	High

important statistics are the measure of dispersion or variability in the numerical data. The range (difference between the largest and smallest observations), interquartile range (e.g., difference between the 75th centile and 25th centile), interpercentile range, variance (quantifies the amount of spread about the sample mean), and standard deviation (SD, square root of variance) are all the measures of dispersions. Note that, standard error (also known as SE or SEM) is the variation of the mean if we repeat sampling the data many times; this is not part of descriptive statistics. Mean and variance are generally used with symmetrical data while the median and percentiles are used with asymmetrical data.

Another useful descriptive statistic is when interest in assessing the size of the variation relative to the size of the observation is the coefficient of variation which is defined as $CV\% = 100 \times SD/(\text{sample mean})$. It has the advantage that the coefficient of variation is independent of the units of observation. This is, for example, while the standard deviation of a set of abdominal circumflex measures for a fetus will be different depending on whether they are measured in inches or centimeters, the coefficient of variation, however, will be the same in the two units and thus comparable.

Probability Density and Distributions

A probability distribution is a table or graph showing all possible outcomes of a variable with their respective probabilities. Discrete variables such as number of prenatal care visits follows a discrete distribution such as Poisson, binomial, or multinomial while continuous variables such as fetal femoral length follows continuous distributions such as normal, t, or gamma. There are many different distributions and one could look at the histogram of a variable (e.g., fetal abdominal circumflex) to decide on the underlying population distribution of that variable. Knowing the population distribution function is very important since it can be used in comparing the population characteristics as well as using it for model building and prediction.

Normal Distribution

Normal distribution is the widely used distribution in practice. There are several theoretical and logical reasons for that. The most important reason is that it can be shown theoretically by so called *central limit theorem* that the average of almost any random variable including the discrete variables such as number of prenatal care visits follow a normal distribution. This is a very powerful result since it allows us to compare the means of two variables that each may not follow a normal distribution. The normal distribution which is also called Gaussian distribution, normal curve, normal probability function, is a symmetric (around the mean) bell-shaped curve that is uniquely characterized by its mean (μ) and variance σ^2 and has the following mathematical relation and shape.

$$f(x \mid \mu, \sigma^2) = \frac{1}{\sqrt{2\pi}\sigma} e^{-(X^2 - \mu)/2}\sigma^2$$

where Pi (π) approximately equals 3.14159 and e is 2.71828, X is the random variable with normal distribution with mean μ and variance σ^2. Since this is a probability function, the area under the curve is always equal to 1. Under the null hypothesis one could assume a specific normal distribution with a known mean and variance. The question then is whether data supports such hypothesis. For example, suppose the distribution of the time of the first prenatal care visit has a normal distribution with a mean of 10 weeks and variance of 9 weeks. With this information we can uniquely define the distribution and could test whether a patient who has her first prenatal care visit at 28 weeks of gestation belongs to this population. To answer this we need to compute the probability of

$$P(X \geq 28 \text{ weeks}) = \int_{28} f(x) \, dx \qquad (2)$$

If this is too small (e.g., less than .05), then we say that this patient has a small chance of coming from a normal distribution with the mean of 10 and variance of 9 weeks.

Standardized Normal Distribution

For a given set of observations, it is extraordinarily time consuming to apply the above in-

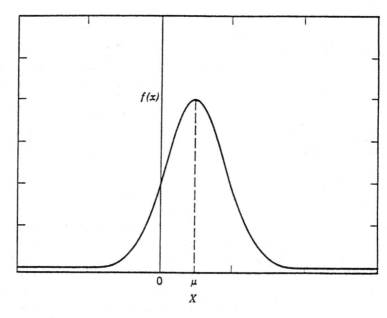

Figure 23-1. Graph of the normal probability density function with mean μ and variance σ^2.

tegration. One way to solve this problem is to standardize the X variable as

$$Z = \frac{X - \mu}{\sigma} \qquad (3)$$

and use the table available for Z, standardized normal curve. Here, Z has a unit normal distribution, which always has a mean of 0 and variance of 1 and is also called Z-statistics.

Graphs of Some Distributions

I. Example of Discrete Variable: For a discrete random variable, the probability distribution is equal to the probability of occurrence of each possible outcome. For example, the probability distribution of number of prenatal care visits may follow the following probability function (factious data).

X	$f(x)$
0	0.08 (8%)
1	0.17 (17%)
2	0.20 (25%)
3	0.30 (30%)
4	0.15 (15%)
5	0.06 (6%)
>5	0.04 (4%)

1.1. Binomial Distribution. This is the most used discrete distribution in practice. In general the number of successes or failures in n independent trials would follow a binomial distribution. For example, suppose the chance of preterm delivery in a population of women is 30% (in general called p). If we study 1000 patients from such a population the number of women actually delivering preterm would be a random variable, X, which can vary between 0 to 1000 (from no preterm to all preterm). As long as these 1000 patients are independent then we should expect 300 preterm deliveries (1000 × .30 = 300). While under the null (H_0:$p = 0.30$), we expect to observe 300 but in reality we could observe any number. However, if the number of observed preterm births is too small (e.g., less than 200) or too large (e.g., more than 400) then one would suspect that the hypothesized pre-

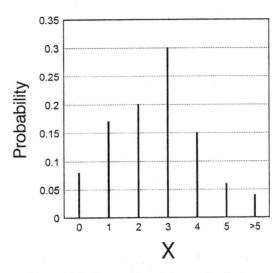

Figure 23-2.   Presentation of discrete distribution.

term rate of 30% is not attainable with the available data. For testing the null, the exact P value can be computed from the binomial distribution or approximate P value can be computed from normal distribution for which the variance is required and can be computed from $\sigma^2 = np(1 - p)$ which for the above example is equal to $\sigma^2 = [1000 \times .30 \times .70 = 210]$. The following figure shows the probability function of three binomial distributions.

Multinominal and Poisson are the other widely used discrete distributions in practice.

II. Examples of Continuous Variables
    a. Normal Distributions
    b. Standardized Normal Distribution
    c. Nonnormal Distributions
        1. t-distribution
        2. Chi-square Distribution
        3. Exponential and Gamma Distributions

STATISTICAL INFERENCE

Statistical inference is a formal process that uses information from collected data to draw conclusions about the population. The terms statistical inference, hypothesis testing and significance testing are often used interchangeably.

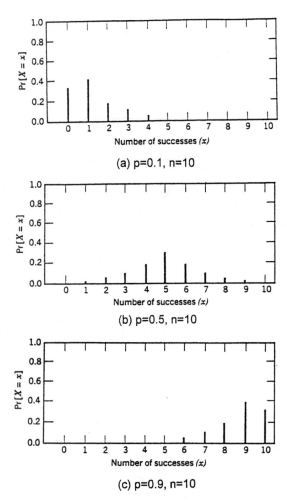

(a) p=0.1, n=10

(b) p=0.5, n=10

(c) p=0.9, n=10

Figure 23-3. Probability function of binomial distribution with varying proportion of successes.

Statistical Hypothesis Testing

Statistical hypothesis testing is a several step procedure that needs to be followed carefully. First, the null and alternative hypothesis must be scientifically stated and formulated and the proper test statistics calculated from the data. Second, the relevant distribution for the test statistics (e.g., Z-distribution, t-distribution, Chi-Square distribution) must be identified so the proper comparison can be made (Tables 23-2–23-4). This is a most critical step in hypothesis testing since a choice of improper distribution could change the final conclusion. Third, the level of significance (referred to as alpha, α)

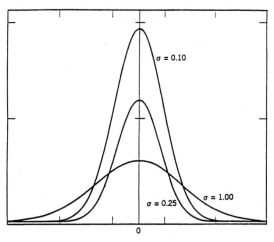

Figure 23-4. Normal distributions with mean (μ) = 0 and standard deviation (σ) = 0.1, 0.25 and 1.

must be selected and therefore the critical region or region of rejection could be identified. Here, α is the area in the tail or tails (dependent on the one-sided or two-sided alternative) of the distribution of the test statistics. The rejection region (RR) contains values of test statistics that are relatively improbable to occur if the null hypothesis is true. Since the values in RR deviate sufficiently from what is expected under the null hypothesis, we will reject the null in favor of the alternative hypothesis if the value of test statistics falls in this region. If the value of the statistic falls inside the region (region of retention) we say there was no evidence to reject the null. In fact the total value of areas fallen outside a region created by the test statistics is called P value.

Figure 23-11 shows the P value under the null. By tradition, α is considered to equal 0.05.

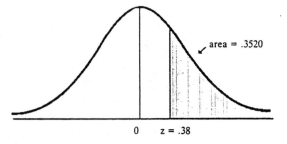

Figure 23-5. Standard normal distribution (Z); mean (μ) = 0, variance (σ^2) = 1; area beyond a z-value of 0.38.

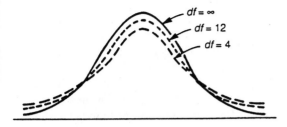

Figure 23-6. *t*-distribution with 4, 12, and ∞ degrees of freedom.

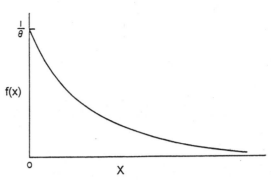

Figure 23-8. Density function of the exponential distribution with mean θ.

Although this is purely arbitrary, it is widely accepted in the literature. In practice, the value of α should not be set by tradition but rather by the context of the experiment.

Errors in Hypothesis Testing

In hypothesis testing two errors are possible: a true hypothesis can be rejected or a false hypothesis can be retained. These are labeled as Type I and Type II errors, respectively. Simply put, a Type I error occurs when a true null hypothesis is rejected. The probability of making such an error is equal to α, the value of all rejection regions as we discussed before. Note that when the value of α is low, one makes fewer Type I errors. That is when α is small, there is a small chance that you will mistakenly call a result significant. One could see that there is a close relationship between the *P* value and α. We set α in advance based on the Type I error

and use it as a threshold for *P* value which is calculated from data and test statistics.

The Type II error (sometimes called β error) occurs when a false null hypothesis is retained. This is the error of accepting the null hypothesis when in fact it is false. Note that, if the null hypothesis is true, there can be no Type II error and in general the Type II error is inversely related to the Type I error. The probability of making a Type II error is called β. The complement of a Type II error is called power of the test (Power = 1 − β). This information can be summarized as:

Null Hypothesis	Decision on Hypothesis	
	Accept	Reject
True	Correct conclusion	Type I or α error
False	Type II or β error	Correct decision

TYPES OF INFERENTIAL STATISTICS

Basic Concept

The distribution of individual observation is generally different from the distribution of the test statistics that are being used to test the null hypothesis. If we are dealing with the mean of a population the relevant distribution may be either normal or *t* distributions but also the distribution of test statistics could be chi-square, *F* or other distributions which should clearly be identified. In Table 23-5, we provide some sum-

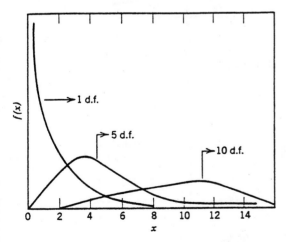

Figure 23-7. Chi-square distribution for 1, 5, and 10 degrees of freedom.

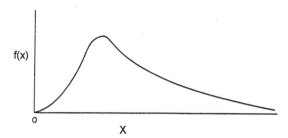

Figure 23-9. Gamma density function.

mary statistics used in specific cases and for further reading see.[2-4]

Confidence Intervals

From a single data set, population parameters such as population mean (μ) or variance (σ^2) could be estimated as the *point estimates*. Obviously these estimates will change if the parameters estimated from a second sample are taken from the same population. Because of random variations in these estimates, it is customary to provide so-called *interval estimates*, or

confidence interval in addition to *point estimates*. The process of calculating confidence intervals is quite simple if we know the distribution of point estimates. For example, a population parameter for mean femoral length for a 30-week gestation fetus can be estimated by an arithmetic mean of femoral length for 20 fetuses measured by ultrasound. However, if we repeat the same measurements on 20 different fetuses, we are more likely to find a different estimate for the mean and variance. Now, if we know the distribution of a sample mean (say normal), then we can compute the confidence interval (*CI*) or confidence limits for a true population mean of femoral length at 30 weeks gestation. For example, for the sample mean of X and known variance of σ^2, with $\alpha = 0.05$, the 95% *CI* for the true population mean (μ) would be $X \pm 1.96$ $\sigma/\sqrt{n}$, where 1.96 corresponds to .025 area of Z-distribution. This can be explained that, we are 95% sure that the true population mean of femoral length at 30 weeks gestation is bounded by $X - 1.96\ \sigma/\sqrt{n}$ and $X + 1.96\ \sigma/\sqrt{n}$.

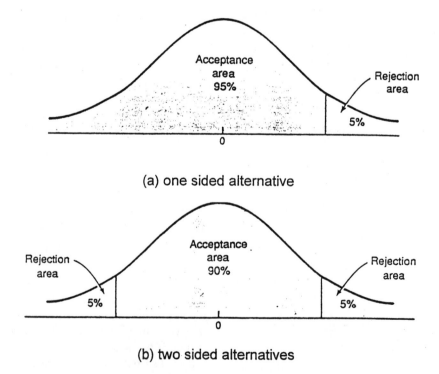

Figure 23-10. Distribution of test statistics under the null hypothesis and rejection regions (RR).

Table 23-2. Methods of Analysis of Single (One) Sample

Type of Measurement	Type of Hypothesis	Parameter Tested	Test Statistics	Sample Size Requirement
Categorical				
1. Nominal	H_0: $p = p_0$	Proportion rate	Binomial test, Z-test approximation, chi-square test	Large
2. Ordinal or Ordered	H_0: $p = p_0$	Proportion/rate	Same as above	Large
	H_0: $\theta = \theta_0$	Median	Sign test, Wilcoxon signed rank test	Moderate
	H_0: $\sigma^2 = \sigma_0^2$	Variance	Chi-square test, Siegel-Tukey test	Moderate
Continuous				High
Interval/ratio	All the above	All the above	All	Large
	H_0: $\mu = \mu_0$	Mean	Paired test, Z-test	Small
	H_0: $\sigma^2 = \sigma_0^2$	Variance	Chi-square test, Bartlett F-test, Moses rank-like test	Moderate

t-test

In the above example, if the population variance (σ^2) was not known then the test statistics

test statistics

$$= \frac{\text{sample statistics} - \text{hypothesized value}}{\text{standard error of the sample statistics}} = \frac{X - \mu_0}{S/\sqrt{n}}.$$

had a t-distribution with $n - 2$ degrees of freedom than Z distribution, where X and S^2 are the sample mean and variance respectively, μ_0 is a known value and n is the sample size used in the study.

Unlike the normal distribution which is dependent on the mean and variance, the t-distribution depends only on the degree of freedom.[4] It is unimodal, symmetric, and bell-shaped about a mean of zero. However, the variance of t-distribution is greater than standard normal distribution. As a result it is flatter and has slightly wider tails than Z-distribution. When n

Table 23-3. Methods of Analysis of Two Sample Cases

Type of Measurements	Sample Size	Parameter	Two Related Samples (Paired or Matched Data)	Two Independent Samples
Categorical				
1. Nominal	Small	Proportion	—	Fisher's exact test
	Moderate/large	. . .	McNemar Test	Chi-square test
2. Ordinal	Small	Proportion	All of above	All of above
	Moderate/large	. . .	McNemar test	Chi-square test
	Small/moderate/large	Median/mean	Paired t-test	Two-sample t-test
			Sign test I	Two-sample Wilcoxon test
			Wilcoxon signed rank test	
	Moderate/large	Variance	—	Siegel-Tukey test
				Bartlett F-test
Continuous				
Interval/ratio	Small/moderate/large	Median/mean	All the above	All the above
			Permutation test	Permutation test
		Variance	—	F-test
				Moses rank-like test

Table 23-4. Methods of Analysis of K-Sample Cases ($K > 2$)

Type of Measurements	Types of Test	K-Related Samples	K Independent Samples
Categorical			
1. Nominal	Nonparametric	Cochran Q test	Chi-square test, log-linear
		Log-linear categorical model	categorical model
2. Ordinal	Parametric	All the above	All the above
		Repeated measure analysis	ANOVA
		Random effect model	
		Generalized estimating equation	
	Nonparametric	Freidman test	Kruskal-Walls test
		Page test for ordered alternative	Jonckheere for ordered alternative
Continuous			
Interval/ratio	Parametric	All the above	All the above
	Nonparametric	All the above	All the above

is very large, the *t*- and *Z*-distribution become identical.

The *t*-distribution is the distribution of choice when comparing the paired data, means or proportion of two (or single) populations with unknown variances. For more reading and degrees of freedom and *t*-distribution see.[1-5]

Chi-Square Test

Chi-square (χ^2) test is used frequently to test the association between two criterion applied to a sample of observations including a 2×2 table. The reason this is called a chi-square test is because the corresponding test statistic has a chi-square distribution. Similar to *t*-distribution, a chi-square distribution can be uniquely identified by its degree of freedom. In fact, if we square a standardized normal variable Z, the new variable Z^2 will have a chi-square distri-

bution with one degree of freedom. The distribution is asymmetric as shown in the following figures.

Most of the goodness of fit tests would follow a chi-square distribution. However, the most references to chi-square test were made when testing the independent assumption in contingency tables (tables of r rows and c columns). For more detail see.[1-5]

Analysis of Variance

Analysis of variance (ANOVA) and analysis of covariance (ANCOVA) are used to compare the means of more than two populations without and with adjusting for confounding parameters. There are many different types of ANOVA and ANCOVA models and a typical graduate student in a statistics program spends more than a year studying this subject. In short, ANOVA involves partitioning the total sums of squares (total variance) into many distinct components of sums of squares and the ratio of these sums of squares form the test statistics and the F-distribution predominately used for testing null hypotheses and calculating the P-values.

Association and Correlation

Another parameter often reported in medical studies is the correlation between two variables. The association between two variables can be

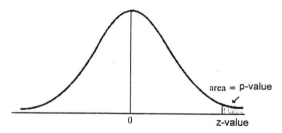

Figure 23-11. Distribution of test statistics under the null hypothesis and P value.

Table 23-5. Measures of Association Between Two Variables

Type of Measurements Variable 1	Type of Measurements Variable 2	Types of Statistics
Binary/Dichotomous	Binary/Dichotomous	Cramer coefficient C Phi coefficient for a 2×2 table
Nominal/Categorical	Nominal/Categorical	Cramer coefficient C Phi coefficient for a 2×2 table The kappa coefficient of agreement, asymetrical association, the lambda statistic,
Nominal/Categorical	Ordinal/Interval/Ratio	All the above
Ordinal/Interval/Ratio	Ordinal/Interval/Ratio	Pearson correlation Spearman rank-order cc Kendall rank-order cc Gamma statistic Somer's index of asymmetric association

shown by a scatter plot for continuous variables and by contingency tables for a nominal or ordinal variable (Table 23-5). The measures of linear association can be measured by Pearson correlation coefficients for continuous variables and the Cramer coefficient C for contingency tables. For an association between one variable (dependent variable) and several independent variables one may use multiple or logistic regression when the dependent variable is continuous or binary respectively. If we are interested in the association between a set of several variables (e.g., clinical and socioeconomic variables) we can use multivariate techniques such as canonical correlation.[7]

Regression Analysis

To predict one variable (dependent variable) from another(s) (independent or explanatory variable(s)), we rely on statistical procedures called regression. Although there are many similarities between the regression and correlation analyses each serves different purposes. Namely, the strength of the relationship between variables is measured by correlation procedures while regression analyses are used to predict one variable from others through the relationship developed by regression analysis. An example of a regression model can be development of a regression model to predict birth

weight for an infant from abdominal circumflex of fetuses measured by ultrasound during 25–30 weeks gestation.

In regression analysis we have only one dependent variable but the predictors can be just one variable (simple regression) or several variables (multiple regression). The dependent variable can be either quantitative or binary (e.g., preterm vs term; cesarean delivery: yes or no, etc.). For continuous numerical values we normally apply ordinary regression analysis while for the binary dependent variables we use so called logistic regression models. In practice fitting a model is only 20% of the model building effort since one must check the goodness of fit (e.g., using a statistic called R^2) to verify the required assumptions and validate the model before reporting the model. Unfortunately we cannot explain this important topic in the space allowed us and refer readers to references.[1–5] However, we list a few simple steps that should be followed when using this model.

- To construct a scatter diagram for the dependent and independent variable.
- Inspect a scatter diagram and assess whether it developed a linear relationship.
- Understand and explain why the relation is important.
- Fit the regression model.[5]
- Check the goodness of fit statistics (R^2); is it clinically useful?

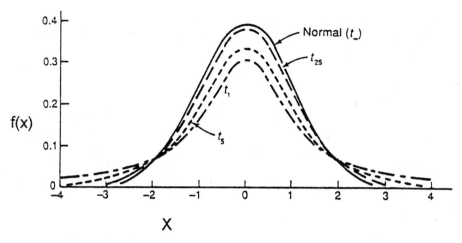

Figure 23-12. The *t*-distribution as function of its degrees of freedom.

- If yes, check the residuals and vary the required assumptions.[5]
- If the requirements are met, validate the model by testing on a new set of data.

Sensitivity, Specificity, and Predictive Value

Many studies of medical testing and medical decision making involve reports of sensitivity, specificity, and predictive values. These are all descriptive statistics and can be calculated from a 2 × 2 (two by two) table as described in the many biostatistics text books (e.g., see[9]). These measures are closely related to the measures of risk in epidemiological studies. With the following 2 × 2 table which predicts the presence or

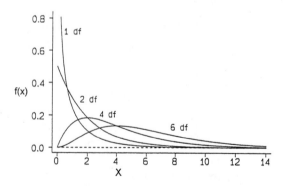

Figure 23-13.   Chi-square probability distribution with varying degrees of freedom.

absence of a particular disease we will define these measures.

	True Disease or Condition		
	Present	Absent	Total
Test Result: +	A	B	$A + B$
−	C	D	$C + D$
Total	$A + C$	$B + D$	$A + B + C + D$

By definition A, B, C, and D are: A = true positives, B = false positives, C = false negatives, and D = true negatives. Using A, B, C, and D one may define the following descriptive measures:

1. Sensitivity = $[A \div (A + C)]$: is the ability to correctly identify a diseased individual.
2. Specificity = $[D \div (B + D)]$: is the ability to correctly identify a nondiseased individual.
3. False-positive rate = $[B \div (B + D)]$: is the proportion of false positives among nondiseased.
4. False-negative rate = $[C \div (A + C)]$: is the proportion of false negatives among diseased.
5. Positive predictive value = $[A \div (A + B)]$: is the proportion of true positives among all test positives.
6. Negative predictive value = $[D \div (C + D)]$:

is the proportion of true negatives among all negatives.

7. Accuracy of a test = $[(A + D) \div (A + B + C + D)]$: is the proportion of all true positives and negatives among all the individuals.

A useful diagnostic test is one that improves our guess about the patient's disease status over the guess that could be made on just the general prevalence of the disease. While sensitivity and specificity are characteristics of the test itself, the predictive values are very much influenced by how common the disease is. The primary interest of a clinician, is the predictive value of a positive test $(PV+)$, which is the proportion of people having a positive test who really have the disease: $A/(A + B)$, and the predictive value of a negative test $(PV-)$, which is the proportion of people with a negative test who really don't have the disease: $D/(C + D)$. Sensitivity and specificity are characteristics of the test itself, but the predictive values are very much influenced by how prevalent the disease is. For further readings see.[5-6]

Epidemiological Measures

Epidemiology is defined as the study of the distribution and determinants of disease in populations. Epidemiological research typically seeks to understand the causes of disease, plan treatment and contribute to the development of public health policies. To do that the epidemiologist uses epidemiology measures when describing the pattern of a disease. The epidemiological measures vary with the type of the study undertaken.

Prospective or Cohort Study

In a prospective or cohort study which is also known as longitudinal or incidence study a group of individuals with and without exposure to a risk factor (e.g., smoking) but otherwise having similar characteristics are followed for a specified period of time and the presence or absence of a specific disease (e.g., gestational diabetes) was observed. Data then can be summarized in a table similar to the one given below.

		State of Disease or Condition		
		Present	Absent	Total
Risk factor:	Present	A	B	$A + B$
	Absent	C	D	$C + D$
	Total	$A + C$	$B + D$	$A + B + C + D$

Then the appropriate statistics would be:

1. Incidence rate among individuals with positive risk factor = $[A \div (A + B)]$. This is also called the absolute risk for individuals with risk factor.
2. Incidence rate among individuals with no risk factor = $[C \div (C + D)]$. This is also called the absolute risk for individuals without risk factor.
3. Relative risk = $\{[A \div (A + B)]/[C \div (C + D)]\}$: incidence rate among individuals having risk factor $\div$ incidence rate among individuals not having risk factor.
4. Attributable risk = $AR = [A \div (A + B) - C \div (C + D)]$.
5. Attributable risk percent = $100 \times AR/[A \div (A + B)]$: attributable risk is a percent of absolute risk.

In these types of studies measure of relative risk is a most popular statistic. It is a scaleless number that gives the risk of developing disease for individuals who have been the exposed risk factor (having risk factor) relative to individuals without risk factor (unexposed to risk factor).

Retrospective or Case Control Study

Retrospective or case control studies begin with the presence (cases) or absence (controls) of an outcome (e.g., gestational diabetes) and look backward in time to try to detect possible causes or risk factors that were possibly responsible for the onset of the disease. Data from this type of study can also be summarized in a 2 $\times$ 2 table discussed before but the descriptive statistics would be different. For instance, in a case control study, it is not possible to determine either the incidence rate or a relative risk because of the retrospective nature of the study. However, in practice this has been estimated by the odds ratio which is equal to *AD/BC*. Epidemiological measures such as birth rate, fertility rate, perinatal mortality rate, neonatal mortality rate, infant mortality, and postneonatal mortality rate are all descriptive statistics. The important issue here is to distinguish between the true rates in a mathematical sense and probability of occurrence of certain events (risk of an event). Also important is the difference between the incidence rate and incidence risk. For detailed study see Kirkwood,[5] chapter 15.

SAMPLE SIZE AND POWER

The basic question in any medical study is "How many subjects do we need?" Unfortunately, in practice, the sample size is determined by more gut feeling than scientific calculation. On one hand, we do not want to study more subjects than are necessary therefore saving time, money and other resources. On the other hand, by studying too few subjects we are unlikely to be able to answer the questions in a reasonable manner. Thus, knowing the required sample size before the start of the study is essential and statistical methods could help in calculating that.

However, investigators should realize that there are no universal formulas for calculating the required sample size and it depends on many factors including the hypothesis of interest, type of the variable, statistics of interest, variation of the data, clinically meaningful differences that one would likely detect as a significance difference, and type I (α error) and type II (β error) error (note that power of the test is equal to 1 − β). For example, it would not be sufficient to state simply that the objective is to demonstrate whether or not smokers are at greater risk of a premature birth than nonsmokers. It is necessary to state the size of the increased risk that it was desired to demonstrate since, for example, a smaller sample would be needed to detect a fourfold increase rather than a twofold one. Although the computation can be simple in some

cases,[1,4] it is not always a straightforward procedure and requires a close communication between the investigator and the statistician. First of all, for calculating the sample size, the statistician needs to know what is the primary hypothesis of interest since a separate sample size can be calculated for each hypothesis. Second, the statistician needs to know the type of the variable of interest (e.g., discrete, continuous, etc.), and some specific information about the variable. The statistician needs to know what the statistics of interest are (e.g., proportion, mean, median, regression parameter, survival curves, etc.). Probably the most critical information needed which should be supplied by the investigator is the effect size or the size of differences we want to detect. This is the minimum size of the differences that you are willing to miss detecting. Suppose, for example, that in the control group 80% of the patients without any treatment recover while 90% of the treated group recover. Also, there is consensus that this 10% difference (=90% − 80%) in recovery rate is clinically important and we want to be sure that this difference would also be statistically significant. This means that if the treatment group recovery rate was 86% you would be willing to miss finding that small an effect. However, if the treatment rate were 90% or more, you would want to be sure to be statistically significant. How sure we would like to be depends on the power of the statistical test (1 − β) which is the probability of finding a significant difference when the null hypothesis is false. Using the above information and $\alpha = 0.05$, $\beta = 0.90$ (power = 90%), we can calculate the required sample size from one sample proportion formula (Kirkwood[5]), we have

$$n \geq \frac{[Z_\alpha\sqrt{p_0(1 - p_0)} - Z_\beta\sqrt{p_1(1 - p_1)}]^2}{(p - p_0)^2}$$

$$= \frac{\{1.28\sqrt{[0.8(1 - 0.8)]} + 1.96\sqrt{[0.9(1 - 0.9)]}\}^2}{(0.80 - 0.90)^2}$$

$$= \frac{(0.512 + 0.588)^2}{0.01} = 121 \qquad (4)$$

where

n = 121 = minimum required sample size;
p_1 = 0.8 = proportion of interest;
p_0 = 0.9 = hypothesis proportion;
Z_β = 1.28 = one-sided percentage point of the Z-distribution corresponding to Type II error, β = 0.1 (power = 90%);
Z_α = 1.96 = two-sided percentage point of the Z-distribution corresponding to Type I error (α = 0.05).

Note that this formula is valid only when we require a sample to compare a proportion to a hypothesized proportion. There are different sample size formulas for other situations; some are simple and some are very complex. There are several computer software packages [e.g., SOLO Power Analysis, BMDP Statistical Software, Inc., Los Angeles, CA] which aid us in calculating the required sample for simple studies. For more complex designs such as repeated measures and random effect models there is no help available. Table 23-6 offers several sample

size calculation formulas. For more details see.[5,7]

META-ANALYSIS

Combining the results of several studies is called meta-analysis. This idea is not new in medical literature. In the past, review articles written by knowledgeable authors have played an important role in helping busy clinicians by reporting the summary of many studies on a single issue. Meta-analysis takes the review article a step further by using statistical procedures in combining various studies and thus provides a more scientific and uniform summary. A meta-analysis does not simply add the means or proportions across studies to determine an average or proportion. There are several different methods for combining results which use the principle called effect size. In general, meta-analysis is not a simple task to carry out and requires a team of investigators including a competent stat-

Table 23-6. Some Simple Formula for Sample Size Calculations to Demonstrate Significant Differences

Type of Model	Null Hypothesis	Sample Size Formula	Comment
Single Sample Proportion	H_0: $p = p_0$	$N \geq [Z_\alpha \sqrt{p_0(1 - p_0)} - Z_\beta \sqrt{p_1(1 - p_1)}]^2 / (p_1 - p_0)^2$	p_1 is the desired value p_0 is the value of null hypothesis
Mean	H_0: $\mu = \mu_0$	$N \geq [(Z_\alpha - Z_\beta)\sigma]^2/(\mu_1 - \mu_0)^2$	$(\mu_1 - \mu_0)$ is the desired clinical difference σ is the population standard deviation or a "good" sample estimate of σ.
Two Sample Two Proportions	H_0: $p_1 = p_2$	$N \geq [Z_\alpha \sqrt{2p_1(1 - p_1)} - Z_\beta \sqrt{p_1(1 - p_1)} + p_2(1 - p_2)]^2/(p_2 - p_1)^2$	p_1 is the proportion in group 1 (i.e., control) p_2 is the proportion in group 2 (i.e., treatment)
Two Means	H_0: $\mu_1 = \mu_2$	$N \geq 2[(Z_\alpha - Z_\beta)\sigma]^2/(\mu_2 - \mu_1)^2$	$(\mu_2 - \mu_1)$ is the magnitude of differences to be detected in two groups σ is the population standard deviation in the population or a "good" pooled sample estimate of σ.

Z_α is the two-tailed critical value from standard normal table. For example, for α = 0.05, the two-tailed $Z_{0.05}$ is equal to 1.96 which corresponds to one tail critical value of .025; Z_β.

istician. Nevertheless, when reading a meta-analysis study, several important questions should be asked: (1) How the literature search was conducted? (2) How much effort was made to find all the published and unpublished studies? (3) How did the authors have select papers to study? (4) How many papers initially were selected? (5) Did the authors state the inclusion and exclusion criteria clearly? (3) Were the studies all clinical trials? (4) How many studies were kept in the final analysis? (5) Why did they exclude the others? (6) Who were the patients in each study? (7) How similar were the diagnoses and treatments? How were the results pooled? (8) Did they look at various patient subgroups separately? (9) How each study was weighted? and why? (10) Who paid for the study? (11) How similar were the results in the studies?

REFERENCES

1. Dawson-Saunders B, Trapp RG. *Basic and Clinical Biostatistics*, 2nd Ed. Norwalk, CT: Appleton & Lange, 1990.
2. Motulsky H. *Intuitive Biostatistics*. Oxford, UK: Oxford University Press, 1995.
3. Altman DG. *Practical Statistics For Medical Research*. London: Chapman and Hall, 1991.
4. Pagano M, Gauvreau K. *Principles of Biostatistics*. Belmont, CA: Wadsworth Publishing Company, 1993.
5. Kirkwood BR. *Essentials of Medical Statistics*. London: Blackwell Scientific Publications, 1988.
6. Sacket DL, Haynes RB, Tugwell P. *Clinical Epidemiology: A Basic Science and Clinical Medicine*, 2nd Ed. Boston: Little Brown and Company, 1991.
7. Pocock SJ. *Clinical Trials A Practical Approach*. London: John Wiley & Sons, 1983.
8. Thompson SK. *Sampling*. New York: John Wiley & Sons, Inc., 1992.
9. Dunn G, Everitt B. *Clinical Biostatistics—An Introduction to Evidence-Based Medicine*. London: Edward Arnold, 1995.
10. Johnson RA, Wichern DW. *Applied Multivariate Statistical Analysis*, 3rd Ed. New York: Prentice Hall, 1992.

QUESTIONS

1. Measures of centrality include all of the following except.
    a. Mean
    b. Median
    c. Mode
    d. Coefficient of variation
    e. Midrange

2–6. The following table gives the result of screening tests and status of disease ABC of the population being tested

Disease ABC

Screening Test	Yes	No	Total
Positive	100	400	500
Negative	50	600	650
Total	150	1000	1150

Match each screening test parameter listed below to the appropriate numerical value.
    a. 20%
    b. 66.7%
    c. 92.3%
    d. 60.9%
    e. 60%

2. Sensitivity
3. Specificity
4. Positive predictive value
5. Negative predictive value
6. Accuracy of test
7. The most appropriate statistical test to compare the mean of two distributions of laboratory values in women with and without gestational diabetes is:
    a. Chi-square
    b. The paired *t*-test
    c. Two-sample *t*-test
    d. Correlation
    e. Regression
8. A study was undertaken to evaluate any increased risk of breast cancer among women who use birth control pills. The relative risk was calculated. A type I error in this study consists of concluding:
    a. A significant increase in the relative risk when the relative risk is actually greater than 1

b. A significant increase in the relative risk when the relative risk is actually 1

c. No significant increase in the relative risk when the relative risk is actually 1

d. No significant increase in the relative risk when the relative risk is actually greater than 1

e. No significant increase in the relative risk when the relative risk is actually less than 1

9. The scale used in measuring serum creatinine (mg/dL) is:
   a. Nominal
   b. Ordinal
   c. Continuous
   d. Discrete
   e. Qualitative

10. The scale used in measuring presence or absence of a risk factor for premature birth is:
    a. Nominal
    b. Ordinal
    c. Continuous
    d. Quantitative
    e. None of the above

11–12. In an epidemiological study of the effect of vaginoses in premature births, an investigator selected 500 postpartum mothers with vaginosis during their prior pregnancy and 200 postpartum mothers with no vaginosis during their pregnancy. The investigators obtained a history of all previous pregnancies in both groups of workers. Among the women with vaginosis, 120 gave birth to a preterm infant; among the 200 women with no vaginosis in their previous pregnancy, 40 gave birth to preterm infants.

The odds ratio is:
a. 0.5
b. 1.0
c. 2.0
d. 3.0
e. Not determinable from the above information

This study is best described as a:
a. Cross-sectional study
b. Cohort study
c. Case-control study
d. Controlled experiment
e. Randomized clinical trial

13. An investigator wishes to study whether having vaginal infection during pregnancy (vaginosis) is associated with subsequent preterm delivery. If, in reality, the presence of vaginosis leads to a relative risk of disease of 2.0, the investigator wants to have a 95% chance of detecting an effect this large in the planned study. This statement is an illustration of specifying:
    a. A null hypothesis
    b. A type I, or alpha, error
    c. A type II, or beta, error
    d. Statistical power
    e. An odds ratio

Answer Key

Chapter 1
1. C
2. B
3. A
4. B
5. A
6. C

Chapter 2
1. C
2. B
3. E
4. E
5. E

Chapter 3
1. A
2. C
3. D
4. C
5. B

Chapter 4
1. C
2. D
3. B
4. D
5. C

Chapter 5
1. C
2. B
3. B
4. B
5. B
6. C

Chapter 6
1. A
2. C
3. A
4. D
5. C
6. D
7. C
8. A

Chapter 7
1. B
2. A
3. C
4. D

Chapter 8
1. D
2. B
3. B
4. A
5. C

6. B
7. C
8. D

Chapter 9
1. D
2. B
3. C
4. E
5. C
6. B
7. D
8. E
9. C
10. A

Chapter 10
1. C
2. B
3. A
4. D
5. B
6. D
7. D
8. D
9. E
10. A

Chapter 11
1. D
2. D
3. C
4. B
5. D

Chapter 12
1. E
2. C
3. D
4. C
5. C
6. D
7. A
8. C
9. A

Chapter 13
1. D
2. A
3. D
4. A
5. E

Chapter 14
1. D
2. A
3. D
4. True
5. True

Chapter 15
1. C
2. D
3. C
4. A
5. C

Chapter 16
1. C
2. D
3. B
4. B
5. D
6. D
7. B
8. B
9. C
10. A

Chapter 17
1. C
2. D
3. D
4. E
5. D
6. C
7. D
8. E

Chapter 18
1. E
2. C

3. A
4. B
5. D
6. B
7. C
8. C

Chapter 19

1. B
2. C
3. A
4. D
5. E
6. B
7. D
8. B
9. B
10. E

Chapter 20

1. B
2. D
3. B
4. D
5. B

Chapter 21

1. 32
2. D
3. placenta (subamnionic, chorionic sample)
4. A & B

5. A, B, and C
6. False

Chapter 22

1. appropriate charting
2. (1) standard of care
   (2) breach of the standard of care
   (3) proximate cause
   (4) damages
3. Failure to perform an act which should have been done, or performance of an act which should not have been done.
4. The casual relationship between a negligent act to the sustained injury.
5. Outline your discussion with the patient in your progress notes and have the patient sign their name.

Chapter 23

1. D
2. B
3. E
4. A
5. C
6. D
7. C
8. B
9. C
10. A
11. D
12. A
13. D

Glossary

acceleration phase—The first phase of active labor, identified by rapid cervical dilation in association with regular uterine contractions.

acrocentric—A chromosome with its centromere close to one end.

acute tubular necrosis (ATN)—The most common cause of acute renal failure. It is usually associated with damaged renal tubules secondary to aminoglycosides, sepsis, or hypotension.

acyclovir—Purine nucleoside analog active against herpes simplex and varicella.

Addison's disease—Addison's disease is primary adrenal insufficiency that results from the destruction of the adrenal cortex by any cause. The low cortisol production causes elevated ACTH levels, and aldosterone deficiency results in increased renin production.

AEDV—Absent end-diastolic velocity usually refers to Doppler of the umbilical artery and suggests increased risk of fetal disease.

AFI—Amniotic fluid index is a way of evaluating amniotic fluid by dividing the uterus into quadrants and adding together the sum of the four vertical pockets (normal 50–200 mm; > 240 mm is hydramnios).

allele—Refers to different forms of a gene (normal and mutant).

amniocentesis (routine)—Inserting a needle into the uterine cavity and through the amnion at 15 weeks menstrual weeks or greater.

analgesia—The augmentation or elimination of painful sensations in the conscious patient.

anencephaly—A major defect of the cranial vault incompatible with viability and usually easily diagnosed after 16 weeks gestation.

aneuploidy—A chromosome number that is not an exact multiple of the haploid number. Usually refers to a trisomy or monosomy.

antiphospholipid antibodies—Anticardiolipin antibodies and the lupus anticoagulant.

antiphospholipid syndrome—Occurrence of antiphospholipid antibodies with arterial or venous thrombosis, recurrent fetal loss, thrombocytopenia, or neurological disorders.

anxiolytic—A medication that decreases anxiety.

arrest—The cessation of cervical dilation or descent of the presenting part during active labor.

asynclitic—An anterior or posterior deflection of the fetal parietal bone with the saggital suture in the transverse plane.

attitude—The degree of extension of the fetal cervical spine from fully flexed (vertex presentation) to fully extended (face presentation).

autosome—Any nonsex chromosome. There are 22 pairs of autosomes in humans and one pair of sex chromosome.

basal metabolic rate—Minimal energy expenditure for circulation, respiration, and heat exchange, about 20 kcal/kg.

bilateral renal cortical necrosis—A cause of renal failure associated with anuria. Usually it is associated with severe complications of pregnancy such as abruption or severe preeclampsia.

blastomere—One of the cells resulting from the cleavage or segmentation of a fertilized ovum.

blood dyscrasias—Leukopenia and agranulocytosis.

BOO—Fetal bladder outlet obstruction is a lower urinary tract obstruction that can result in progressive fetal renal dysplasia and pulmonary hypoplasia. BOO caused by posterior urethral valves in male fetuses in selected cases can be treated with antenatal shunt procedures or in inuterosurgery.

BPD—Biparietal diameter is the maximal distance between the two fetal parietal bones and an important component of equations to estimate fetal gestational age and weight.

brachiocephaly—A round head. May make the BPD unreliable.

breach—The breaking or violating of a law, right, or duty, either by commission or omission.

bupivicaine—A long acting aminoamide local anesthetic. Normal concentrations are 0.25% to 0.5%. Duration of action for epidural analgesia is 1.5 to 2.5 hours. At toxic dose levels, it can cause prolonged cardiac arrest. Pregnancy itself may increase suscepibility to the cardiotoxic effects of bupivicaine.

cardiac output—Whole blood volume pumped into the aorta per minute; termed cardiac index when expressed per square meter of body surface. Cardiac output equals stroke volume times heart rate, about 5 L/min; measured by thermal dilution, O2 consumption (Fick).

centromere—A region in the chromosome where spindles attach during mitosis or meiosis.

cervical incompetence—Painless cervical dilatation in the midtrimester without preterm labor, resulting in pregnancy loss.

choriocarcinoma—A highly malignant gestational trophoblastic neoplasia (GTN). Choriocarcinoma is characterized by the absence of villi and is a pure sheet of epithelial neoplasia derived from syncytial trophoblasts and cytotrophoblasts.

choroid plexus cysts—Central nervous system cysts associated with chromosomal abnormalities and increased perinatal consults.

chromosome—Structure containing genetic information stored in DNA in the nucleus of eukaryotic cells.

chronic hypertension—BP > 140 mm Hg systolic or >90 mm Hg diastolic antedating pregnancy or before 20 weeks gestation (except with hydatidiform mole) or persisting beyond 6 weeks postpartum.

civil injury—Injuries to person or property, resulting from a breach of contract, deceit, or criminal offense, which may be redressed by means of a civil action.

codon—The triplet nucleotides that code for an amino acid.

colloid osmotic pressure—Force regulating the diffusion of solutes and water through capillary membranes exerted by (anionic) proteins like albumin. Nonpregnant values: 28 mm Hg.

colposcopy—Examination of the vagina and cervix by means of a binocular endoscope (colposcope) that magnifies cells to allow direct observation, use of filters (green filter) and directed biopsy to evaluate abnormal lesions on the genitalia.

combined spinal epidural (CSE)—A technique where an epidural needle and an intrathecal injection are given. The spinal needle is then removed, the epidural catheter is threaded through the epidural needle into the epidural space. The epidural needle is then removed and the catheter is then secured. Combines the benefits of both techniques into one procedure.

complete mole—A gestational trophoblastic neoplasia (GTN) formed by the partly developed products of conception characterized by trophoblastic proliferation, hydropic degeneration, absence of central vessels and absence of the fetus.

congenital adrenal hyperplasia (CAH)—This is the most common cause of female pseudohermaphroditism. It results from inherited defects in enzymes required in the biosynthetic pathways of steroid hormones. Cortisol synthesis is diminished, and there is accumulation of intermediate metabolites due to the absence or reduced activity of an enzyme required for their further processing.

continuous epidural anesthesia (CEA)—A continuous infusion of an anesthetic solution into the epidural space to provide pain relief. Local anesthetics, narcotics or the combination of the two are generally used. CEA is used commonly for labor pain as well as postoperative pain relief.

cordocentesis—Antenatally sampling fetal blood from the umbilical cord. Also termed percutaneous umbilical cord sampling (PUBS) and fetal blood sampling.

CPAP—Continuous positive airway pressure. This is obtained by applying a tight seal on the face with the mask.

creatinine clearance—Volume/time relationship describing renal elimination of creatinine from plasma; a common marker of renal function, usually 100 cc/min.

CRL—Crown rump length, measured from the fetuses head to rump to determine estimate of fetal gestational age.

Cushing's syndrome—This syndrome describes the combination of symptoms and signs caused by excessive exposure to glucocorticoids.

CVS—Chorionic villus sampling. A transcervical or

transabdominal technique, usually performed between 9 and 12 weeks to obtain samples of placental tissue for antenatal testing.

damages—A pecuniary compensation or indemnity, which may be recovered by the courts by any person who has suffered loss, detriment, or injury, whether to his person, property, or rights, through the unlawful act or omission or negligence of another.

dead space—Respiratory tree constituents with no ability to exchange gases, for example, oropharynx, trachea, bronchi; approximated at 2 cc/kg ideal body weight.

diabetic ketoacidosis—Acidosis in diabetes is caused by the enhanced production of ketones. The increase in serum ketones is due to a lack of insulin or an excess of glucose counterregulatory hormones such as glucagon.

diploid—The number of chromosomes in most somatic cells. In humans the diploid number is 46.

discovery—In a general sense, the ascertainment of that which was previously unknown; the disclosure of coming to light of what was previously hidden; the acquisition of notice or knowledge of given acts or facts; as, in regard to the "discovery" of fraud affecting the running of the statute of limitations, or the granting of a new trial for newly "discovered" evidence.

dolichocephaly—An elongated (fetal) head. May make the BPD unreliable.

Duhrssen's incision—An emergency cervical incision at 2:00, 6:00 and 10:00 o'clock to assist delivery of the entrapped aftercoming fetal head.

dystocia—A general term meaning "difficult labor."

early amniocentesis—An amniocentesis performed prior to 15 menstrual weeks.

eclampsia—Preeclampsia plus a seizure.

embryo—Stage in early human development from the second to the eighth week post conception inclusive.

embryo transfer—Transferring the pre-implantation embryo to the uterus or fallopian tube.

embryoscopy—Observing an embryo through an intact amnion via endoscope (4–10 weeks).

engagement—The fetal biparietal diameter has passed below the pelvic inlet.

exon—A segment of DNA that is present in the mature mRNA of eukaryocytes (as contrasted to intron).

expiratory reserve volume (ERV)—The extra amount of air expelled with forced exhalation.

expressivity—The degree of phenotypic expression of a gene or genotype.

fetal hydrops—Subcutaneous edema with pleural and/or pericardial effusion and ascites which may indicate fetal heart failure.

fetal reduction—Reducing the number of fetuses within the uterus in a multifetal pregnancy. The procedure is performed with the anticipation of improved survival of the remaining fetuses.

fetoscopy—A technique for obtaining fetal blood and skin through an endoscope inserted within the uterus.

fetus—The stage in human development from roughly the third month to birth. Prior to that time the human is referred to as an embryo.

four-chamber view—Classic view of fetal heart with left and right atria and ventricles that rules out most cardiac anomalies.

functional residual capacity (FRC)—The volume of gas that is left in the lung after passive exhalation. If FRC is reduced, induction of anesthesia is more rapid as well as the development of arterial hypoxemia with apnea.

gamete intrafallopian transfer (GIFT)—Transfer of a mixture of eggs and sperm into the fallopian tube.

gastroschisis—An abdominal defect with small bowel herniation to the right of the cord insertion with a low risk of other anomalies or chromosomal abnormalities.

general anesthesia (GA)—The pharmacologic induction and maintenance of a depressed state of consciousness or unconsciousness with impairment of airway reflexes. The ability to maintain ventilation and the ability to respond appropriately to physical or verbal stimuli is inhibited or lost.

gestational diabetes (GDM)—Carbohydrate intolerance that is diagnosed during the index pregnancy.

gestational trophoblastic neoplasia (GTN)—A term that includes hydatidiform mole, invasive mole and choriocarcinoma. An invasive mole is characterized by the presence of chorionic villi with hydropic degeneration, trophoblastic proliferation and invasion of the myometrium.

glomerular filtration rate (GFR)—Rate of solute transfer from renal plasma to urine by the nephron, often determined for inulin because of lack of tubular resorption or secretion.

glomerulonephritis—Renal disease associated with hematuria, proteinuria, and usually hypertension and edema.

glycosylated hemoglobin—A sugar moiety that is permanently attached to the N-terminal valine of each beta chain (HbA1c is the largest fraction) and is expressed as a percentage of total hemoglobin.

This is a measure of glucose control over the previous 2 months.

Grave's disease—Grave's disease is the most common cause of hyperthyroidism during pregnancy. It is an autoimmune process. The hypersecretion of thyroid hormones is caused by stimulation of the thyroid gland by circulating immunoglobin, which bind to the TSH receptor and stimulate thyroid hormone biosynthesis and secretion.

haploid—The chromosome number of a normal gamete (one from each chromosome pair). In humans the haploid number is 23.

Hashimoto's thyroiditis—This is an autoimmune disease of unknown etiology. It causes a rubbery, diffuse goiter and, in most cases, hypothyroidism.

HELLP syndrome—A disease of pregnancy associated with hemolysis, elevated liver enzymes and a low platelet count.

heterotopic pregnancy—Simultaneous intrauterine and ectopic pregnancy.

hydrocephalus—Central nervous system (CNS) defect seen with increased CNS fluid. CNS atrial enlargement is usually over 1 cm.

hydrops—Diffuse edema. In obstetrics, it refers to edema of fetus and placenta, usually accompanied by polyhydramnios (excessive volume of amniotic fluid).

hypertension—BP > 140 mm Hg systolic or >90 mm Hg diastolic.

hypotonic uterine dysfunction—Contractions occurring at regular intervals during active labor without adequate intensity to effect cervical dilation or descent of the presenting part. Associated with obstructed labor.

indicated preterm delivery—Preterm delivery because continuation of the pregnancy is deemed life-threatening to the mother or fetus.

infertility—Inability to conceive within one year of unprotected heterosexual intercourse.

interstitial nephritis—A cause of acute renal failure associated with damage to the renal parenchyma resulting in an inactive urine sediment (no RBCs or casts). Commonly associated clinical causes include some antibiotics classes such as the penicillins or sulfa agents.

intron—A segment of non-coding DNA within a gene. It is transcribed but removed from the primary RNA transcript prior to translation.

in vitro fertilization (INF)—Fertilization of an egg by sperm in culture media.

IUGR—Intrauterine growth restriction. Can be symmetrical or asymmetrical (head sparing). Impaired fetal growth resulting in abnormally low weight for gestational age, on the basis of a variety of causes. Lower limit of weight for gestational age has been defined variously as the 5th or 10th percentile or 2 S.D. below the mean.

Jarisch-Herxheimer reaction—Allergic-type reaction which occurs within 48 hours of treatment of syphilis probably due to rapid release of antigens from dying spirochetes.

ketones—Acetone, B-hydroxybutyrate, and acetoacetate formed through hepatic oxidation of fatty acids in the setting of insulin deficiency.

LEEP—Loop electrosurgical excision procedure of the cervix which can substitute for cone biopsy.

lie—The relation of the fetal long axis to that of the mother.

litigen—An agent that does not increase the risk of congenital malformations but increases medical-legal risks.

local anesthesia—The elimination of painful sensations by the application or injection of a drug into a part of the body.

Low birth weight (LBW)—Infants born with birth weights less than or equal to 2500 g.

MAC or minimum alveolar concentration—This is the alveolar concentration of a gas which prevents movement in 50% of individuals in response to a noxious stimulus. MAC is used to compare potency of the various inhaled anesthetic gases.

macrosomia—Fetal weight greater than 4000 kg of greater than the 90th percentile for gestational age.

malpractice—Any professional misconduct, unreasonable lack of skill of fidelity in professional or fiduciary duties, evil practice, or illegal or immoral conduct.

McRoberts maneuver—Hyperflexion of the maternal hips to effect delivery of an impacted fetal shoulder.

mean arterial pressure (MAP)—Time-averaged arterial pressure, approximated by adding diastolic pressure to one third the difference between systolic and diastolic measures.

meconium adapter—Device used with an endotracheal tube and wall suction for removal of meconium-stained fluid from the trachea.

meiosis—Cell division in germ cells resulting in the production of gametes with a haploid number of chromosomes from diploid cells.

minute alveolar ventilation—Air volume entering pulmonary sacs each minute; always a subset of total ventilation which also includes dead space.

mitosis—Cell division resulting in two cells with the same number of chromosomes as the parent cell.

Montevideo units—Total pressure generated by uterine contractions in a 10-minute period. Calculated by subtracting baseline pressure from peak concentration pressures, in mm Hg.

mosaicism—Condition where an individual has two or more distinct genetic cell lines.

MSF—Meconium-stained fluid.

multifactorial—Determined by multiple factors both genetic and non-genetic (environmental, eco-genetic).

nephropathy—Excretion of greater than 300 mg of protein in a 24-hour period without other causes.

NRP—Neonatal resuscitation program sponsored by the American Academy of Pediatrics and the American Heart Association.

NTD—Neural tube defect refers to a class of defects such as anencephaly, cephaloceles, and spina bifida (myelomenigocele meningocele).

nuchal fold thickening—Over 6 mm from skin edge to skull at the posterior fossa (15–20 weeks) seen with chromosome abnormalties.

nuchal translucency—Membrane at neck associated with chromosome abnormalities (11–14 weeks).

OETT—Oral endotracheal tube.

oligohydramnios—Decreased amniotic fluid as determined clinically or by a decreased AFI. Seen with IUGR or fetal renal abnormalities.

omphalocele—A major abdominal wall defect at the cord insertion which can often be associated with other anomalies or chromosome abnormalities.

oocyte donation—The oocytes from one female individual are retrieved by sperm and implanted into the uterus of a different female individual.

oxygen dissociation curve—The sharp sinusoidal curve describing the relationship between tissue oxygen saturation (y-axis) and oxygen tension (x-axis).

P/P—Peak inspiratory pressure/peak end expiratory pressure.

partial mole—A gestational trophoblastic neoplasia (GTN) formed by the partly developed products of conception characterized by fetal trophoblastic changes that affect the syncytial layer only. The fetus is present and usually dies in the first trimester. Rarely, a living infant is born in the second or third trimester.

pathophysiology—Derangement in normal physiologic function.

PIH—New onset of hypertension, or a BP rise of >30 mm Hg systolic or >15 mm Hg diastolic after 20 weeks gestation or earlier with hydatidiform mole.

PIP—Peak inspiratory pressure. The highest pressure obtained with inflation during bag and mask ventilation.

placental site trophoblastic neoplasm—A gestational trophoblastic neoplasia (GTN) that is char-acterized by the absence of villi, proliferation only of the intermediate cytotrophoblast cells and rare metastasis.

polyhydramnios—Increased amniotic fluid clinically or by AFI. Seen with maternal diabetes mellitus or fetal gastrointestinal obstruction.

polymerase chain reaction (PCR)—Method of DNA amplification which can detect specific sequences in minute quantities and thus can be useful to detect some pathogens.

position—The relation of an arbitrary fetal anatomic landmark to the maternal pelvis: the occiput in cephalic and the sacrum in breech presentation.

postdural puncture headache—A "spinal head-ache" is thought to be due to the loss of CSF through a break in the dura resulting from a spinal or epidural needle. It is one of the most common complications of epidural or spinal anesthesia. It is classically described as occipital of frontal in location, occurs or worsens with an erect posture, and is relieved when supine.

postpartum acute renal failure—A disease associated with microangiopathic hemolytic anemia, hypertension, seizures, acute renal failure, and thrombocytopenia.

postpartum thyroiditis—Postpartum thyroiditis is usually caused by painless lymphocytic thyroiditis that may be identified in 5–9% of women about 12 months following delivery. The hallmark of a postpartum thyroiditis, is its transient nature.

PPROM—Preterm, premature rupture of the membranes is rupture of the membranes without the onset of labor between 20 and 37 completed weeks of gestation.

PPV—Positive pressure ventilation.

preeclampsia—PIH with proteinuria or generalized edema.

pre-embryo—Stage in early human development up to 14 days postconception.

pregnancy-aggravated hypertension—Chronic hypertension plus pregnancy induced hypertension.

prerenal azotemia—An elevation of the BUN with relative sparing of the serum creatinine. It is usually due to clinical disorders associated with a decreased renal blood flow such as volume depletion or congestive heart failure.

presentation—The portion of the fetus that is foremost in or nearest to the birth canal; what is palpated through the vagina.

pressor—Any substance that, upon administration, causes a rise in BP.

preterm birth—Delivery of a fetus prior to 37 completed weeks of gestation.

preterm labor—Regular uterine contractions associated with cervical change prior to 37 weeks completed of gestation.

protraction—Slower than expected rate of progress in active labor.

proximate cause—That which, in a natural and continuous sequence, unbroken by any efficient intervening cause, produces the injury, and without which the result would not have occurred.

pulmonary capillary wedge pressure—Approximating left atrial pressure, PCWP is measured by obstructing a pulmonary artery branch with a balloon catheter; usual value is 6–8 mm Hg.

residual lung volume—Air remaining after forced expiration, about 1–1.5 L.

restriction fragment-length polymorphism (RFLP)—A DNA fragment that is not the cause of a genetic disease but segregates with a genetic disorder and can be used to diagnose the disorder.

S/D ratio—The ratio of systolic to diastolic Doppler velocity of blood flow. Usually refers to the umbilical artery and used to evaluate IUGR.

Sheehan's syndrome—This syndrome of postpartum pituitary necrosis is associated with postpartum hemorrhage and hypotension. It is presumably the hyperplastic gland in pregnancy that is more vulnerable to an inadequate blood supply.

spiramycin—Macrolide antibiotic used to prevent fetal toxoplasmosis when maternal infection is demonstrated.

standard—Stability, general recognition, and conformity to established practice.

statute of limitations—A statute prescribing limitations to the right of action on certain described causes of action; that is, declaring that no suit shall be maintained on such causes of action unless brought within a specified period after the right accrued.

stroke volume—The volume of blood pumped into the aorta per beat.

stuck twin—A twin with little or no surrounding amniotic fluid that may appear fixed to the side of the uterus. A stuck twin can occur in diamnionic monochorionic twins who develop a twin to twin transfusion syndrome (hydropic recipient twin with hydramnios, growth restricted donor twin with oligohydramnios).

supine hypotensive syndrome—The result of aortocaval compression by the gravid uterus usually occurring after 20 weeks gestation. Severe obstruc-

tion of venous return causing hypotension. May cause symptoms consistent with shock. Fetal distress can be precipitated.

systemic vascular resistance—Total impedance to flow of all vessels outside the pulmonary bed, the quotient of mean arterial minus central venous pressures multiplied by 80 dynes-sec cm2/cardiac output. Approximate SVR: 1500 dynes-cm-5.

telomere—End(s) of chromosome arms.

teratogen—A physical or chemical agent that increases the risk of congenital malformations.

tidal volume (TV)—Volume of air exchanged with each breath, usually about 400–500 cc.

tocolytic agents—Agents that decrease uterine contractile activity.

total lung capacity (TLC)—All the air in the lungs with forced inspiration; usually about 5–6 L. Vital capacity plus residual volume.

toxemia—A nonspecific term referring to any hypertensive disorder in pregnancy. No longer an accepted medical term.

triple check—A test using maternal serum levels of alpha-fetoprotein (MSAFP), human chorionic gonadotropin (hCG), and unconjugated estriol (uE3) to screen for genetic abnormalities. The triple check is recommended between 15 and 20 weeks and can detect 60% of Down syndrome fetuses.

Type I diabetes mellitus (insulin-dependent)—Characterized by an absolute deficiency of endogenous insulin.

Type II diabetes mellitus (noninsulin-dependent)—Characterized by insulin resistance and relative insulin insufficiency.

vertical transmission—Passing on of a pathogen from mother to offspring.

very low birth weight (VLBW)—Infants born with birth weights less of equal to 1500 g.

volatile inhalational anesthetics—A group of anesthetic gases that include isoflurane, enflurane, halothane, methoxyflurane, sevoflurane, and desflurane.

Woods screw maneuver—An attempt to dislodge an impacted anterior shoulder by rotating the posterior shoulder anteriorly 180 degrees.

zidovudine—Thymidine analog used in management of HIV disease as it inhibits viral reverse transcriptase. Also known as AZT.

Index